Dr. med. Dipl. Biol. M. Pruggmayer
Facharzt f. Humangenetik
Facharzt f. Frauenheilkunde
Herm.-Ehlers-Str. 9 • D-31224 Peine
Tel. 05171 / 37 75 • Fax 05171 / 1 21 71

Spina bifida –
neural tube defects

Spina bifida – neural tube defects

Basic research, interdisciplinary diagnostics and treatment, results and prognosis

Edited by
D. Voth and P. Glees

In collaboration with
J. Lorber

W
DE
G

Walter de Gruyter
Berlin · New York 1986

Prof. Dr. med. Dieter Voth
Klinikum der Johannes-Gutenberg-Universität
Neurochirurgische Klinik und Poliklinik
Langenbeckstr. 1 · D-6500 Mainz

Prof. Dr. med. Paul Glees
University of Cambridge
Department of Anatomy
Downing Street
Cambridge CB2 3DY · Great Britain

This book contains 105 illustrations and 66 tables

CIP-Kurztitelaufnahme der Deutschen Bibliothek

Spina bifida neural tube defects : basic research, interdisciplinary
diagnostics and treatment, results and prognosis / ed. by D. Voth
and P. Glees. In collab. with J. Lorber. – Berlin ; New York :
de Gruyter, 1986.
   ISBN 3-11-010768-6
NE: Voth, Dieter [Hrsg.]

Library of Congress Cataloging in Publication Data

Main entry under title:
Spina bifida – – neural tube defects.
   Based on the 5th workshop held in Mainz, Sept. 1984. Includes
   bibliographies and indexes.
     1. Spina bifida – – Congresses. 2. Dysraphia – – Congresses.
I. Voth, D. (Dieter), 1935 –   . II. Glees, Paul. III. Lorber, John.
[DNLM: 1. Spina Bifida – – congresses.
WE 730 S7573 1984]
RJ496. S74S69 1986   617'.482   85-29183
ISBN 0-89925-149-8 (U.S.)

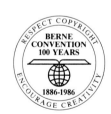

Dedicated in cordiality to
Professor Dr. Heinrich Bredt,
my academic teacher in pathology,
on the occasion of his 80th birthday.

Mainz, January 1986   *D. V.*

Preface

Malformations resulting from a defective or delayed closure of the embryonic neural tube contribute a significant portion of malformations to human pathology. Although morbidity of the most severe type is decreasing, the presence of dysraphia is a serious medical challenge for modern treatment of the accompanying symptoms, such as for internal hydrocephalus which can preserve life into maturity.

The interdisciplinary multitude of problems caused by dysraphia is bound to involve a number of clinical disciplines such as genetics, pathology, gynecology, neuro- and pediatric surgery, pediatry, orthopedics and urology.

The main purpose of our 5th autumn workshop in Mainz (Sept. 1984) was the combination of these disciplines. Special attention was paid to fundamental aspects and to experimental pathology, the present tools used in antenatal diagnostics and to get an up to date insight of the therapeutic standard.

We express the hope that these published reports of well known specialists in this field will provide a basis for a modern approach both for the benefit of the patient and for the clinician in his decision for the best possible available therapy.

February 1986

D. Voth, Mainz
P. Glees, Cambridge
J. Lorber, Sheffield

Contents

I Pathology and morbidity of neural tube defects

Spina bifida — a vanishing nightmare?

J. Lorber

Introduction

The object of this communication is to draw attention to the declining incidence of spina bifida in many parts of the world, especially in Great Britain, and to outline the role that antenatal diagnosis followed by termination of pregnancies has played in this phenomenon. It is now possible that spina bifida is a disappearing disorder.

In the past, increases in spina bifida births occurred during war, famine or economic disasters. Correspondingly, there was a tendency to steady decline when the circumstances have improved.

Unfortunately, reliable official national statistics over a prolonged period, based on population surveys are still rare. Such statistics are still not available even for many of the medically most advanced countries, including the United States of America. However, from 1980 onwards monitoring was started by the International Clearinghouse for Birth Defects in which more and more countries or groups of hospitals participate. From this some useful short-term information regarding trends is already available. In Europe a beginning has been made by the EEC Concerted Action Project ("Eurocat") which started publishing figures from 1979. These are local, rather than national statistics and so far relatively few centres have contributed their data. Much of the information, as yet, is incomplete.

England and Wales

Fortunately, accurate information has been available for England and Wales for over 20 years from the publications of the Office of Population Censuses and Surveys. These indicate that in the last 10 years a precipitous decline occurred, of a degree which was never experienced in the past.

Concurrently, the selective non-treatment of the most severely affected has substantially decreased the number of profoundly handicapped survivors, which was such a prominent fate for many who were born in the 1960s.

In England and Wales the incidence of spina bifida was high, both absolutely and by international comparisons up to 1972. There were only minor fluctuations in the rate which was on average 20 per 10,000 total births each year. In 1972, 1473 babies or 21 per 10,000 were born with spina bifida. This was the last year before antenatal diagnosis became a possibility.

Since then there has been a rapidly progressive decline in the births of spina bifida babies to 880 (14.9 per 10,000) in 1976 and to 422 (6.7 per 10,000) in 1983.

An even greater reduction occurred in anencephalic births from 13.1 per 10,000 total births in 1974 to only 1.8 in 1983. This substantial decrease can be largely accounted for by antenatal diagnosis followed by termination of pregnancy, although accurate figures for terminations are not available, as yet.

During the same period there was also a considerable decrease in the birth of hydrocephalic infants (unassociated with spina bifida) from 4.8 to 3.1 per 10,000, although antenatal diagnosis and terminations played no part in this decline. Possibly this is a true change in the incidence of the disorder and of similar degree to what might have been observed in the case of neural tube defects, had there been no medical interference. This suggestion is supported by the fact that in Ireland, where therapeutic abortions are not carried out, the incidence of spina bifida decreased to a similar proportion as is the case for hydrocephalus in England and Wales. Caution is necessary not to take the figures for hydrocephalus too literally, because many cases are not diagnosed in the neonate and so cases diagnosed later may not be included in the figures.

The exact role of antenatal diagnosis in the decrease of neural tube defects in the country as a whole is not fully clear: notifications of terminations of pregnancy because the foetus had a neural tube defect are almost certainly incomplete. Further, the official data merely give a total of terminations for *all* neural tube defects, without separating those for spina bifida and for anencephalus. With these provisos in mind, the figures indicate a rapidly increasing number from 34 in 1974 to a peak of 481 in 1980, but since then there has been no significant change in the notifications. As it is probable that most terminations were carried out because the foetus had anencephaly, the number terminated because of spina bifida was unlikely to have exceeded 150 in any one year, yet in 1982 some 1000 fewer babies were born with spina bifida than only 10 years earliers. The rate fell to on-third of the 1972 figure.

Selective terminations could, and should, play a bigger role in the prevention of spina bifida than was the case in the whole of England and Wales. This is shown for example by the experience in Sheffield in England, and Glasgow in Scotland.

Other congenital defects

Whatever are the cause, or causes, of the decline in CNS defects, these are not applicable to any other type of congenital malformations. On the contrary, the prevalence of all congenital malformations, other than CNS defects, is on the increase. The rate for *all* congenital defects, including the CNS was 197 in 1974 and progressively increased to 221 per 10,000 total births in 1983. Excluding CNS defects the increase was from 159 to 209.

The experience in Sheffield

Sheffield is an industrial city with a population of 550,000 and an annual average of 6,500 births. An accurate congenital anomalies registry was established some 20 years ago, and it is a most valuable source of information. The information is abstracted from the birth certificates, on which every evident congenital abnormality is recorded.

Like elsewhere, there were no measures known to prevent spina bifida births until about 1965 [8] when my large scale study established that there was an approximate 5% risk of neural tube defects in a family after they had a baby with spina bifida. Prevention of recurrences, however, was only possible by avoiding further pregnancies. This made no measurable impact on the number of spina bifida births.

In 1972, after Brock's [1] first paper on the value of alphafetoprotein estimation in the amniotic fluid, it was in Sheffield in 1973 that the first termination was carried out because the foetus had an open neural tube defect. Since then, amniocentesis was offered to all high risk couples. Although this was most valuable to such couples, it made no measurable difference to the spina bifida births, because over 95% of such births are the first event in their families. Soon after came the possibility of discovering a much higher number of families at high risk with the estimation of the routine serum alphafetoprotein level in pregnant women and since then more and more „normal" pregnancies were monitored by serum tests. Routine serum tests started in January 1977 on women who presented at the antenatal clinic in good time and in 1983 over 90% of the pregnant population has been screened. When indicated, serum test was followed by amniocentesis.

Concurrently, increasing use was made of diagnostic ultrasound monitoring of pregnancies and now ultrasound monitoring of pregnancies is part of the routine management. The economic status of the city was improving in the 1960s. As the then Prime Minister, Sir Harold MacMillan, said "You've never had it so good." There was little unemployment and the diet of the population was probably as good as has ever been. Yet, the incidence of spina bifida was around 20 per 10,000 births. The late 1970s saw a progressive deterioration in the standard of living for those who became unemployed and by the 1980s some 15% of the population were jobless. It is not known wether this fact affected the nutrition of pregnant women.

During the 1970s and 1980s the annual *number* of spina bifida births fell progressively from an average of 18 in 1968 – 1970 to 10 in 1971 – 1973; 8 in 1974 – 1976; and 6 in 1977 – 1981. There were 2 in 1982 and 3 in 1983. The *rate* per 10,000 total births was 21 in 1968 – 1970 and only 4 per annum in 1982 – 1983. Further, in recent years a larger proportion than usual of these births had simple meningocele, so it was the more severe cases whose numbers declined most steeply. However, not all this decline was due to therapeutic terminations of pregnancy.

I carried out a detailed examination for 1979 to 1983 inclusive, of all the notifications of births; all the antenatal tests; and all the relevant obstetric records in the 3 large neonatal units where almost all births in Sheffield take place.

During these 5 years 8 babies were born with meningocele; 18 with myelomeningocele and 3 with encephalocele. In the same 5 years, 14 terminations were carried out because the foetus had myelomeningocele. Consequently, an average of 6 myelomeningocele *conceptions* occurred during these years which is about one-third compared with the experience in the 1960s but the number of *births* fell to an average of 3.6 per year. Antenatal diagnosis, therefore, reduced the number of such births by about 40%. The results are even more encouraging in 1982 and 1983. In these years there were only 4 myelomeningocele births and 9 terminations.

There are several reasons why there were still 18 births with myelomeningocele in the last 5 years. In 2 diagnosis was made antenatally but the parents refused termination; in a further 4 instances a suggestive positive serum result was not followed up by amniocentesis; and in another 4 instances the serum gave false negative results and ultrasound was not used. Finally, 8 were not screened, largely because the mothers attended too late for the first antenatal visit. In this group there was an undue proportion of immigrant women from the Asian sub-continent.

The problem of a large number of babies surviving with major multiple handicaps has been practically eliminated. There were only 18 babies born with myelomeningocele in the last 5 years, as compared with some 90 in 5 years in the 1960s. Thirteen of the 18 had severe permanently handicapping lesions at birth within the criteria for non-treatment. They were not treated and all 13 died early in infancy. Two others who were borderline cases were not treated at birth but were operated on later. These 2 and only these 2 are those who survived with severe handicaps. The last 3 were far less severe cases, were treated and survived with only mild to moderate handicap.

Antenatal screening was even more successful in contributing to the elimination of anencephalic births in Sheffield. No such births occurred in the last 3 years (1981 – 1983). During the same 3 years there were 15 terminations of anencephalic foetuses. This comparses with an average of 13 such births per annum between 1968 and 1973.

If the currently available preventive measures were even more fully used, then the elimination of all myelomeningocele births becomes a practical possibility and the painful decision of selective non-treatment will hardly ever have to be used. The prospect would be even brighter if true prevention with adequate diet or vitamin supplementation of the entire pregnant population would prove to be of value and could be achieved by practical means.

Other English cities and Wales [10]

The general trend of decrease in the major cities in England was similar to that experienced in Sheffield. In 1983 the rate for 9 provincial cities with births of over 5000 in each was an average of 4.1, compared with the national average of 6.7. The only exception was *Bradford* (rate 8.7) which has a very large minority of Asian origin. In *Nottingham*, with 7657 births in 1983 not a single baby was notified of having been born with spina bifida.

This lower incidence in the cities must be balanced with the higher prevalence in smaller communities and suggests that the provision of antenatal services is better in the cities (where all the University units are located) than in rural areas.

The population of *"London"* is incorporated in to 4 different regions and includes large surrounding areas. In these 4 regions the rate was similar to the national average.

In *Wales* the incidence of spina bifida was always higher than in England. It still remains higher, but is falling fast. In 1983 37 babies were notified or 10.4 per 10,000 total births. This figure is now as low as in East Anglia. Interestingly, because East Anglia was a low incidence area, major efforts with routine antenatal tests were considered unnecessary [9]. The incidence is now higher there (10.3) than in any other English region.

Scotland

In the *West of Scotland*, with an average of 37,000 births a year, the major role played by antenatal diagnosis by serum alphafetoprotein tests was shown by Ferguson-Smith (1983) [5]. By 1981 73% of the pregnant population had routine serum tests; 1% only needed amniocentesis and 56 terminations of pregnancy were carried out where the foetus had spina bifida. Yet more cases of spina bifida were detected antenatally, but the mothers refused to agree to termination.

Greater Glasgow is within Western Scotland and is Scotland's largest city with an average of 13,000 births a year. Spina bifida births declined from 56 (40 per

10,000) in 1974 to only 10 in 1981 and to 7 (5 per 10,000) in 1983 [6]. Some 21 terminations were carried out in 1981 because of spina bifida, suggesting that 31 spina bifida conceptions took place, in contrast to the 56 7 years earlier. Terminations were responsible for about half of the decline in spina bifida births. Again, there must be additional explanations for the remainder of the six-fold reduction in a mere 7 years.

It is interesting that in Glasgow there was an equally rapid decrease in the births of babies with hydrocephalus unassociated with spina bifida from 16 in 1975 to 2 per 10,000 total births in 1983, although antenatal diagnosis and terminations for this condition were not practised [6].

Ireland

Ireland is divided into two countries: the smaller Northern Ireland, which is largely protestant and the larger Eire which is predominantly Roman Catholic. In both countries the incidence of neural tube defects, including spina bifida was always very high, possibly the highest in the world.

In *Northern Ireland* with an average of 30,000 births per year the annual rate of spina bifida births was 36 between 1964 and 1968 [3] and 33 between 1969 and 1973 [4], but in 1975 it even rose to 45 per 10,000 total births. Subsequently, a major drop occurred, down to 20 in 1980, about the same as was in England 10 years earlier.

In the capital, *Belfast*, the trend was similar but the rate was even higher, though by 1982 this dropped to 23. As only high risk women were offered antenatal tests, it is not surprising that according to Professor Nevin's estimate only 2% of this decrease can be attributed to selective abortions [9].

In *Eire* selective antenatal tests are rare and officially abortions are forbidden. Detailed birth statistics are available only for the capital, *Dublin*. Here the rate fell steeply from 32 in 1979 to 22 by 1982 but was still at least as high as it was in England & Wales or Sheffield in the 1960s. In contrast, the rate in Sheffield was 3 per 10,000 in 1982.

International data

Hungary

Detailed comprehensive national records are available from Hungary from the studies of Czeizel. Interestingly, the trend here is different to that seen in Great Britain. There was a steady decline in the incidence of spina bifida from 12 per 10,000 in 1970 to 7.5 in 1976[2], but then it started to rise again and there were 8.6 per 10,000 conceptions with a spina bifida foetus in 1982.

Antenatal diagnosis and termination of pregnancies on a small scale started in 1977. In 1982 spina bifida births were reduced, slightly, because of 9 selective terminations. It is not clear what proportion of the population are offered antenatal diagnosis but it is clear that the natural decline in Hungary has stopped and that, so far, selective abortions have made little impact on the birth incidence.

Even anencephalic births are only slightly on the decline.

The Federal Republic of Germany (Bundesrepublik Deutschland)

In the Bundesrepublik there is compulsory notification of congenital malformations detectable within the first 3 days of life. The results are published by the Statistisches Bundesamt in Wiesbaden, but it is probable that there is under-reporting. A further source of error is that the figures do not include stillbirths. For example, in 1983 only 86 babies were reported to have been born with spina bifida, that is 1.4 per 10,000 births and only 12 liveborn with anencephalus. Yet, Koch and Fuhrmann [7] estimate that the current prevalence of NTD defects is about 10 to 15 per 10,000 births, with about equal distribution for spina bifida and anencephalus. The latter estimate, based on hospital statistics, is also liable to considerable error. Consequently, the regrettable conclusion is that there are no reliable data for the Bundesrepublik. Personal communications from various treatment centres and mortality statistics suggest, however, that there is a considerable recent decrease.

First-year deaths for the last 6 years, from 1978 to 1983 inclusive do indicate a substantial and year-by-year progressive decline from 114 in 1978 to 43 in 1983 (Statistisches Bundesamt, Wiesbaden). Methods of treatment are unlikely to have contributed to this decline, because during these years there have been no major changes in technique or in policies of selective treatment. Consequently, even if the data are incomplete, there are reasons to believe that the incidence of spina bifida in the Bundesrepublik is declining.

I could find no information, after extensive search, whether and to what extent are antenatal diagnosis and termination of pregnancy practised.

Other Countries

The International Clearinghouse for Birth Defects Monitoring Systems only provide data for 1980 to 1982 and so can give little firm idea, as yet, about the long term trends in the participating countries.

If the published figures are accurate, then within 3 years decreases of the order of 15–20% have taken place in *Czechoslovakia*, *Denmark* and *New Zealand*, none in *Finland* or *Norway*, while in *Hungary* and *Sweden* spina bifida may be on the increase.

Taking at their face value, the incidence in all the countries mentioned, except for Hungary, appear to be lower than in Great Britain even in 1982, but one is dubious whether the notifications are complete and whether the reporting is accurate. One can find widely differing figures relating to the same years for the same countries.

In the *United States* there are hospital-based statistics. Their birth defects monitoring programme records live and stillbirths based on 1,200 self-selected US hospitals and monitors some one million births yearly, this being approximately one-third of all births in the country. In 1970–1971 the rate per 10,000 births was 7.5, in 1976–1977 it was 5 and in 1980 it remained 5 [13]. Clearly, antenatal diagnosis has not made its impact yet in the United States but the overall incidence of spina bifida in the earlier years was much lower than in Great Britain. The gap had closed substantially by 1980.

From a small hospital-based statistics Stein and his colleagues from the Brooklyn Hospital, New York, were able to give a title to their paper "Is Myelomeningocele a Disappearing Disease?" [12].

Conclusion

In conclusion, in spite of the absence of reliable figures worldwide, and in spite of the different classifications used in various countries, there appears to be a general decline in the incidence of spina bifida which is particularly noticeable in the United Kingdom, possibly because it is easier to see a major decline in countries where the incidence was very high.

The total disappearance of spina bifida from much of the medically advanced and liberally-minded communities is now a real, none-too-distant possibility. Nevertheless, failure to use the existing and perhaps future preventive measures could lead to disaster and might still bring back conditions which existed in the past. We must be on guard against such events and not lull ourselves into false security, because just now spina bifida is on the decline for unknown epidemiological reasons.

Acknowledgements

1. Dr. A. Milford-Ward, Director of the Department of Immunology, The University of Sheffield, who carried out all the alphafetoprotein estimations and for allowing his records to be used for this paper.

2. Doctors Weatherhill and Alderson of the Office of Population Censuses and Surveys for valuable statistical information regarding England.

3. Dr. F. Hamilton and Mr. T. Sinclair of the Greater Glasgow Health Board who provided information for Scotland.

4. Dr. Proebsting of the Statistisches Bundesamt in Wiesbaden who provided information for West Germany.

5. Professor Ian Cooke of the University of Sheffield and Dr. B. A. M. Smith of the Northern General Hospital in Sheffield for valuable information regarding terminations and the outcome of pregnancies following antenatal tests.

6. The Richard Fund, Sheffield for secretarial assistance.

References

[1] Brock, D. J. H, R. G. Sutcliffe: Alphafetoprotein in the antenatal diagnosis of anencephaly and spina bifida. Lancet, 29th July (1972) 197 – 199.

[2] Czeizel, A.: Letter to British Medical Journal, vol. 287, 6th August (1983) 429.

[3] Elwood, J. H.: Major central nervous system malformations notified in Northern Ireland 1964 – 68. Dev. Med. and Child Neurol. **14** (1972) 731.

[4] Elwood, J. H.: Major central nervous system malformations notified in Northern Ireland 1969 – 73. Dev. Med. and Child Neurol. **18** (1976) 512 – 520.

[5] Ferguson-Smith, M. A.: The reduction of anencephalic and spina bifida births by maternal serum alphafetoprotein screening. Brit. Med. Bull., vol. 39, **4** (1983) 365 – 372.

[6] Hamilton, F. M. W., T. Sinclair: Greater Glasgow Health Board. Personal communication (1984).

[7] Koch, M., W. Fuhrmann: Epidemiology of Neural Tube Defects in Germany. A review.

[8] Lorber, J.: The family history of spina bifida cystica. Pediatrics **35** (1965) 589.

[9] Nevin, N. C.: Prevention of neural tube defects in an area of high incidence. In: Prevention of spina bifida and other neural tube defects (J. Dobbing, ed.), pp. 127 – 144. Academic Press Inc., Ltd., London 1983.

[10] Office of Population Censuses and Surveys Monitor 1984 (M3 84/5).

[11] Standing, S. J., M. J. Brindle, A. P. MacDonald et al.: Maternal alphafetoprotein screening: 2 years' experience in a low-risk district. Br. Med. J., vol. 283, 12 September (1981) 705 – 707.

[12] Stein, S. C., J. G. Feldman, M. Friedlander et al: Is myelomeningocele a disappearing disease? Pediatrics, vol. 69, **5** (1982) 511 – 513.

[13] Winham, G. C., L. D. Edmonds: Current trends in the incidence of neural tube defects. Pediatrics, vol. 70, **3** (1982) 333 – 337.

In much of this paper references were obtained from the official statistics of the Office of Population Censuses and Surveys; the Sheffield Congenital Anomalies Register; the International Clearinghouse for Birth Defects Monitoring Systems; Eurocat and the Statistisches Bundesamt, Wiesbaden.

Comparative aspects of dysraphic malformations in domestic animals

M. Vandevelde

Dysraphic malformations such as anencephaly, encephalocoele, meningocoele and myelocoele, have all been described in most domestic and laboratory animals [2, 6, 7].

Spontaneously occurring malformations of the nervous system, have been closely studied in cattle with the primary purpose to decrease their incidence by breeding measures. The frequency of all malformations in this species is 0.3% of which one third also involve the nervous system. Spina bifida with or without neurospinal dysraphism is one of the most common congenital defects in calves. In most cases, spina bifida is associated with other CNS anomalies especially the Arnold Chiari malformation. Another frequent combination is spina bifida, neurospinal dysraphism and articular rigidity also known as the bovine congenital arthrogryposis syndrome. Extensive teratologic studies on large numbers of newborn calves suggest that genetic factors play an important role in the pathogenesis. These results were based on systematic analysis of the offspring from parental animals used for artificial insemination [19]. Although some parental animals have a much higher malformation frequency in their offspring than others, the genetic mechanism is difficult to explain in most cases because calves often exhibit multiple, apparently unrelated malformations. Therefore the concept of genetic burden is applied: by exceeding a certain critical number of deletary cooperating genes in the population, malformations occur. Environmental factors, especially infectious agents can not be excluded as possible causes. However, although many viruses are known to produce development defects in the CNS of domestic animals ranging from hydrocephalus to deficient myelin development, infectious agents specifically causing dysraphic malformations have not been identified.

In companion animals (dogs, cats) dysraphic malformations have been described mostly as sporadic cases [3, 4, 8, 10]. Spina bifida and associated cord malformations are the most common defect. In contrast to cattle these lesions in small animals are usually not combined with other malformations. The most common site is the lumbosacral area with bladder, colon and sphincter problems but rarely locomotor signs. Spina bifida in dogs has a very high incidence in the English Bulldog which would suggest genetic factors.

Reproducible hereditary neural tube defects have been studied in the Manx cat and the Weimaraner dog. The dysraphic malformation in Manx cats is genetically associated with the absence of the tail, including sacrococcygeal dysgenesis, spina bifida with or without meningo-myelocoele and incomplete development of the sacral spinal cord and cauda equina. α-feto-protein has been demonstrated in the amniotic fluid of Manx cats with neural tube defects. The mode of inheritance is autosomal dominant with incomplete penetration.

Neurospinal dysraphism in Weimaraner dogs is clinically characterized by a hopping gait; other, less common, signs are thoracolumbar scoliosis, koilosternia and abnormal hair streams in the cervical area. In all clinically affected animals more or less subtle spinal cord malformations may be found at all levels and include: lack of a dorsal septum; absent, enlarged or abnormally shaped central canal; abnormal position and fusion of the ventral horns; absent or incompletely penetrating ventral median fissure. In adult dysraphic Weimaraner dogs syringomyelia, especially in the central areas and along the dorsal midline is common.

Neurospinal dysraphism in Weimaraner dogs has a partially dominant mode of inheritance with incomplete penetration and variable expression. By mating clinically dysraphic animals 70−80% of the embryos or fetuses exhibit spinal cord anomalies. True closure defects of the neural tube have not been observed in developmental studies; abnormal migration patterns appear to be the underlying defect whereby parts of the mantle layer are displaced ventrally and invagination of the ependyma appears to result in a duplication of the caudal neural tube.

References

[1] Cho, D. Y., H. W. Leipold: Spina bifida and spinal dysraphism in calves. Zbl. Vet. Med. A, 24 (1977) 680−695.
[2] Done, J. T.: Developmental disorders of the nervous system in animals. Adv. Vet. Sci. and comp. Med. Academic Press, New York, San Francisco, London, vol. 20 (1976) 69−114.
[3] Engel, H. N., D. D. Draper: Comparative prenatal development of the spinal cord in normal and dysraphic dogs: embryonic stage. Am. J. Vet. Res. 43 (1982) 1729−1734.
[4] Engel, H. N., D. D. Draper: Comparative prenatal development of the spinal cord in normal and dysraphic dogs: fetal stage. Am J. Vet. Res. 43 (1982) 1735−1743.
[5] Herzog, A.: Embryonale Entwicklungsstörungen des Zentralnervensystems beim Rind. Habilitationsschrift, Gießen 1971.
[6] Kalter, H.: Teratology of the central nervous system. The University of Chicago Press, Chicago−London 1968.
[7] Kitchen, H.: Spina bifida. In: Spontaneous animal models of human disease. Vol. II. (E. J. Andrews, B. C. Ward, N. H. Altman, eds.). Academic Press, New York−London−Toronto−Sydney−San Francisco 1979.

[8] McGrath, J. T.: Spinal dysraphism in the dog. Pathologia Veterinaria, vol. 2, Suppl. S. Karger, Basel – New York 1965.

[9] Rieck, G. W., A. Herzog, W. Schade: Modell Hessen: Populationsweites Kontrollsystem zur pathologischen Überwachung des Besamungsbullen. Tierärztl. Umschau 6 (1977) 305 – 314.

[10] Wilson, J. W., H. J. Kurtz, H. W. Leipold et al.: Spina bifida in the dog. Vet. Pathol. 16 (1979) 165 – 179.

[11] Frauchiger E., R. Fankhauser: Vergleichende Neuropathologie des Menschen und der Tiere. Springer Verlag, Berlin 1957.

The embryology and pathology of dysraphias

U. Roessmann

Following the gastrulation phase, the cells of the dorsal region are induced through the chordomesoderm to form the neural plate. This neuroepithelium, which is to form the central nervous system proliferates and expands into the neural groove. The fusion of the dorsal rims of the neural groove − neurulation − begins approximately 20 days after the fertilization of the ovum. Failure of closure or its disruption after it has closed are presumed to be the basic events in the formation of the dysraphic malformations.

Myelomeningocele is the prototype of the schisis of the neural tube. The spinal cord is formed as if the neural groove never closed and the cells simply matured in the normal sequence. The neural arch above remains open and the attached muscular structures are poorly, if at all, developed. In most instances the entire lesion is covered by a layer of very simply structured epidermis. This sequence can be considered as a primary failure of induction to close the neural tube, which in turn fails to induce the formation of mesenchymal elements. Since the caudal neuropore is the last site to close, it seems natural that its failure to close should lead to the most commonly occurring lesion. There is, however, evidence that the involved segments of the spinal cord in the lumbo-sacral region are formed only after the caudal neuropore has already closed. They arise from the so-called end-bud through coalescence and canalization of several proliferating cell groups [5]. Since the end-bud organization is a much more complex event than the actual neuropore closure, it is somewhat easier to think in terms of improper induction through the closely involved chordal tissue rather than of failure of closure or reopening of the already closed tube. In the majority of the surgical specimens following the repair of the myelomeningocele, the neural elements consist primarily of disorganized islets rather than exhibiting the classical open cord picture. This suggests that the neuroepithelial tissue in the most involved area never reached the neural groove stage of organization.

In contrast, true dysraphic spinal cord is usually found at higher levels. The lesion consists of a bifid spine and a well organized but split spinal cord, which are enclosed by normal subcutaneous tissue and covered by intact skin. The rachischisis fails to induce the disruption of the overlying skin and muscle. The most logical explanation for such a lesion is that the neural groove develops normally but fails to close and that it secondarily induces the vertebral anomaly. Presumably, the spinal cord in such lesions should be structurally and functionally intact, save for the split. Such a presumption, however, must not be accepted without further evaluation, both through more exact anatomical observations as well as through physiological studies. With new diagnostic capabilities it should be possible to identify individuals with such lesions that may be minimally symptomatic and study the physiological parameters of the split spinal cord. No observations from such cases are available at present on the segmental organization of the spinal cord or on the skeletal muscle in the involved region, although Barson [1] has emphasized that a kyphosis does not occur with the lesions above low thoraco-lumbar levels. Furthermore, such lesions may be associated with symptoms related to lower segments which still need explaining.

Another interesting problem is the longitudinal splitting of the spinal cord which may or may not be associated with skeletal malformations. These changes are described under the names of diplomyelia or diastematomyelia. The two terms used are interchangeable in the literature. Confusion could be avoided by use of words such as duplication and splitting (Verdoppelung or Spaltung). The split cord is of considerable clinical interest since the frequent presence of a dural septum containing bony or cartilagenous spicules interferes with the proper relationship between the neural elements and the vertebral column during the development, particularly during the rapid growth phase of the adolescent. This misalignment results in stretching of the spinal cord and of the rootlets, causing symptoms and requiring surgical intervention. The doubled spinal cord is of more interest to the physiologist who would like to know the functional aspects of this abnormality. From an anatomical point of view the two malformations are most confusing because of the lack of the distinguishing criteria and the multiple overlapping aspects of the anatomical findings. From an embryological viewpoint the cause of this remains unclear. To explain the split cord, Bremer [2] has postulated a persistent neurenteric canal as the basic pathogenetic mechanism. The dorsal fistula should result, in an anterior division of the neural tube. It is not possible, however, to find such a neurenteric canal or an anterior vertebral defect in every case of diastematomyelia or diplomyelia. Furthermore, there are so many problems of overlapping between these malformations and the failure of the closure type of malformations that it is difficult to envisage a single pathogenetic mechanism for the entire group. We have examined a case in which duplication of the spinal cord occurred together with the duplication of the pituitary gland. Since the neurulation and the development of the hypophyseal anlage take place at approximately the same time and, since both probably are induced by the chordomesenchymal tissue, it seems reasonable to suggest that such malformations can occur under the perturbed influence of the notochord. There is experimental evidence available to support the view that notochordal disturbance induces proliferation of the cells in the neural plate which could result in duplication.

Anencephaly is the most frequent dysraphia, but because of its lethal outcome it is of no interest to neurosurgeons. Because of its peculiar geographic and ethnographic distribution it has initiated epidemiological studies searching for a causative agent. Anatomically, the most significant findings are those of Marin-Padilla [6], who demonstrated convincingly that the skeletal malformation is an integral part of the problem. While it is again not possible to say which structure induces the other, it seems clear that the extent of the brain destruction depends on the extent of the bony defect. It is not possible to explain the entire complex with a simple failure of closure of the anterior neuropore. It is more likely, that the failure of the mesenchymal tissue elements results in the destruction of the more or less normally induced neural components which have reached a fairly advanced state of organization. This is shown by the development of the eyes and other parts of the system which remain preserved in such cases where the bony defect allows it. The problem of exencephaly seems to contradict this idea, yet careful examination actually support it. The exencephalic brain shows no evidence of any failure of closure. The changes seen in such brains are more consistent with interference with the cell multiplication. This occur at considerable time after the neuropore closure, and are most likely due to external factors acting on the growing brain in the absence of the protective skeleton.

The Chiari complex is of greatest interest to the clinical branches. It is most amenable to corrective measures and even offers possibilities for intrauterine treatment, but it presents a most confusing problem due to its anatomical complexity. This malformation has at least two components, which at first sight seem to differ in their embryological derivation. The first is myelomeningocele, most commonly in the lumbo-sacral area, which was discussed above. The second component consists of the major malformation at the foramen magnum. Here, instead of the neural tube defect, there is a massive caudal displacement of the structures of the brain stem. Not only is there a shift in relation to the surrounding bones, but also between the ventral and dorsal components of the brain stem, further complicated by the involvement of the cerebellar structures. All theories to explain these complex events on purely mechanistic grounds are clearly inadequate. The first study to use an embryological approach is that of Jennings et al. [4]. The authors propose a downward displacement of the brain-cord transition zone during the initial fusion of the neural folds. This could result in a displacement of the "anlage" forming the caudal rhombcncephalon and of the somites programmed to develop the cervical vertebrae. While there may be missing parts in the story, the proposal has considerable merit in providing a unified explanation for the entire complex. A downward shift in the brain-cord transition zone could also result in a downward shift in the induction of the remainder of the neural tube leading to the schisis in the lumbo-sacral area.

The severity of the shift may also vary, resulting in variations in the extent of the malformation in the posterior fossa and foramen magnum region. This variation results in clinically less severe problems and allows for a variety of symptom complexes. To alleviate confusion in the nomenclature a simplified classification is proposed [3]. It is based on decreasing severity of the anatomical malformation and correlates with the clinical course of the patients. In the adult the Chiari malformation is characterized by survival before the symptoms become manifest and anatomically consists of a downward herniation of the cerebellar tonsils, the medulla oblongata and the fourth ventricle. Chronic tonsillar herniation is a self-defining term. In both groups the spinal dysraphism is virtually non-existent, but in both instances segmental malformation of the cervical spine, cervico-occipital misalignment and syringomyelia frequently occur. Both groups are of great clinical interest since they respond well to simple posterior fossa decompression.

References

[1] Barson, A. J.: Spina bifida: The significance of the level and extent of the defect to the morphogenesis. Dev. Med. Child Neurol. 12 (1970) 129–144.
[2] Bremer, J. L.: Dorsal intestinal fistula; Accessory neurenteric canal; Diastematomyelia. Arch. Pathol. 54 (1952) 132–138.
[3] Friede, R. L., U. Roessmann: Chronic tonsillar herniation. An attempt at classifying chronic herniations at the foramen magnum. Acta Neuropathol. (Berl.) 34 (1976) 219–235.
[4] Jennings, M. T., S. K. Clarren, V. G. Kokich et al.: Neuroanatomic examination of spina bifida aperta and the Arnold-Chiari malformation in a 130-day human fetus. J. Neurol. Sci. 54 (1982) 325–338.
[5] Lemire, R. J.: Variations in development of the caudal neural tube in human embryos (Horizons XIV to XXI). Teratology 2 (1969) 361–370.
[6] Marin-Padilla, M.: Morphogenesis of anencephaly and related malformations. Curr. Top. Pathol. 51 (1970) 145–174.

Neural tube defects: Experimental findings and concepts of pathogenesis

R. C. Janzer

Introduction

It is generally accepted that the aetiology and pathogenesis of neural tube defects (NTD) are multifactorial. They include genetic predisposition as well as environmental factors [1, 12]. A recent advance in prophylaxis has been achieved by the clinical finding that periconceptional administration of multivitamins, especially folic acid, can significantly reduce recurrences of NTD [10, 24]. Despite this progress the basic mechanisms leading to NTD remain for the most part hypothetical. For testing concepts of pathogenesis the use of animal models and substances with known sites of action are essential. Of the more than 30 agents known to produce dysraphic lesions [3] most are effective only around the restricted time of fusion of the neural folds [9]. Therefore, the most probable common mode of action of several teratogenic agents lies in the disturbance of cell adhesion and recognition mechanisms during neural fold fusion. Glycosylated membrane proteins and lipids are generally known to play an important role in these mechanisms [2, 6]. We therefore investigated the normal distribution of Concanavalin A binding sites during neurulation in the chick embryo by light-, scanning- and transmission-electron-microscopy and induced NTD by topical application of Concanavalin A.

Material and methods

A more detailed description of the methods employed is given elsewhere [8]. Briefly, stage 6 to 10 chick embryos [5] were divided in two main groups. Group A (for investigation of normal distribution of Concanavalin A binding sites) was either fixed in 2% glutaraldehyde, exposed to ferritin-conjugated Concanavalin A and processed for scanning or transmission electron microscopy (SEM and TEM), or treated first with FITC-conjugated Concanavalin A, freeze-dried and examined by fluorescence microscopy. In controls, Concanavalin A (Con A) was replaced by Ringer's solution. Group B (for induction of NTD) was treated in ovo by a single subgerminal injection of native Con A (or Ringer's solution in controls). After various time intervals the embryos were fixed in 2% glutaral-dehyde and processed for SEM or TEM. The processing for SEM was the same for both groups A and B. The specimens were glued onto a stainless steal grid and the whole preparation either postfixed in OsO_4 or 2% glutaraldehyde. After dehydration in acetone and critical-point-drying in liquid CO_2 the specimens were mounted onto object holders. A gold coating was applied in a sputtering device. After SEM-examination the specimens were transfered to ethanol, emb-edded in araldite and further processed according to standard TEM procedures. The ultrastructure of specimens previously processed for SEM was comparable to that of embryos processed directly for TEM.

Results

Normal distribution of Concanavalin A binding sites

The normal distribution of Con A binding sites, described elsewhere in more detail [7], showed a predilection for the leading edges of the neural folds prior to fusion. The greatest amount of binding sites was seen on a few cell layers of the opposing neural folds in the fusion zone. At the luminal surface of the basal portion of the closing neural tube there was only weak staining. This pattern could be similarly observed in the fusion zone of stages 7, 8, 9 and 10. Older stages were not investigated. Rostrally and caudally from the fusion zone sig-nificant amounts of Con A binding sites were observed at the edges of the elevating neural folds but were not found in the adjacent neural groove or lateral surface ectoderm.

Dysraphic lesions induced by Concanavalin A

Dysraphic lesions in the cervico-thoracic region were obtained in about 40% of the animals treated by subgerminal injections of Con A. Twentyfour hours after treatment the extent of the dysraphic lesion was greatly variable. Small lesions measured about 200 microns while larger ones occupied the whole length of the cervico-thoracal spinal cord (fig. 1A, 1B). The lumbosacral region was not affected in any of these animals. The dysraphic lesion was covered cranially and caudally by normal ectoderm. Specific changes were seen at the lateral edges of the open neural tube selectively at the junction between neural folds and lateral ectoderm at the level of the dysraphic lesion. These changes consisted of malorien-tated filopodia and excessive blebbing (fig. 2B). Blebs consisted of rounded cells or cell portions attached by intermediate type cell junctions to the underlying

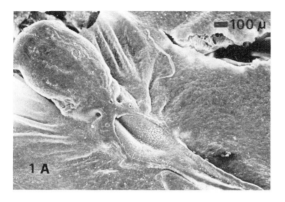

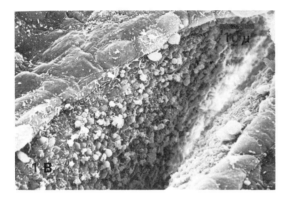

Fig. 1   SEM of dysraphic chick embryo treated with Concanavalin A at stage 8. Widely open neural tube (A). Intact lateral surface ectoderm with microvilli at cell borders; open neural tube with blebbing on neuroepithelial cells (B).

normal neural fold cells (fig. 3). These elements contained intact nuclei with abundant nucleopores and the normal range of cell organelles found at these stages in the underlying normal neural tube cells. However, neither cytoskeletal elements nor cilia were present in these blebs. At earlier stages (90 min after treatment with Con A) small blebs were already present at the prospective fusion zones. In addition, some cells had a smooth and bulging cell surface with loss of their single central cilium, normally present at these stages in neuro-epithelial cells. Generally the cilia on the cells of the prospective fusion zone had an abnormal, randomly arranged orientation. At the cranial and caudal end of the dysraphic lesion, which was mostly covered intact by surface ectoderm, there was in some specimens an overfolding and overgrowth of the neural folds leading to early stages of diastematomyelia (fig. 2A).

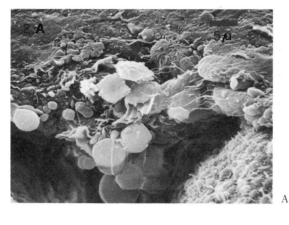

A

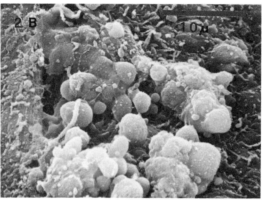

B

Fig. 2   SEM of dysraphic lesion. Rostral part of the NTD: Covering of normal surface ectoderm and neuroepithelium with abnormal aberrant filopodia and multiple smooth blebs at the dorsal aspect of the neural tube (A). Lateral edge of the NTD: At left normal surface ectoderm, at right normal neuroepithelial cells of the neural groove. In the junction zone small and large smooth blebs (B).

Discussion

The pathogenesis of neural tube defects (NTD) is still controversial. The earliest possible disturbance of nervous system development is by interference in the induction of neural plate formation. The mechanisms for neural induction have not yet been elucidated, but in other developmental systems the necessity for transport of macromolecular substances by diffusion, by direct cell to cell contact or by vesicular transport has been demonstrated [25]. Based on the observation that not only neuroectodermal but also mesodermal elements are severly disturbed in NTD, some authors have postulated defective induction [13]. The evidence,

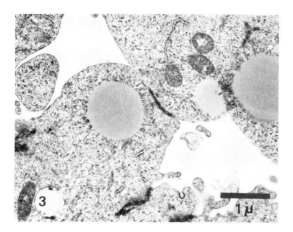

Fig. 3   TEM of blebbing regions (topography showed in fig. 2B). Blebs are attached to the underlying apical surface of the neural tube cell by intermediate type junctions and contain polyribosomes, lipid drop lets, mitochondria and rough endoplasmic reticulum, but no cytoskeletal elements.

however, is indirect, and has not been supported by experimental findings. The next step in neurulation involves elongation of cells in the neural plate, brought about by the orientation of microtubules in parallel. This step in differentiation can be inhibited by agents, which interfere with the function of microtubules, eg. Vinka-alkaloids or colchicine. Using these agents NTD have been produced experimentally [14]. Also important in early neural development is the folding mechanism by which the neural plate is elevated to form the neural folds and the neural groove. This process is apparently mediated by the constriction of apical microfilaments. NTD have also been successfully induced by inhibition of this constriction process with cytochalasin B [27] or papaverin [15]. The fusion process itself, is the most complex step in neurulation and involves cell recognition as well as nonspecific and specific adhesion mechanisms. These are mediated by species- and stage-dependent specialized cell surface structures such as lamellipodia, filopodia, cilia, ruffles, etc. [4, 23, 26], by the presence of an extracellular matrix [18, 20], and by integral membrane glycoproteins and glycolipids [2]. However, the attention of most authors was focused on the elucidation of the normal fusion process, rather than on the morphogenesis of NTD.

Our results show that interference with Con A binding sites, present in high amounts at the leading edges of the opposing neural folds just prior to fusion [7], leads initially to a desorientation of surface extensions. The smooth cell surfaces bulge and form rounded blebs. These consist of portions of cells, partly containing a normal nucleus. While still attached to the apical surfaces of underlying neural fold cells, they protrude into the lumen and apparently inhibit proper contact and adhesion with the opposing edge. The folding process thus remains ongoing, leading in some cases to an overfolding and overgrowth and potentially to diastematomyelia [8]. The stage of normal intercellular junction formation is never reached. By these morphological changes, adhesion and recognition mechanisms are disturbed and the fusion process prevented. It is noteworthy that in a genetic mouse model where spontaneous NTD occurs in 60% of the offspring, application of cytostatic agents reduces the occurrence of NTD, but only when applied during the critical period of the fusion process itself [22]. It is not entirely clear why cytostatic substances, which interfere with DNA metabolism are only effective during the fusion process in preventing NTD. One can speculate that by altering the cell cycle the time for the production and action of substances essential for adhesion or recognition may be sufficiently increased to overcome the deficient fusion process observed in the untreated animals.

Additional theories invoke a reopening of an already closed neural tube as the primary mechanism for NTD. Support for these theories comes from experiments with cytostatic agents applied after neural tube closure [11, 20] and mechanical reopening [18]. In addition, there have been a few findings in normal human embryos, which suggest the concept of secondary "neuroschisis" [16]. Some human dysraphias may be due to neural fold overgrowth following fusion [17]. There are undoubtedly selected specimens, which support the reopening hypothesis, but most of the experimental findings, including those presented here, point to the importance of a disturbed fusion process.

Conclusion

Experimental agents known to produce NTD are most effective during fusion of the neural folds. Our experiments demonstrate specific morphologic changes induced by occupation of Concanavalin A binding sites in the prospective fusion zone, which proceed to NTD. These findings indicate that the disturbance of adhesion and recognition mechanisms during neural fold fusion may be one of the most important pathogenetic factors for the evolution of NTD in some laboratory animals and possibly also in humans.

References

[1] Carter, C.O.: Clues to the aetiology of neural tube malformations. Dev. Med. Child Neurol. **16** (1974) 3–15.
[2] Edelman, G.M., S. Hoffman, C.-M. Chuong et al.: Structure and modulation of neural cell adhesion molecules in early and late embryogenesis. Cold Spring Harbor Symposia on Quantitative Biology **23** (1983) 515–526.

[3] Elwood, J. M., J. H. Elwood: Epidemiology of anencephalus and spina bifida. Oxford University Press, Oxford 1980.

[4] Geelen, J. A. G., J. Langman: Ultrastructural observations on closure of the neural tube in the mouse. Anat. Embryol. **156** (1979) 73 – 88.

[5] Hamburger, V., H. L. Hamilton: A series of normal stages in the development of the chick embryo. J. Morph. **88** (1951) 49 – 92.

[6] Ivatt, R. J. (ed.): The biology of glycoproteins. Plenum Press, New York 1984.

[7] Janzer, R. C., B. Walker: Concanavalin A binding sites are predominantly expressed on neuroepithelial cell surfaces at the leading edge of the elevating neural folds. Acta anat. (submitted).

[8] Janzer, R. C., B. Walker: Concanavalin A induced neural tube defects in the early chick embryo. Neuropathol. Appl. Neurobiol. (submitted).

[9] Kalter, H.: Teratology of the central nervous system. Univ Chicago Press, Chicago 1968.

[10] Laurence, K. M., N. James, M. H. Miller et al.: Double-blind randomised controlled trial of folate treatment before conception to prevent recurrence of neural tube defects. Br. Med. J. **282** (1981) 1509 – 1511.

[11] Lee, H. Y., R. S. Hikida, M. A. Levin: Neural tube defects caused by 5-Bromodeoxyuridine in chicks. Teratology **14** (1976) 89 – 98.

[12] Lemire, R. J., J. B. Beckwith, J. Warkany (eds.): Anencephaly. Raven Press, New York 1978.

[13] Marin-Padilla, M., V. H. Ferm: Somite necrosis and developmental malformations induced by vitamin A in the golden hamster. J. Embryol. Exp. Morphol. **13** (1965) 1 – 8.

[14] Messier, P. E.: Microtubules, interkinetic nuclear migration and neurulation. Experientia **34** (1978) 289 – 296.

[15] O'Shea, K. S.: Calcium and neural tube closure defects: an in vitro study. Birth Defects **18** (1982) 95 – 106.

[16] Padget, D. H.: Neuroschisis and human embryonic maldevelopment. J. Neuropathol. Exp. Neurol. **29** (1970) 192 – 216.

[17] Patten, B. M.: Overgrowth of the neural tube in young human embryos. Anat. Rec. **113** (1952) 381 – 393.

[18] Rokos, J., J. Knowles: An experimental contribution to the pathogenesis of spina bifida. J. Path. **118** (1976) 21 – 24.

[19] Sadler, T. W.: Distribution of surface coat material on fusing neural folds of mouse embryos during neurulation. Anat. Rec. **191** (1978) 345 – 350.

[20] Sadler, T. W., R. R. Cardell: Ultrastructural alterations in neuroepithelial cells of mouse embryos exposed to cytotoxic doses of hydroxyurea. Anat. Rec. **188** (1976) 103 – 124.

[21] Schoenwolf, G. C., M. Fisher: Analysis of the effects of Streptomyces hyaluronidase on formation of the neural tube. J. Embryol. Exp. Morphol. **73** (1983) 1 – 15.

[22] Sellner, M. J.: The cause of neural tube defects: some experiments and a hypothesis. J. Med. Gen. **20** (1983) 164 – 168.

[23] Silver, M. H., J. M. Kerns: Ultrastructure of neural fold fusion in chick embryos. SEM/1978/II, pp. 209 – 215. III Research Institute, Chicago 1978.

[24] Smithells, R. W., M. J. Seller, R. Harris et al.: Further experience of vitamin supplementation for prevention of neural tube defect recurrences. Lancet I (1983) 1027 – 1031.

[25] Toivonen, S., D. Tarin, L. Saxen: The transmission of morphogenetic signals from amphibian mesoderm to ectroderm in primary induction. Differentiation **5** (1976) 49 – 55.

[26] Waterman, R. E.: Topographical changes along the neural fold associated with neurulation in the hamster and mouse. Am. J. Anat. **146** (1976) 151 – 172.

[27] Webster, W., J. Langman: The effect of cytochalasin B on the neuroepithelial cells of the mouse embryo. Am. J. Anat. **152** (1978) 209 – 222.

Occlusion of the Lumen of the neural tube, and its role in the early morphogenesis of the brain

M. H. Kaufman

Formation of the spinal and cephalic regions of the neural tube: primary and secondary neurulation

Innumerable studies have been carried out which have attempted to investigate the various factors involved in neurulation. Both descriptive and experimental reports are now available that shed light on the underlying mechanisms involved and how these are temporally interrelated. To date, most of the researchers in this field have examined the sequential changes that take place in amphibian and avian embryos, but more recently similar studies have been carried out with mammalian embryonic material.

While the sequence of events involved in the establishment of the primitive brain and spinal cord was until quite recently considered to be a relatively simple progression, involving the transition of the neural plate into the neural tube via the process of neurulation, even this series of events is now seen to be an oversimplification. The basic morphological changes that take place during neurulation, with the initial formation of the neural groove and neural folds, and their subsequent elevation, apposition and eventual fusion across the dorsal midline are well known [6, 7, 27, 31, 62, 67, 68], and our understanding of these events has been greatly facilitated with the availability of transmission and scanning electron microscopy [2, 3, 54, 60, 79]. This sequence of events has now been termed primary neurulation, and it is by this process that the cephalic and most of the spinal part of the neural tube is formed. However, it now appears that the caudal portion of the spinal cord forms by a quite different process, and the series of events which take place during this second phase has been termed secondary neurulation. The latter process, which appears to be much less precise than primary neurulation, results in a slight lengthening of the spinal axis. Descriptive accounts are available of secondary neurulation in the chick embryo, and these events are first observed at about the time that the caudal neuropore closes [12, 30, 36, 56, 59, 63].

Unlike the situation in primary neurulation, in secondary neurulation the prospective neural tissue is located subcutaneously when the dorsal region of the embryo is completely covered with ectoderm. Initially, a solid medullary cord forms by the aggregation of cells in the dorsal region of the tail bud, and these cells subsequently differentiate into peripheral and central components. This stage is followed by the process of canalization in which a single central cavity forms within the medullary cord which eventually unites rostrally with the lumen of the neural tube. Histologically the caudal neural material is slightly difficult to interpret, as in the prospective lumbosacral region of the avian embryo primary neurulation progresses dorsally while secondary neurulation occurs ventrally. An approximately similar sequence of events has also been described in several mammalian species [human: 5, 26, 40, 41; mouse: 62]. However the principal difference between these events in avian and mammalian embryos relates to the fact that in the latter the lumen formed by canalization (during secondary neurulation) appears always to be continuous rostrally with the lumen of the previously formed neural tube. As indicated above, secondary neurulation appears to lack the precision of primary neurulation, and in the caudal region accessory lumens and cellular proliferation into the main lumen are frequently observed.

The canalization phase in the human embryo is followed by a more precise phase associated with the disappearance of the tail region. The latter phase is termed retrogressive differentiation [72], and this phase continues until after birth and results in the formation of the coccygeal medullary vestige, the filum terminale and the ventriculus terminalis [41].

Concomitant with the occurrence of these events in the caudal part of the embryonic axis, may be observed major changes in the morphological appearance of the cephalic region of the embryo. While there are only slight differences in the overall pattern of closure of the neural folds in the cephalic region of rodents and related species [mouse: 20, 32, 78; hamster: 35, 42, 69, 77, 78; rat: 1, 4, 8, 17, 34], with approximately simultaneous closure at various sites, this pattern is in marked contrast to the events described in the human embryo. In man [48, 73], as well as in the macaque embryo [24], fusion of the neural folds proceeds rostrally as a continous zipper-like process from the prospective cervical region to the region of the rostral neuropore.

Some time after the neural tube has closed in the cephalic region, the caudal neuropore closes. The exact timing of this event varies between species [rat: 81; human: 41, 43, 73], and even between strains within a single species [mouse: 9, 57, 75]. This event also results in the closure of the neural tube at both of its extremities, so that the neural tube may now be considered as a completely sealed system for the first time during its morphogenesis. Desmond and Jacobson [14] therefore related the timing of the initiation of rapid brain enlargement with the closure of the caudal neuropore. This event occurs in most chick embryos by about stage 12 [22, 76]. It was argued that once the neural canal closed, a positive fluid pressure could build up within the system which would then enable rapid brain enlargement to occur. However, more recent studies have indicated

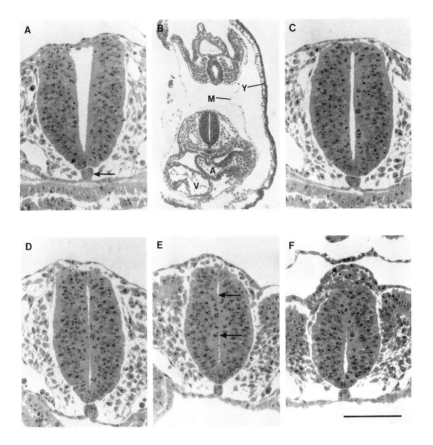

Fig. 1   Representative transverse sections through the neural tube of an 'unturned' embryo with
10 – 12 pairs of somites present, isolated in the afternoon on the 9th day of gestation. Sections
stained with meythylene blue.

a) Section through the neural tube at the mid-cardiac level. Note that the neural lumen is
widely patent, and the notochord (arrowed) clearly seen; b) low magnification view through
the 'thoracic' region of this embryo. The section is taken through the caudal one third of
the heart, and through the mid-tail region. Key: A = atrium, V = ventricle, Y = yolk sac,
M = amnion; c) higher magnification view through the neural tube in the 'thoracic' region
at a level identical to that illustrated in b). A slight indication of side-side apposition is
apparent at this level; d) section through the neural tube at the level of the sinus venosus,
at the caudal extremity of the heart. A considerable degree of side to side apposition is seen,
particularly in the central region of the neural tube, though the neural lumen is still patent
at this level; e) section through the neural tube about half way between the sections illustrated
in *d* above and *f* below, some distance proximal to the U-shaped lordotic segment in this
'unturned' embryo. The middle third of the neural lumen (region between arrows) appears
to be completely occluded. f) Section through the neural tube just proximal to the lordotic
segment; the dorsal half of the lumen appears to be completely occluded whereas the ventral
segement is still patent. Bar = 100 μm.

[33, 62] that rapid brain enlargement may be initiated before the caudal neuropore closes, and that a totally enclosed system is in fact achieved at this time via a quite separate process termed neural luminal occlusion. This mechanism enables a considerable proportion of the neural lumen along the spinal axis to be completely occluded. In all of the species so far studied, the rostral extent of occlusion is either to the prospective cervical region, or may even extend to the level of the otocysts. Any increase in luminal pressure which results either from an increase in fluid production, or its decreased removal from this site, is therefore associated with selective dilatation of the prospective brain region. The timing of these events, and the underlying changes that take place during the occlusion process, forms the basis of the present paper. I have decided to concentrate on this aspect of the early morphogenesis of the neural tube because its significance has only recently been appreciated.

Occurrence of neural luminal occlusion

Most of the information in the literature regarding the occurrence of this phenomenon has been obtained from analyses of histological sections through the neural tube of the developing chick embryo [23, 37, 51, 54, 66], and no doubt many others, and indeed are even hinted at in the diagrams of mid-somite level sections of the neural tube illustrated in Duval [16], though the significance of these findings was apparently not appreciated until quite recently.

Though attention had not necessarily been drawn to the presence of neural luminal occlusion, histological evidence of this phenomenon is available not only in the chick (where it has long been known to occur, see above, and discussion

---

Fig. 2   Representative transverse sections through the neural tube of an almost completely 'turned' embryo with about 20 pairs of somites present, isolated in the evening on the 9th day of gestation. Sections stained with methylene blue.
a) Section through the cephalic region just rostral to the otic pits and slightly distal to the origin of the 1st branchial arches (arrowed). Some degree of dorsal and particularly ventral side to side apposition is apparent in the hindbrain region (H). Key: F = forebrain, G = foregut; b) section through the hindbrain at the level of the otic pits (arrowed). Note that the neural lumen is completely occluded. Key: F = foregut, 1 = first branchial arch, 2 = origin of the second branchical arch, Bar = 300 μm. c) Section through the 'thoracic' region at the level of the distal one-third of the heart. The ventral two-thirds of the neural lumen is occluded at this level. Key: A = atrium, prior to division into right and left sides, V = ventricle; d) section through embryo at the level of the two horns of the sinus venosus (S). The neural tube is virtually completely occluded at this level; e) slightly oblique section through embryo just above the forelimb bud (arrow). The lumen in the ventral half of the proximal region of the neural tube (upper) is almost completely occluded, while in the distal region (lower) the lumen, though narrow, is completely patent; f) section through embryo just below the forelimb bud. The middle two-thirds of the neural tube shown here represents the occluded proximal ventral segment of the lumen illustrated in e) above. The paraxial blocks of somites are clearly seen at this level.

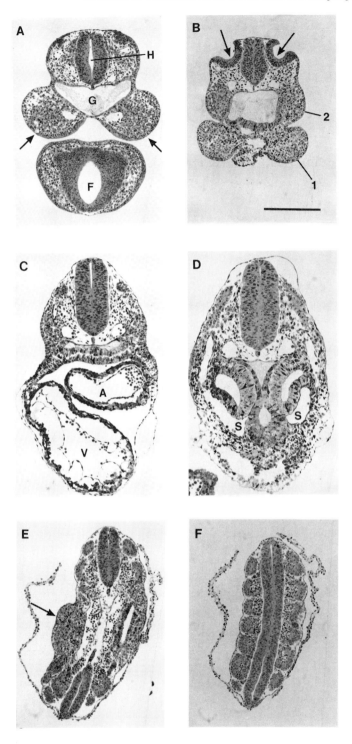

in [3]), in the human [13] and mouse [33, 49], but also in *Xenopus* [67], the quail [37], and in the rat [18] at approximately comparable stages of embryonic development. Appropriate scanning of the literature would probably reveal further evidence of this phenomenon in a host of other vertebrate species. Possibly the most significant recent finding in this regard is the observation that the neural lumen almost invariably becomes completely occluded *prior to* the closure of the caudal neuropore. Of the 3 species in which this phenomenon has so far been studied in some detail, complete neural luminal occlusion first occurs in a proportion of mouse embryos at an even earlier stage, that is, prior to the closure of the rostral neuropore [33] (see fig. 1). In the human embryo, neural luminal occlusion is first seen in embryos in which the rostral neuropore has already closed [13]. In the chick the situation appears to be slightly different, in that occlusion begins in a proportion of embryos at the level of the more rostral somites near the time that the neural folds become apposed in the dorsal midline [64].

Neural luminal occlusion occurs in the 2 mammalian species so far studied some considerable time after neurulation is completed along the spinal axis (see figs. 2–4), rather than concomitant with it as appears to occur in some chick embryos. It is possible that this difference in the timing of the occlusion event in relation to axial neurulation may in some way reflect the apparent decreased degree of complexity of the avian compared to the mammalian neural plate and neural tube. Alternatively, this difference may merely reflect species variability in the underlying mechanism of achieving neural luminal occlusion. However, it

---

Fig. 3   Representative transverse sections through the neural tube of a parasagittally sectioned mouse embryo isolated at about midday on the 11th day of gestation. In this embryo, the neural lumen is partially occluded. The occluded segment extends caudally from the lower trunk region almost to the tip of the tail. Embryo embedded in paraffin wax and sections stained with haematoxylin and eosin.

a) Parasagittal section through the cephalic region which also cuts through the proximal part of the tail region at the level of the hindlimb buds. Key: L = lens vesicle, R = rhombencephalon, O = otocyst, F = forelimb bud, H = hindlimb bud, N = neural tube; b) parasagittal section through the cephalic, thoracic and mid-trunk regions. Note that the neural lumen is partially occluded in the lower trunk region and at the base of the tail. Key: F = forebrain, O = optic stalk, H = heart, S = somites, N = neural tube; c) transverse section through the neural tube in the proximal part of the tail region. Note that about two-thirds of the lumen is occluded at this level; d) longitudinal slightly oblique section through the neural tube at a slightly deeper level than that illustrated in figure b); e) transverse section through the neural tube at the level of the hindlimb buds. Note that the middle one-third of the neural lumen is occluded at this level; f) transverse section through the neural tube at a level slightly distal to that illustrated in figure e); g) higher magnification view of neural tube at same level as that illustrated in figure f). Note that the ventral half of the neural lumen is still patent, and a small channel is also patent dorsally; h) transverse section through the neural tube at a level slightly distal to that illustrated in figures f) and g). Note that the dorsal segment of the neural canal is not patent at this level.

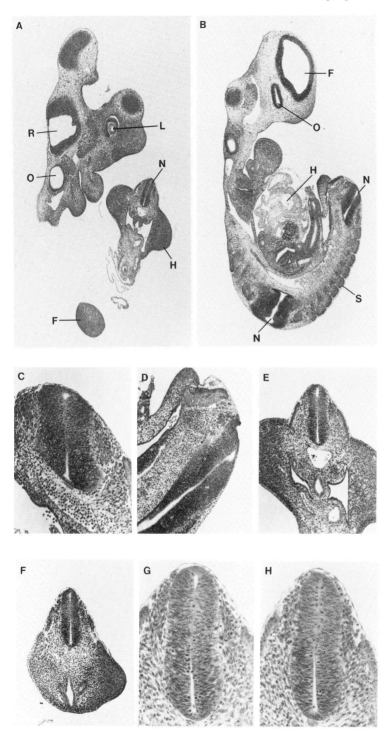

should be noted that in many chick embryos occlusion undoubtedly occurs after the completion of neurulation in the spinal region.

What does appear to be extremely curious is the fact that despite numerous descriptive accounts of avian neurulation over nearly 100 years since the classic account of Duval [16] on the embryology of the chick, the significance of this phenomenon has only recently been appreciated. Some authors assumed luminal occlusion was an artefact of fixation [80], whereas others working with seemingly identical material either failed to observe it or simply ignored it.

While it is possible that occlusion may not be observed in histological sections of poorly fixed material, it is likely that the latter phenomenon, though frequently encountered, was generally disregarded because it had no obvious role to play during either neurulation or the early development of the nervous system. This apparent deficiency in reporting this phenomenon is all the more curious since luminal occlusion is particularly marked in chick embryos at stage 9 of Hamburger and Hamilton [22], during the apposition phase shortly before neural tube closure, and in embryos as they progress between stages 10–19 when the spinal canal is virtually completely occluded in most embryos [64].

Morphological features of neural luminal occlusion

It is of interest at this juncture to discuss the current information available on the ultrastructural morphology of the neuroepithelial cell surfaces in regions of very close apposition or complete occlusion. What little information is available on the reopening of the neural canal along the neural axis will then be discussed.

Various approaches have been employed to analyse in detail the ultrastructural changes that occur both prior to and during the occlusion phase. The most detailed account of the events that occur in the chick embryo is undoubtedly

---

Fig. 4   Scanning electron micrographs showing the appearance of the neural tube at various locations in embryos isolated on the 10th (figs. a – c) and 12th day (fig. d) of gestation.
a) Appearance of the neural tube in the mid-trunk region of an embryo isolated in the afternoon on the 10th day of gestation. Note that the ventral half of the neural lumen appears to be occluded. The notochord is arrowed; b) appearance of the neural tube in the proximal part of the tail region of the same embryo as that illustrated in figure a). The ventral half of the neural lumen appears to be occluded. The notochord is arrowed; c) appearance of the neural tube in the mid-trunk region of an embryo that appeared externally to be at approximately the same stage of development as the embryo illustrated in figures a) and b). Note that the neural lumen is completely patent at this level; d) appearance of the neural tube sectioned through the proximal part of the tail region. This embryo was isolated at about midday on the 12th day of gestation. Note that while a small channel is present dorsally, elsewhere the lumen is almost completely occluded.

that of Schoenwolf and Desmond [64], while the morphological appearance of the neuroepithelial cell surface in the mouse embryo (see fig. 5) has recently been described by Kaufman [33].

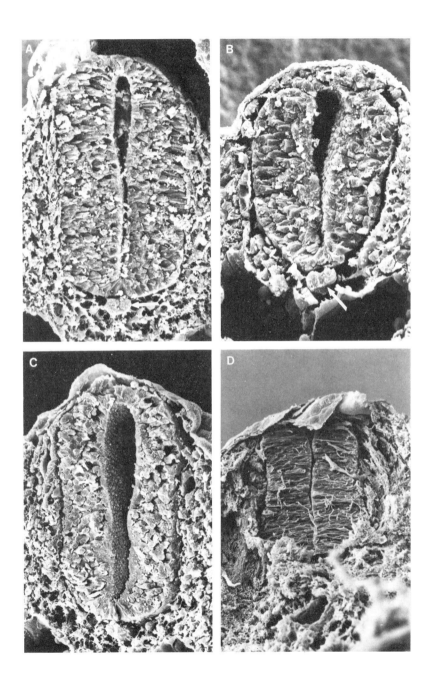

Despite the considerable differences found in these 2 studies regarding the overall relationship between neurulation and neural luminal occlusion, at the ultrastructural level the findings are remarkably similar. Indeed, the changes which are thought to occur in the neuroepithelial cell surfaces of closely apposed cells during the occlusion process are almost identical in these 2 species.

The various ultrastructural changes that are thought to underlie the occlusion process probably occur in the following sequence: Initially, a segment of the apical regions of the neuroepithelial cells along the lateral walls of the neural tube become closely apposed across the midline. In the mouse embryo the actual segment involved may be relatively limited in length or may be quite extensive, whereas in the chick embryo where the neural groove is distinctly V-shaped, apposition tends to occur along the entire dorsoventral axis, so that the whole neural lumen is rapidly obliterated like the closing of a hinge. In the mouse embryo [33] as well as in the human embryo [13], luminal occlusion always appears to take place after the completion of neurulation, whereas in some chick embryos occlusion takes place concomitant with the apposition of the neural folds, prior to the completion of neurulation. In many chick embryos, however, the pattern is apparently closer to that seen in the mouse, with occlusion following the completion of neurulation.

When the apices of the neuroepithelial cells on the lateral walls of the neural folds (or neural tube) are examined, no obvious specialised structures are observed that might facilitate the apposition process. It is possible, however, that the first contact may be established across the midline by the interdigitation of relatively small diameter projections that protrude from the surfaces of the neuroepithelial cells whose apices abut on the spinal lumen. In locations where cellular contact has been made across the midline, the initial contacts are usually established between relatively small or occasionally quite large cellular protuberances. Characteristically, the majority of the apposing cell surfaces are either completely flattened or have a few small undulations. At locations of very close apposition,

---

Fig. 5   Transmission electron micrographs illustrating appearance of neuroepithelial cell surfaces at sites of cell-cell apposition and luminal occlusion. These are representative thin sections from various sites along the neural axis of an embryo with about 25 pairs of somites present a) and b). Apposing neuroepithelial surfaces bridged by relatively large cellular protrusions. Between these sites of initial contact, the cell surfaces are either completely flattened or only slightly undulating. Both micrographs × 2600;   c) extensive region of close apposition in which a narrow luminal channel is still visible. Note the occasional presence of coated pits (large arrow) and coated vesicles (small arrows) × 3700;   d) extensive regions in which the neural lumen is completely obliterated, interspersed with small lacunae containing 'spinal' fluid × 3100;   e) higher magnification view of region in which the neural lumen is completely obliterated. Note the presence of coated pits and vesicles with granular contents (arrowed) in close proximity to the neuroepithelial cell surfaces, and the absence of junctional complexes between the apposed neuroepithelial cell surfaces. In this, and in *a-d* above, apical junctional complexes (white arrows) are observed between adjacent neuroepithelial cells × 12,500.

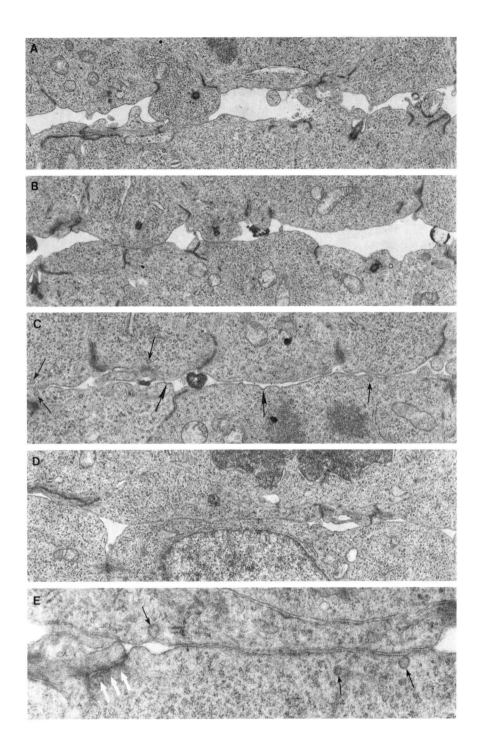

only a few areas where minimal 'point' contact is established are generally seen. Cellular contact is generally established between two non-dividing cells, but is not uncommonly observed between a non-dividing and a dividing cell.

While areas of minimal membrane specialisation in the form of localised areas of increased electron density have been reported in the chick in regions of close apposition, no *well-defined* intercellular junctional complexes have been reported in either the chick or the mouse embryo, even though the apical complexes between adjacent neuroepithelial cells are clearly apparent. While this does not unequivocally exclude the possibility that some type(s) of specialised complexes are in fact formed, clearly other techniques eg. freeze fracture analysis, would be required to demonstrate them. The absence of obvious junctional complexes is presumably a reflection of the temporary and reversible nature of the occlusion process.

In areas where extensive cellular contact is established, only small pockets of luminal fluid remain in areas of neuroepithelial cellular fusion. The absence of pinocytic vesicles in the subcortical region tends to suggest that absorbtion of the luminal fluid probably plays only a minor role in its removal from this site. This is probably a reasonable assumption, since apposition and fusion (in the mouse and chick embryo, though possibly not in the human embryo) is first apparent when both the rostral and caudal neuropores are still widely open. Under these circumstances most of the luminal fluid is probably displaced caudally or rostrally into the amniotic cavity rather than resorbed locally.

The initial contact and adhesion between apposing neuroepithelial cells in the mouse may be facilitated by the presence of extracellular material at the luminal surface of these cells, though Schoenwolf and Desmond [64] were unconvinced that surface coating material played any significant role in the occlusion process in the chick embryo. However, the presence of coated pits and vesicles at and subjacent to the cell surface noted by Kaufman [33] may be indicative of their role-possibly facilitating the removal of excess extracellular matrix material at the fusion site [53] during the final stages of luminal occlusion. This should not be altogether surprising, as an increase in ruthenium-red-positive material has been demonstrated along apical neural fold borders and on the overlying ectoderm cells in regions immediately prior to and at the time of neurulation [44, 55, 58], and its removal at this time can interfere with neural tube closure [38, 50]. The presence of similar surface coat material is also observed along prospective zones of fusion in the palate [21, 52] and during fusion of the medial and lateral nasal processes [19, 70]. In all of these locations, a decrease in the distribution of surface macromolecules is observed after fusion.

The other intrinsic factors that have to be taken into consideration are the shape changes that take place in neuroepithelial cells. It is unclear at the present time whether these various shape changes – such as cellular elongation and apical cell constriction play a role in the occlusion process. These changes undoubtedly play a critical role in neurulation [7, 27, 31, 67, 68], and it would seem reasonable to suggest that these cytoskeletal-mediated cell shape changes probably also play a vital (but as yet undefined) role in the occlusion process.

A variety of extrinsic factors presumably also play a vital role in the occlusion process, and a range of hypothetical 'forces' have been proposed some of which may be involved in pushing the 2 sides together – possibly generated by the somites or surfaces ectoderm [61], or by the subjacent extracellular matrix material [chick: 66, rat: 45, 46, 71]. However it is easier to list these hypothetical 'forces' than demonstrate them, and much more experimental work has to be carried out before the morphogenetic mechanisms underlying these various processes are clearly understood.

Significance of neural luminal occlusion in relation to rapid brain enlargement

Various measurements have been made of the avian cerebrospinal fluid pressure in the prospective brain region [28, 29], and this information coupled with the experimental findings following intubation of the brain [11, 14, 65] and eye [10] strongly suggests that intraluminal pressure within the developing nervous system is essential for its normal morphogenesis. Direct measurements of the fluid pressure within the mesencephalon in the chick embryo following caudal neuropore closure has revealed the presence of a positive pressure of 2.5–3.0 mm of water in this location [28, 29]. However, other factors including differential cellular proliferation must also be borne in mind in relation to brain morphogenesis. For example, prior to the earliest evidence of complete neural luminal occlusion in most mouse embryos (when about 15 pairs of somites are present) the optic vesicles and fore- and midbrain vesicles have already become moderately dilated, while the rhombencephalon, which has yet to close over its dorsal aspect is also rounded in appearance [32]. These observations strongly suggest that while luminal occlusion undoubtedly facilitates the dilatation of these various brain and related vesicles, neither occlusion nor necessarily the presence of an enclosed chamber need to be present to initiate the dilatation process. It seems likely therefore that the initiation of dilatation can be brought about in the absence of increased intraluminal pressure. As long as the cellular cytoskeletal system of the neuroepithelial cells is functioning normally, this factor alone enables sheets of cells to roll up and form either tubes (as occurs in the case of the neural tube) or develop into vesicles (as occurs in the case of the optic, otic and lens vesicles). Numerous experimental studies are also available to confirm that interference with the normal functioning of the cellular cytoskeletal system undoubtedly leads to abnormal morphogenesis [49]. Clearly no single factor can account for the changes that take place during neurulation, and numerous extrinsic as well as intrinsic factors are known to play a vital role in these events. For example, there is experimental evidence to suggest that the shape of the neural tube and its lumen depend on the type of mesoderm that surrounds it [25, 74]. Curiously, in *Triton* the neural lumen only becomes slit-like when the neural tube is in close proximity to the notochord [39]. The fact that it is the ventral half of the neural lumen that is more commonly occluded than the dorsal half may reflect the earlier differentiation of the cellular components within the ventral rather than the dorsal horns. It has also been suggested [3] that the shape of the lumen may be related to the water content of the neural tube and subjacent tissues in the embryo, as large fluid volume movements occur from the albumen through the tissues of the embryo into the sub-blastodermic fluid during the early stages of embryogenesis in the chick [47].

Following closure of the caudal neuropore in the mouse, which normally occurs on the 11th day of gestation when the embryo possesses 30 − 34 pairs of somites [9], one might expect that there would no longer be a requirement for neural luminal occlusion. For whatever reason, partial and often complete obliteration of the neural lumen is frequently seen on the 11th and even on the 12th day of gestation (see figs. 3 and 4). On the 11th day, the occluded segment is usually found in the lower trunk region, and extends caudally from the level of the forelimb buds into the proximal part of the tail region. On the 12th day, the partially or completely occluded segment is usually located in the region of the hindlimb buds and extends caudally into the tail region.

It is possible that the regions of complete or partial occlusion may serve to protect the extremely thin plate of neuroepithelium in the region of the caudal neuropore from bulging and possibly even bursting as a result of the elevated hydrostatic pressure needed to complete the morphogenesis of the various cerebral vesicles. In the light of these observations, it would be of considerable interest to obtain direct measurements of the pressure within this system at different stages of gestation, in order to compare the values thus obtained with the readings of Jelínek and Pexieder [28, 29] during their studies of the stages of rapid brain enlargement in the chick embryo. Desmond and Jacobson [14] have emphasized that normal brain enlargement involves an interplay between cerebrospinal fluid pressure and an increase in cellular proliferative activity at this time − in the absence of one or other factor, the outcome is likely to be deficient or disorganised growth. These factors are also involved in shaping the brain during later stages of its development when the enlarging hemispheres are subjected to localized resistance due to regional variations in brain tissue morphology, or to the extrinsic pressures imposed by surrounding tissues. It may well be that the relatively uniform tubular architecture of the axial part of the neural tube resists deformation under conditions of increased neural luminal pressure, whereas the partially dilated rostral extremity may be less capable of resisting the forces that arise within its much modified lumen.

It was briefly mentioned in an earlier section that no convincing evidence has so far been obtained of well-defined junctional complexes that cross the midline that might facilitate the apposition of the two sides of the neural tube during the period of luminal occlusion, though their absence would, of course, enable the two sides to separate rapidly when required. The latter is said to occur in the chick embryo [15], but information is so far lacking regarding the reopening phase in other species. It can only be speculated that whatever intrinsic or extrinsic 'forces' are present that help to maintain the occluded state, these are either overcome or are induced to disappear. How the neural lumen reopens, and the factors that induce it do so, will undoubtedly provide the experimental embryologist with many additional fertile areas for research.

Acknowledgements

The work described here was supported by a grant from the National Fund for Research into Crippling Diseases (Action Research for the Crippled Child).

References

[1] Adelmann, H.B.: The development of the neural folds and cranial ganglia of the rat. J. Comp. Neur **39** (1925) 19 – 171.
[2] Bancroft, M., R. Bellairs: The onset of differentiation in the epiblast of the chick blastoderm (SEM and TEM). Cell Tiss. Res. **155** (1974) 399 – 418.
[3] Bancroft, M., R. Bellairs: Differentiation of the neural plate and neural tube in the young chick embryo. A study by scanning and transmission electron microscopy. Anat. Embryol. **147** (1975) 309 – 335.
[4] Bartelmez, G.W.: The proliferation of neural crest from forebrain levels in the rat. Contr. Embryol. Carneg. Inst. **37** (1962) 1 – 12.
[5] Bolli, P.: Sekundäre Lumenbildungen in Neuralrohr und Rückenmark menschlicher Embryonen. Acta Anat. **64** (1966) 48 – 81.
[6] Burnside, B.: Microtubules and microfilaments in newt neurulation. Devl Biol. **26** (1971) 416 – 441.
[7] Burnside, B.: Microtubules and microfilaments in amphibian neurulation. Am. Zool. **13** (1973) 989 – 1006.
[8] Christie, G.A.: Developmental stages in somite and post-somite rat embryos, based on external appearance, and including some features of the macroscopic development of the oral cavity. J. Morph. **114** (1964) 263 – 286.

[9] Copp, A. J., M. J. Seller, P. E. Polani: Neural tube development in mutant (*curly tail*) and normal mouse embryos: the timing of posterior neuropore closure *in vivo* and *in vitro*. J. Embryol. exp. Morph. **69** (1982) 151 – 167.

[10] Coulombre, A. J.: The role of intraocular pressure in the development of the chick eye. I. control of eye size. J. exp. Zool. **133** (1956) 211 – 225.

[11] Coulombre, A. J., J. L. Coulombre: The role of mechanical factors in brain morphogenesis. Anat. Rec. **130** (1958) 289 – 290 (Abstract).

[12] Criley, B. B.: Analysis of the embryonic sources and mechanisms of development of posterior levels of chick neural tubes. J. Morph. **128** (1969) 465 – 501.

[13] Desmond, M. E.: Description of the occlusion of the spinal cord lumen in early human embryos. Anat. Rec. **204** (1982) 89 – 93.

[14] Desmond, M. E., A. G. Jacobson: Embryonic brain enlargement requires cerebrospinal fluid pressure. Devl Biol. **57** (1977) 188 – 198.

[15] Desmond, M. E., G. C. Schoenwolf: Ultrastructural studies of occlusion and re-opening of the lumen of the spinal cord during rapid brain enlargement. Anat. Rec. **208** (1984) 44 (Abstract).

[16] Duval, M.: Atlas d'Embryologie. G. Masson, Paris 1889.

[17] Edwards, J. A.: The external development of the rabbit and rat embryo. In: Advances in Teratology (D. H. M. Woollam, ed.), vol. 3, pp. 239 – 263. Logos Press, New York 1968.

[18] Freeman, B. G.: Surface modifications of neural epithelial cells during formation of the neural tube in the rat embryo. J. Embryol. exp. Morph. **28** (1972) 437 – 448.

[19] Gaare, J. D., J. Langmann: Fusion of nasal swellings in the mouse embryo. Surface coat and initial contact. Am. J. Anat. **150** (1977) 461 – 476.

[20] Geelen, J. A. G., J. Langman: Closure of the neural tube in the cephalic region of the mouse embryo. Anat. Rec. **189** (1977) 625 – 640.

[21] Greene, R. M., D. M. Kochhar: Surface coat on the epithelium of developing palatine shelves in the mouse as revealed by electron microscopy. J. Embryol. Exp. Morph. **31** (1974) 683 – 692.

[22] Hamburger, V., H. L. Hamilton: A series of normal stages in the development of the chick embryo. J. Morph. **88** (1951) 49 – 92.

[23] Hay, E. D.: Embryologic origin of tissues. In: Histology (R. O. Greep, ed.), p. 64. McGraw-Hill, New York 1966.

[24] Heuser, C. H., G. L. Streeter: Early stages in the development of pig embryos, from the period of initial cleavage to the time of the appearance of limb-buds. Contr. Embryol. Carneg. Inst. **20** (1929) 1 – 29.

[25] Holtfreter, J.: Formative Reize in der Embryonalentwicklung der Amphibien, dargestellt an Explantationsversuchen. Arch. exp. Zellforsch. **15** (1934) 281 – 301.

[26] Ikeda, Y.: Beiträge zur normalen und abnormalen Entwicklungsgeschichte des caudalen Abschnittes des Rückenmarks bei menschlichen Embryonen. Z. Anat. Entw. Gesch. **92** (1930) 380 – 490.

[27] Jacobson, A. G., R. Gordon: Changes in the shape of the developing vertebrate nervous system analyzed experimentally, mathematically and by computer simulation. J. exp. Zool. **197** (1976) 191 – 246.

[28] Jelínek, R., T. Pexieder: The pressure of encephalic fluid in chick embryos between the 2nd and 6th day of incubation. Physiol. Bohemoslovaca **17** (1968) 297 – 305.

[29] Jelínek, R., T. Pexieder: Pressure of the CSF and the morphogenesis of the CNS. I. Chick embryo. Folia Morphol. (Praha) **18** (1970) 102 – 110.

[30] Jelínek, R., V. Seichert, E. Klika: Mechanism of morphogenesis of caudal neural tube in the chick embryo. Folia Morphol. (Praha) **17** (1969) 355 – 367.

[31] Karfunkel, P.: The mechanisms of neural tube formation. Int. Rev. Cytol. **38** (1974) 245 – 271.

[32] Kaufman, M. H.: Cephalic neurulation and optic vesicle formation in the early mouse embryo. Am. J. Anat. **155** (1979) 425 – 444.

[33] Kaufman, M. H.: Occlusion of the neural lumen in early mouse embryos analysed by light and electron microscopy. J. Embryol. exp. Morph. 78 (1983) 211 – 228.

[34] Keibel, F.: Normentafel zur Entwicklungsgeschichte der Wanderratte (Rattus norvegicus Erxleben). Fischer, Jena 1937.

[35] Keyzer, A.: The development of the diencephalon of the Chinese hamster. An investigation of the validity of the criteria of subdivision of the brain. Acta Anat. (Basel) Suppl. 59 (1972).

[36] Klika, E., R. Jelínek: The structure of the end and tail bud of the chick embryo. Folia Morphol. (Praha) 17 (1960) 29 – 40.

[37] Le Douarin, N.: The Neural Crest. Cambridge University Press, Cambridge 1982.

[38] Lee, H., J. B. Sheffield, R. G. Nagele et al.: The role of extracellular material in chick neurulation. I. Effects of concanavalin A. J. exp. Zool. 198 (1976) 261 – 266.

[39] Lehmann, F. E.: Die Entwicklung von Rückenmark, Spinalganglien und Wirbelanlagen in chordalosen Körperregionen von Tritonlarven. Rev. Suisse Zool. 42 (1935) 405 – 415.

[40] Lemire, R. J.: Development of the caudal neural tube in human embryos (Horizons XIII – XXI) Teratology 2 (1969) 264 (Abstract).

[41] Lemire, R. J., J. D. Loeser, R. W. Leech et al.: Normal and Abnormal Development of the Human Nervous System, pp. 71 – 83. Harper and Row, Hagerstown, MD 1975.

[42] Marin-Padilla, M.: The closure of the neural tube in the golden hamster. Teratology 3 (1970) 39 – 46.

[43] Marin-Padilla, M.: Clinical and experimental rachischisis. In: Congenital Malformations of the Spine and Spinal cord (P. J. Vinken, G. W. Bruyn, N. C. Myrianthopoulos, eds.). Handbook of Clinical Neurology, vol. 32, pp. 159 – 191. Elsevier/North Holland, Amsterdam 1978.

[44] Moran, D., R. W. Rice: An ultrastructural examination of the role of cell membrane surface coat material during neurulation. J. Cell Biol. 64 (1975) 172 – 181.

[45] Morriss, G. M., M. Solursh: Regional differences in mesenchymal cell morphology and glycosaminoglycans in early neural-fold stage rat embryos. J. Embryol. exp. Morph. 46 (1978) 37 – 52.

[46] Morriss-Kay, G. M., B. Crutch: Culture of rat embryos with β-D-xyloside: evidence of a role for proteoglycans in neurulation. J. Anat. 134 (1982) 491 – 506.

[47] New, D. A. T.: The formation of sub-blastodermic fluid in hens eggs. J. Embryol. exp. Morph. 4 (1956) 221 – 227.

[48] O'Rahilly, R.: The early development of the eye in staged human embryos. Contr. Embryol. Carneg. Inst. 38 (1966) 1 – 42.

[49] O'Shea, S.: The cytoskeleton in neurulation: role of cations. In: Progress in Anatomy (R. J. Harrison, R. L. Holmes, eds.), vol. 1, pp. 35 – 60. Cambridge University Press, Cambridge 1981.

[50] O'Shea, K. S., M. H. Kaufman: Phospholipase C-induced neural tube defects in the mouse embryo. Experientia 36 (1980) 1217 – 1219.

[51] Packard, D. S., A. G. Jacobson: Analysis of the physical forces that influence the shape of chick somites. J. exp. Zool. 207 (1979) 81 – 91.

[52] Pratt, R. M., J. R. Hassell: Appearance and distribution of carbohydrate-rich macromolecules on the epithelial surface of the developing rat palatal shelf. Devl Biol. 45 (1975) 192 – 198.

[53] Pratten, M. K., R. Ducan, J. B. Lloyd: Adsorptive and passive pinocytic uptake. In: Coated Vesicles (C. D. Ockleford, A. Whyte, eds.) pp. 179 – 218. Cambridge University Press, Cambridge 1980.

[54] Revel, J. P., S. S. Brown: Cell junctions in development with particular reference to the neural tube. Cold Spring Harbor Symp. Quant. Biol. 40 (1976) 443 – 455.

[55] Rice, R. W., D. J. Moran: A scanning electron microscopic and x-ray microanalytic study of cell surface material during amphibian neurulation. J. exp. Zool. 201 (1977) 471 – 478.

[56] Romanoff, A. L.: The Avian Embryo. Macmillan, New Yor: 1960.

[57] Rugh, R.: The Mouse – Its Reproduction and Development. Burgess Publishing Company, Minneapolis 1968.

[58] Sadler, T. W.: Distribution of surface coat material on fusing neural folds of mouse embryos during neurulation. Anat. Rec. 191 (1978) 345 – 350.

[59] Schoenwolf, G. C.: Tail (end) bud contributions to the posterior region of the chick embryo. J. exp. Zool. 201 (1977) 227 – 246.

[60] Schoenwolf, G. C.: Observations on closure of the neuropores in the chick embryo. Am. J. Anat. 155 (1979) 445 – 466.

[61] Schoenwolf, G. C.: On the morphogenesis of the early rudiments of the developing central nervous system. Scan. Electron Microsc. I (1982) 289 – 308.

[62] Schoenwolf, G. C.: Histological and ultrastructural studies of secondary neurulation in mouse embryos. Am. J. Anat. 169 (1984) 361 – 376.

[63] Schoenwolf, G. C., J. Delongo: Ultrastructure of secondary neurulation in the chick embryo. Am. J. Anat. 158 (1980) 43 – 63.

[64] Schoenwolf, G. C., M. E. Desmond: Descriptive studies of occlusion and reopening of the spinal canal of the early chick embryo. Anat. Rec. 209 (1984a) 251 – 263.

[65] Schoenwolf, G. C., M. E. Desmond: Neural tube occlusion precedes rapid brain enlargement. J. exp. Zool. 230 (1984b) 405 – 407.

[66] Schoenwolf, G. C., M. Fisher: Analysis of the effects of *Streptomyces* hyaluronidase on formation of the neural tube. J. Embryol. exp. Morph. 73 (1983) 1 – 15.

[67] Schroeder, T. E.: Neurulation in *Xenopus laevis*. An analysis and model based upon light and electron microscopy. J. Embryol. exp. Morph. 23 (1970) 427 – 462.

[68] Schroeder, T.: Mechanisms of morphogenesis: The embryonic neural tube. Int. J. Neuroscience 2 (1971) 183 – 198.

[69] Shenefelt, R. E.: Morphogenesis of malformations in hamsters caused by retinoic acid: relation to dose and stage at treatment. Teratology 5 (1972) 103 – 118.

[70] Smuts, M. S.: Concanavalin A binding to the epithelial surface of the developing mouse olfactory placode. Anat. Rec. 188 (1977) 29 – 38.

[71] Solursh, M., G. M. Morriss: Glycosaminoglycan synthesis in rat embryos during the formation of the primary mesenchyme and neural folds. Devl Biol. 57 (1977) 75 – 86.

[72] Streeter, G. L.: Factors involved in the formation of the filum terminale. Am. J. Anat. 25 (1919) 1 – 11.

[73] Streeter, G. L.: Developmental horizons in human embryos. Description of age group XI, 13 to 20 somites, and age group XII, 21 to 29 somites. Contr. Embryol. Carneg. Inst. 30 (1942) 211 – 245.

[74] Takaya, H.: Two types of neural differentiation produced in connection with mesenchymal tissue. Proc. Imp. Acad. Japan 32 (1956) 282 – 288.

[75] Theiler, K.: The House Mouse. Development and Normal Stages from Fertilization to 4 Weeks of Age. Springer-Verlag, Berlin 1972.

[76] Vaage, S.: The segmentation of the primitive neural tube in chick embryos (*Gallus domesticus*). A morphological, histochemical, and autoradiographical investigation. Advan. Anat. Embryol. Cell Biol. 41 (1969) 8 – 87.

[77] Waterman, R. E.: Use of the scanning electron microscope for observation of vertebrate embryos. Devl Biol. 27 (1972) 276 – 281.

[78] Waterman, R. E.: Topographical changes along the neural fold associated with neurulation in the hamster and mouse. Am. J. Anat. 146 (1976) 151 – 172.

[79] Waterman, R. E.: Scanning electron microscope studies of central nervous system development. Birth Defects: Original Article Series 15 (1979) 55 – 77.

[80] Watterson, R. L.: Laboratory Studies of Chick and Pig Embryos. Burgess Publishing Company, Minneapolis 1955.

[81] Witchi, E.: Development: rat. In: Growth: Including Reproduction and Morphological Development (P. L. Altmann, D. S. Dittmer, eds.), pp. 304 – 314. Federation of American Societies for Experimental Biology, Washington 1962.

The Corpus callosum, an evolutionary and developmentally late crossing midline structure, malformations and functional aspects

P. Glees

Phylogenetically the corpus callosum is a very recent structure and even some mamalian species have no significant callosal commissure. Some marsupials do have a corpus callosum (the kangaroo), while those non-eutherian mammals (echidnas) that do not possess this connexion but have instead an anterior commissure only, which is larger than those found in placentals [14].

Developmental aspects

While spinal cord and lower brain stem have left and right halves interconnected by neural folds closure, the forebrain portions have a paucity of interconnections. The diencephalic portion has a relatively small midline crossing while the paired telencephalic vesicles possess to start with only an anterior and a hippocampal commissure.

The corpus callosum between the cerebral vesicles is formed relatively late in foetal development, after all other crossing midline structures are present.

The first vestige of a link between the two human hemispheres appears in the fourth week of gestation when the cortical plates develop. A thin epithelial layer called the lamina terminalis, which connects the anterior walls of the two hemispheres between the rhinencephalon and the optic chiasma, is the first bridge (fig. 1). This lamina thickens gradually into the commissural plate or lamina reuniens into which grow the fibres of the anterior commissure (fig. 2) the more slender rhinencephalic connexion of the lower animals [10], and also the callosal fibres in the 12th week which than become so formidable in man. By the fifth month of the human foetus, not only are symmetrical points in the anterior parts of the hemispheres connected but also those in the posterior parts, in fact every lobe of the cortex eventually has its communicating bridge of callosal fibres with its counterpart in the opposite hemisphere (figs. 3 – 4). It is not surprising, therefore, that the adult corpus callosum is a structure of considerable size. The sagittal measurements in three brains were found to be between 524.5 mm² and

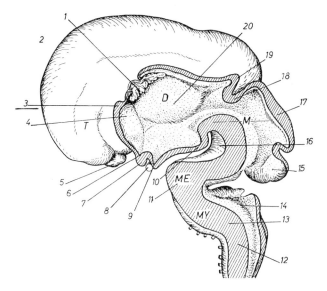

Fig. 1   Median sagittal view of a fetal brain of 3 months. D-diencephalon, M-midbrain, MY-myelencephalon, ME-metencephalon, T-telencephalon.
1 = choroid plexus; 2 = telencephalon; 3 = lamina terminalis, dorsal part; 4 = corpus striatum; 5 = olfactory area; 6 = preoptic recess; 7 = optic chiasm; 8 = hypophyse; 9 = infundibulum of III ventricle; 10 = mamillary body; 11 = pons; 12 = spinal cord; 13 = medulla; 14 = IV ventricle; 15 = cerebellum; 16 = cerebral peduncle; 17 = midbrain; 18 = posterior commissure; 19 = pineal body; 20 = thalamus.

555 mm² [2]. The total number of callosal fibres in these brains varied from 176, 970 to 193, 470 million, of which over 100 million, were myelinated. Myelinization does not occur until after birth, in the third month the fibres joining the central convolutions are myelinated and at six months those of the splenium, but the connexions between the frontal lobes acquire their myelin sheaths later [22] and may not be completed before the 10th year of life. This is relatively similar to the myelination in rat and cat [9].

A thorough and detailed study of the human development of the corpus callosum has been made by Rakic and Yakovlev [15], defining more closely the difference between the ventral lamina terminalis and the dorsal lamina reuniens, which contains the cellular material for future callosal fibres to grow into. *The ventral part* of the lamina reuniens from which eventually the septal nuclei and the paliocortex develops including the anterior commissure. This commissure is in time and location independent of the corpus callosum but may 'show the way' to callosal axons. *The dorsal part* of the lamina reuniens gives rise to the hippocampus (archicortex). The corpus callosum develops in this zone which forms a commissural plate (area or massa pre-commissuralis). In the 11 to 12th

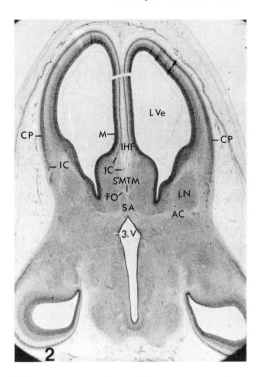

Fig. 2   Embryo 42 mm (author's collection) section showing lateral and third ventricle. At this stage
the anterior commissure is well formed, while the callosal pioneer fibres will cross the midline
in later embryos of 55 – 60 mm stages or 11 – 12 weeks.
AC = anterior commissure; CP = cortical plate; FO = fornix; IC = end of isocortex (medial
and lateral); IHF = interhemispheric fissure; SA = area septalis; LN = lentiform nucleus;
LVe = lateral ventricle; 3.Ve = third ventricle; M = matrix; SMTM = sulcus medianus
telencephali medii.

week pioneer fibres appear in this commissural plate, completing the corpus
callosum between 13 to 20 weeks. It must be emphasized that the axons of neo-
cortical cells form the fibres of the corpus callosum. The commissural plate can
only serve as bridge between the 2 hemispheres. A *comparative* developmental
study has been carried out by Valentino and Jones [21] using rats. These authors
studied with the help of electron microscopy the mode of crossing the midline
gap by callosal axons. The area of fusion of the two hemispheres of the rat
appears to be similar to the massa commissuralis in man, which Rakic and
Yakovlev [15] assume to be a bed of cells for callosal axons. However Valentino
and Jones [21], maintain that this tissue and the surface of the hippocampal
commissure do not provide a pathway for growing callosal axons. What is more
important to realise, is their observation that astrocytes do not form a guidance
or directing channels for the growing axons. Those astrocytic processes present

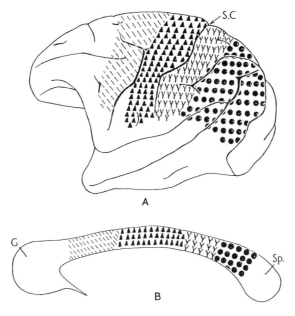

Fig. 3   The origin and major distribution of callosal fibres. (Diagrams from Marchi sections) (see [11]).
(A) The lateral aspect of the left hemisphere; (B) the position of these fibres in sagittal section.
G = genu; Sp = splenium; \ \ \ = premotor cortex; ▲ ▲ ▲ = motor cortex; YYY = sensory cortex; ●●● = parietal cortex; S.C. = central sulcus.
Recent techniques of labelling neuronal processes and cell bodies (Horseradish peroxidase - HPR- and fluorescent dyes) have shown greater details of connexions, s. text.

in the midline show no special orientations before callosal axons cross the midline. For this reason the authors see no evidence for attributing to the neuroglia a *special guiding* function for axonal growth and they refer to their previous studies concerning the problem of pre-existing glial channels for axonal guidance. Dawney and Glees assume in their studies on the descent of corticospinal axons to the spinal cord that the axons themselves are responsible for finding their way and ultimate destination at various cord levels [4].

Clinical observations

The *failure* of the callosal axons to establish inter-hemispheric connexions in man has recently been described by Kendall [13] in a well illustrated radiographically and morphologically informative article. The author reaches the conclusion that cranio-cerebral malformations in pediatric neurological practice are

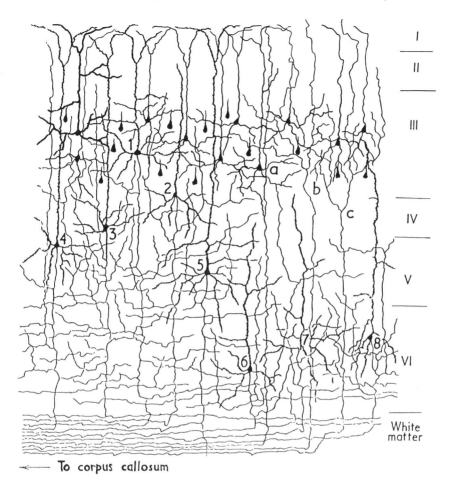

Fig. 4   Diagram showing the origin and terminations of callosal fibres. The Arabic numerals refer
to cells which give rise to callosal fibres, the Roman numerals to layers of the cerebral cortex,
and the letters a, b, c to callosal fibres branching within the layers of the cortex. Note that
most callosal neurons originate in layer III, which also receives callosal afferents.

common. About 20% of the CT scans are required for diagnostic purpose in
these cases and are instrumental in discovering these malformations.

His morphological pictures (figs. 1–4) show the absense of a corpus callosum
very clearly and illustrate furthermore the aberrant callosal fibres as a curled up
big bundle of Probst. This bundle shows clearly that such callosal axons can get
caught inside the lateral ventricle and can be followed posteriorly. The use of
computed tomography for discovering defects in the corpus callosum was recently
demonstrated by Acers and Blackwell, [1]. These authors found in a 3 months

old white male a congenital bilateral ophthalmoplegia associated with a dysplasia of the corpus callosum and suggest that these malformations indicate an embryo-dysgenesis of the mesencephalic tegmentum and the diencephalic lamina reuniens, responsible for bridging the two hemispheres.

Impaired midline cleavage of the embryonic forebrain and midline dysplasia of the face can be associated with agenesis of the corpus callosum. These malformations have been reported by Stewart et al. [19], paying special attention to hormone defiency in the 12 year old girl.

Developmental and experimental observations

It is of interest to note that a number of inbred strains of mice have been examined by Wahlsten [23 – 25] and found to be devective in corpus callosum development. The author stresses the fact that normally the corpus callosum increases in size for many months and declines in size at an age over one year. These findings should be important for researches in heredity. A retardation of corpus callosum fibres in crossing the midline in particular strains of mice has been reported by Wainwright and Deeks [26], while the effect of protein depri-vation (chronic malnutrition) during development of corpus callosum appears to be significant, Wainwright and Stefanescu [28]. A similar effect can be observed in overlapping litters, when agenesis or defiency of corpus callosum was twice as frequent as in non overlapping litters [25].

In a personal communication Dr. Wainwright [29] suggests that the protein deprivation was delaying the growth of the callosal axons and not necessarily stopping them. It is likely that at an extended period of observation the callosal fibres might have crossed the midline. The failure in midline crossing facilities in surgically acallosal mice forcing callosal axons to take an aberrant course can be alleviated by a properly aligned, glia-covered scaffold spanning the hemi-spheres. This observation by Silver and Ogawa [17] is of considerable neurobio-logical interest for the problem of pathway guidance and the role neuroglia might play as the authors speak of 'epigenetic axonal engineering' for the restoration of a malformed fibre pathway in a mammalian brain.

Discussion and summary

Interconnexions in the C.N.S. are of prime importance. It is therefore surprising that neo-cortical connexions between the two hemispheres are established late in evolution reaching their maximal size in primates and man. Evolutionary old connexions from the paleocortex (olfaction) and archicortex (Hippocampus) formed by the anterior commissure and hippocampal commissure appear early in ontogenesis. However the callosal commissure can develop only when the neurons of the neo-cortical plate reach a certain maturation. According to Schwartz, Goldman and Rakic [16], these callosal cells are distinct neuron populations in the monkey having a similar organisation in cortical layers III, IV and V. The authors conclude from their topography and terminal distribution that the callosal system of the posterior parietal cortex and the prefrontal cortex is an integral neural system for spatio-temporal behaviour, especially dense in layer III (see fig. 4). The functions of the callosal connections have been most thoroughly studied in the visual sector and a detailed and exhausting experimental review of the cat's visual system in relation to callosal function has been made by Elberger [7]. In this author's own studies, 1984, it could be shown that if 6% – 16% of intact posterior callosal fibres survive in development these are sufficient for normal visual acuity. Concerning the human callosum the fullest account of patients with divided hemispheres has been given by Sperry [18]. These patients suffered before commissurotomy from severe epilepsy originating in one half of the brain. The interhemispheric connections were cut with the view to prevent spread of the epileptic discharges to the other hemisphere. In this kind of split brain preparation Sperry and his co-workers examined all aspects of visuotactile responses from each hemisphere, paying special attention to the dominant and non dominant or minor hemisphere. Creutzfeldt [3] discussing corpus callosum function and the aspects of the split brain reaches the conclusion that the callosal system is essential for the coordination of the activity of both hemispheres and mental singleness. In view of the emphasis of the meeting on the failure of midline closures in the C.N.S. mainly related to non-fusion of the neural folds, a plea is made in this communication to give due consideration to the failure of a late interhemispheric 'fusion' of a special kind, the corpus callosum. This malformation can now be clearly revealed in the living by computer tomography.

Acknowledgements

The author wishes to thank Mr. I. F. Crane, Dr. A. Continillo and Mrs. F. Glees for their technical assistance.

References

[1] Acers, T. E., C. Blackwell: Oculomotor-corpus callosum dysplasia. Tr. Am. Ophth. Soc. Vol. LXXX (1982).
[2] Blinkow, S. M., I. I. Glezer: The Human Brain in Figures and Tables. Plenum Press, New York 1982.
[3] Creutzfeldt, O. D.: Cortex Cerebri. Springer-Verlag, Berlin – Heidelberg – New York 1983.

[4] Dawney, N. A. H., P. Glees: Somatotopic analysis of fibre and terminal distribution in the primate corticospinal pathway (submitted for publication 1985).

[5] Elberger, A. J., E. L. Smith, J. M. White: Spatial dissociation of visual inputs alters the origin of the corpus callosum. Neuroscience Letters 35 19 – 24 (1983).

[6] Elberger, A. J.: The existence of a separate, brief period for the corpus callosum to affect visual development. Behavioural Brain Res. 11 (1984) 223 – 231.

[7] Elberger, A. J.: The functional role of the corpus callosum in the developing visual system: a review. Progress in Neurobiology 18 (1982) 15 – 79.

[8] Elberger, A. J.: The minimum extent of corpus callosum connections required for normals visual development in the cat. Human Neurobiol. 3 (1984) 115 – 120.

[9] Fleischhauer, K., G. Schluter: Über das postnatale Wachstum des Corpus callosum der Katze (Felis domestica). Z. Anat. Entwick-Gesch. 132 (1970) 228 – 239.

[10] Fox, C. A., R. R. Fisher, S. J. de Salva: The distribution of the anterior commissure in the monkey (Macaca mulatta). J. Comp. Neurol. 89 (1948) 245.

[11] Glees, P.: Experimental Neurology. Clarendon Press, Oxford 1961.

[12] Hajos F., E. Basco: The Surface-Contact Glia. Advances in Anatomy, Embriology and Cell Biology, Vol. 84. Springer-Verlag, Berlin – Heidelberg – New York – Tokio 1984.

[13] Kendall, B. E.: Dysgenesis of the corpus callosum. Neuroradiology 25 (1983) 239 – 256.

[14] Macphail, E. M.: Brain and Intelligence in Vertebrates. Clarendon Press, Oxford 1982.

[15] Rakic, P., P. I. Yakovlev: Development of the Corpus Callosum and Cavum Septi in Man. J. Comp. Neur. 132 (1968) 45 – 72.

[16] Schwartz, M. L., P. S. Goldman-Rakic: Callosal and Intrahemispheric Connectivity of the Prefrontal Association Cortex in Rhesus Monkey: Relation Between Intraparietal and Principal Sulcal Cortex. J. comp. Neurol. 226 (1984) 403 – 420.

[17] Silver, J., M. Y. Ogawa: Postnatally Induced Formation of the Corpus Callosum in Acallosal Mice in Glia-coated cellulose Bridges. Science 220 (1983) 1067 – 1069.

[18] Sperry R. W.: Hemisphere deconnection and unity in conscious awareness. American Psychologist, Vol. 23, No. 10 (1968) 723 – 733.

[19] Stewart, C., M. Castro-Magana, J. Sherman et al.: Septo-optic Dysplasia and Median Cleft Face Syndrome in a Patient with Isolated Growth Hormone Deficiency and Hyperprolactinemia. Am. J. Dis. Child. 137 (1983) 484 – 487.

[20] Treherne, J. E.: Glial-neurone interactions. J. exp. Biol. Vol. 95. Cambridge University Press (1981).

[21] Valentino, K. L., E. G. Jones: The early formation of the corpus callosum: a light and electron microscopic study in foetal and neonatal rats. J. Neurocyt. 11 (1982) 583 – 609.

[22] Villaverde, J. M. de: Beitrag zur Entwicklungsgeschichte des Balkens. Schweiz Arch. Neurol. Psychiat. 45 (1919) 199.

[23] Wahlsten, D.: Deficiency of corpus callosum varies with strain and supplier of the mice. Brain Res. 239 (1982) 329 – 347.

[24] Wahlsten, D.: Mice in utero while their mother is lactating suffer higher frequency of deficient corpus callosum. Develop. Brain Res. 5 (1982) 354 – 357.

[25] Wahlsten, D.: Mode of inheritance of deficient corpus callosum in mice. J. Hered. 73 (1982) 281 – 285.

[26] Wainwright, P., S. Deeks: A comparison of corpus callosum development in the BALB/cCF and $C_{57}BL/6J$ inbred mouse strains. Growth 48 (1984) 192 – 197.

[27] Wainwright, P., M. Gagnon: Effects of Fasting during Gestation on Brain Development in the BALB/c Mice. Exp. Neurol. 85 (1984) 223 – 228.

[28] Wainwright, P., R. Stefanescu: Prenatal Protein Deprivation Increases Defects of the Corpus Callosum in BALB/c Laboratory Mice. Exp. Neurol. 81 (1983) 694 – 702.

[29] Wainwright, P.: Personal communication, 1984.

Diprosopus with craniorachischisis totalis

(Case report)

S. Al-Hami, J. Bohl, K. Becker

Introduction

The association of both incomplete monozygote twinning and neural tube defects was already observed by S. T. Soemmering during the 18th century [18]. About 10 such cases have been reported to date.

The concordance of both malformations is the reason for considering a common pathogenic mechanism. Malformations of the CNS, especially the dysraphic states, are the most common of all congenital abnormalities. They represent a multifactorial or polygenic type of disorder. The striking appearance of incomplete twinning has always commanded the attention and interest of science.

Case report

A 29-year-old patient (already mother of a 3-year-old healthy girl) was admitted to hospital for premature labour. After 3 days the fetal circulation stopped and 6 hours later a spontaneous birth of a dead female fetus took place. Family history is negative.

The female fetus had a length of 34 cm (base of skull to heels), the weight was 1,170 g. External examination showed (fig. 1): the twinned anlage of the head was fused medially; the base of the skull was exposed on both sides, and in the midline where the central anterior edge of the foramen magnum would be expected.

There was no cerebrum, but two separate areae cerebrovasculosae, complete spinal rachischisis together with uncovered double spinal cords, 4 eyes, 2 compressed and rather low-set ears, 2 incompletely separated mouths, 2 separate tongues and an extremely short neck.

Autopsy then revealed two-fold epipharynx with medial fusion, two separate tongues, a single hypopharynx, two mandibles fused medially, normal larynx, trachea and principal bronchi. Additional findings were a normal single eso-

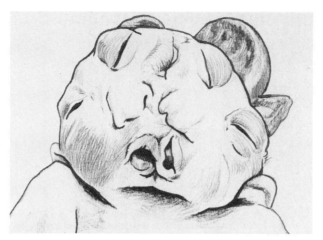

Fig. 1   Facial projection of the diprosopus.

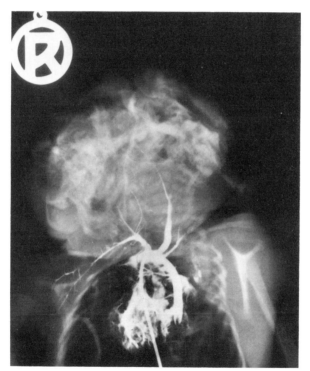

Fig. 2   Arch aortogram.

phagus, an extremely elevated diaphragm (diaphragm on both sides elevated to 2nd intercostal space), and hypoplastic lungs (right lung 2.7 g, left lung 2.6 g).

The heart was clearly hypertrophic and showed several anomalies: Severely dilated right atrium, widely patent foramen ovale ($\varnothing$ 8 mm), dilated and hyper-

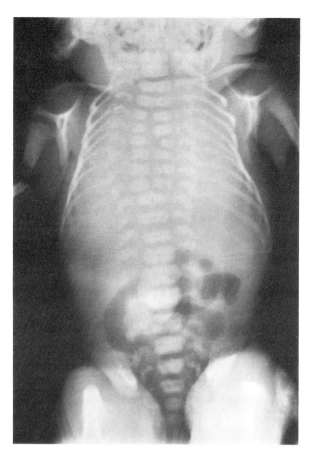

Fig. 3   Radiogram of the whole fetus.

trophic right ventricle (thickness of wall 4 mm). The large blood vessels were completely transposed. The left ventricle was hypoplastic with large defect in the ventricular septum.

The following arteries originated from the aortic arch (fig. 2): brachiocephalic truncus with right subclavian artery, right common carotid artery which again divided into a large vessel running to the exterior side of the right cephalic anlage and giving off assumed internal and external carotid arteries and thyroid artery. Furthermore a vessel passing into the line of fusion of the cephalic anlage which evidently divided into an internal and external left carotid artery of the right cephalic anlage. The aortic arch also gave off a carotid artery on the left dividing into a left external carotid artery and a left internal carotid artery of the left cephalic anlage and also into a right internal carotid artery and right external carotid artery belonging to the left cephalic anlage, furthermore a left subclavian artery branched off from the aortic arch.

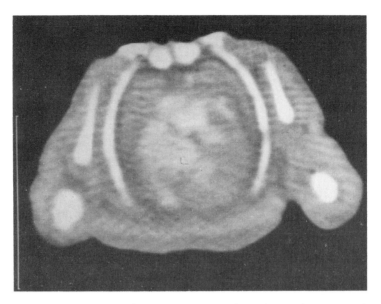

Fig. 4   CT: Horizontal section showing widely opened vertebral archs and two thoracic vertebral bodies.

The abdominal organs showed the following anomalies: The stomach contained a 0.8 cm large pad of ectopic pancreas tissue on the greater curvature. A convolution of large intestine with coecum and appendix (i. e. incomplete rotation of intestine) as well as the common mesentery of both small and large intestine was in the left side of the abdomen.

Radiological examination revealed a single spine with widely open vertebral arches as well as cleft or possibly double thoracic vertebral bodies (fig. 3 and 4) and displastic bases of the skulls with medial fusion.

Histologically we found totally disorganized tissue in both areae cerebrovasculosae with glial and ependymal structures and atypical plexus choroid tissue. Both areae cerebrovasculosae were extremely vascularized. In contrast to Riccardi's case [15] we found a normal anterior pituitary, but no neurohypophysis in each cephalic anlage. The spinal cord was doubled and more widely separated in cervical then in thoraco-lumbal segments (fig. 5). To the naked eye it seemed flat and was severely malformed. The left and right spinal roots of one cord emerged in one direction and formed two spinal roots in each intervertebral foramen; they then united to form a single spinal nerve. Normally constituted small branches communicated with the sympathetic trunk. However, this course of the spinal roots, spinal ganglions, and spinal nerves was by no means encountered constantly in all segments, and considerable variety was observed. In addition, the number of the nerves and vertebral bodies was reduced.

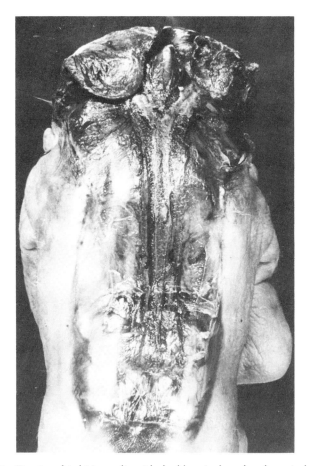

Fig. 5   Craniorachischisis totalis with double spinal cord and atypical course of spinal roots.

Discussion

The incidence of dysraphic states, especially anencephaly, seems comparatively low in completely separated mono- or dizygote twins [12]. James [8] reports a slight increase of incidence in monozygote twins. The association of incomplete twinning (diprosopi) with neural tube defects, however, seems to be quite common and several authors have taken note of this [1, 4, 10, 15]. We intend to add to this observation with our case report.

The cases of diprosopi published until today appear to indicate that the normal development of the neural tube is at least interrupted by the formation of incomplete monozygote twins. Knox's [9] hypothesis proposes an etiological explanation of the origin of neural tube defects by which interaction between one fetus (malformed and later decreased) and the other might be responsible for the incomplete neural tube closure in the survivor.

Summary

We present a case of diprosopus with double craniorachischisis totalis aborted during the 30th week of gestation. The clinical, radiological, and pathological findings are discussed.

References

[1] Arai, T., S. Masaki, M. Nikaido: A case of diprosopus. Acta path. Jap 12 (1962) 407 – 411.
[2] Bell, J. E.: Abnormalities of the spinal meninges in anencephalic fetuses. J. Pathology 133 (1981) 131 – 144.
[3] Bell, J. E., R. J. L. Green: Studies on area cerebrovasculosa of anencephalic fetuses. J. Pathology 137 (1982) 315 – 328.
[4] Fontaine, G., et al.: Anencephaly and twinning (letter). Teratology 18 (1978) 289 – 290.
[5] Friede, R. L.: Developmental Neuropathology. Springer-Verlag, Wien – New York 1975.
[6] Gardner, W. J.: The dysraphic states. Excerpta Medica, Amsterdam 1973.
[7] Harbeson, A. E.: Duplication of the hind-end of an anencephalic fetus. J. obstet-Gynaec. Br. Emp. 45 (1938) 810 – 819.
[8] James, W. H.: Twinning and anencephaly. Ann. Hum. Biol. 3 (1976) 401 – 409.
[9] Knox, E. G.: Fetus-fetus interaction – A model aetiology for anencephaly. Develop. Med. Child. Neurol. 12 (1970) 167 – 177.
[10] Kudo, H., S. Toda: An autopsy case of diprosopus. Acta path. Jap. 20 (1970) 239 – 249.
[11] Langman, J.: Medical Embryology. The Williams & Wilkins Company, Baltimore 1969.
[12] Lemire, R. J., J. B. Beckwith: Anencephaly. Raven Press New York 1978.
[13] Nevin, N. C., J. A. C. Weatherall: Illustrated guide to malformations of the central nervous system at birth. Ferdinand Enke Verlag, Stuttgart 1983.
[14] Persaud, T. V. N.: Advances in the study of birth defects, Volume 7. Central nervous system and craniofacial malformations. MTP Press Limited, Falcon House, Lancaster, England 1982.
[15] Riccardi, V. M., C. A. Bergmann: Anencephaly with incomplete twinning (Diprosopus). Teratology 16 (1977) 137 – 140.
[16] Schwalbe, E.: Die Doppelbildungen. Verlag Gustav Fischer, Jena 1907.
[17] Smith, M. T., et al: Scanning electron microscopy of experimental anencephaly development. Neurology (Ny) 32 (1982) 992 – 999.
[18] Soemmering, S. T.: Abbildungen und Beschreibungen einiger Mißgeburten. Mainz 1791.
[19] Tuchmann-Duplessis, H., M. Auroux, P. Haegel: Illustrated Human Embryology. Volume 3: Nervous system and endocrine glands. Springer-Verlag, New York – Chapman & Hall, London – Masson & Cie., Paris (Editeurs) 1974.
[20] Voth, D., und Mitarbeiter: Hydrocephalus im frühen Kindesalter. Enke-Verlag, Stuttgart 1983.
[21] Warkany, J.: Mental retardation and congenital malformations of the central nervous system at birth. Year Book Medical Publishers, INC., Chicago – London 1981.

"Hindbrain upside-down" in occipital encephalocele — an alternative to the syndrome of Padget and Lindenberg

P. Schmitt

Introduction

In 1972 Padget and Lindenberg [7] reported the observation of an unusual cerebellar malformation which had occurred in an occipital encephalocele and seemed to represent a teratologic link between the Dandy-Walker and the Arnold-Chiari spectrum. The condition was chiefly characterized by agenesis of the cerebellar vermis in a caudally displaced and inverted cerebellum. In the latter, the hemispheres had developed in a ventral direction covering the basal cisternae including the chiasm, midbrain, pons and upper medulla oblongata. The cystic fourth ventricle had been continuous with the occipital encephalocele into which the embryonic tectum and the membranous roof of the rhomboid fossa were herniated. The forebrain was microcephalic with additional malformations such as absence of the corpus callosum and the choroid plexus, almost total atresia of the ventricular system, and thalamic fusion.

Subsequently, the observation of Padget and Lindenberg [7] was confirmed by two further cases reported by Smith and Huntington [9].

Our observation deals with a newborn child which had died shortly after delivery, exhibiting a total inversion of the cerebellum with a huge occipital encephalocele. However, in this observation, the condition of the hindbrain differed significantly from the observations of the authors mentioned above [7, 9] as there was no agenesis of the cerebellar vermis.

Case report

A newborn female infant delivered at the 41st week of gestation presented at birth with a huge occipital encephalocele (fig. 1a) and an abnormally flat neurocranium. There were no records of any exogenous teratogenic events or diseases from the early period of gestation. She died on the 5th day after delivery.

General autopsy was refused. Only removal of the encephalocele was allowed so that the intracranial structures had to be removed through the artificially enlarged cranioschisis.

Neuropathologic findings (A-No. 542/82): The encephalocele measured 23 to 12 to 8 cm and weighed 585 g. It was entirely covered by skin with extensive ulcerations at its top. It was connected with the endocranium by a comparatively narrow stalk about 3 cm in diameter. Except for the small round occipital cranioschisis the neurocranial bones were completely formed. The intracranial space was extremely narrow and flattened. The occipital region beneath the insertion of the encephalocele was bulged in a dorsal direction. The intracranial parts of the forebrain and the cerebellum (fig. 1b, d) altogether weighed 75 g, the cerebellum alone was 20 g. The latter was pressed into a basal excavation of the intracranial forebrain residues to which it was loosely attached by fibrous meninges (fig. 2a). There was no interpeduncular fossa. The olfactory nerves were present. The optic nerves could be traced over a length of 15 mm until they vanished within the strands of cerebral tissue which formed the stalk of the encephalocele, connecting the intra- and extracranial brain structures (figs. 1b, 2a).

The cerebellum was elongated in a horizontal plane and exhibited cone-shaped dorsal extensions (fig. 2b) which had been herniated through the cranioschisis into the stalk of the cele. There was a complete inversion of the cerebellum and the brainstem. The anterior lobe with the streched and irregularly formed vermis faced the base of the skull, and the inferior cerebellar facies including the pons and the rhomboid fossa were at the top, contacting the base of the intracranial forebrain structures which chiefly represented parts of the frontal lobes (fig. 2b, d). The medulla oblongata was located at the rostral border of the cerebellum, bent downward almost at a right angle against the long axis of the cerebellum (figs. 1d, 2c, d). It was embraced by spur-like extensions of the cerebellar tonsils (fig. 2c). Parts of the choroid plexus could be demonstrated in the rostro-cranially located cerebello-pontine angle by light microscopy (fig. 2d, small arrows). Other parts of the plexus were found in a medial position protruding downwards through the foramen of Magendie (fig. 2d, large arrow). The trigeminal nerves and the inferior cranial nerve group were visible in the cranial view of the cerebellum (fig. 2b). The midbrain was changed to cords of neuroectodermal tissue which entered the stalk of the encephalocele.

The major part of the forebrain was displaced extracranially into the large encephalocele (fig. 1b, c). They consisted of two cerebral hemispheres which were surrounded by sclerotic meninges and separated by a falx cerebri (fig. 1c). On coronal sections, enlarged lateral ventricles occurred which were grossly absent from the intracranial forebrain structures. Close to the midline the choroid plexus could be demonstrated on some microscopic sections. Macroscopically,

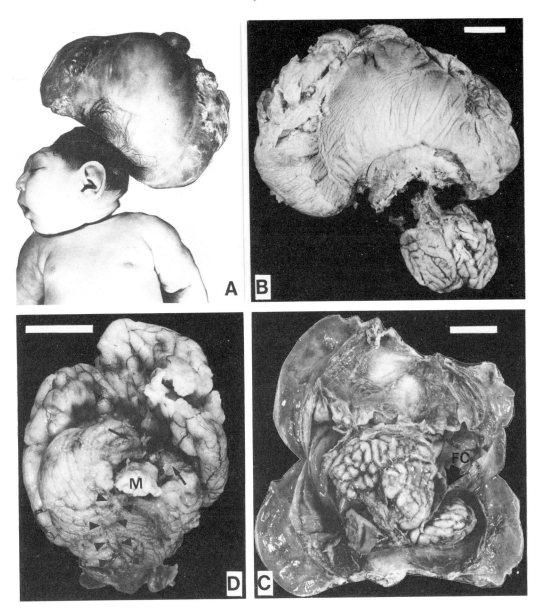

Fig. 1   a) Newborn infant with a huge occipital encephalocele; b) isolated hernial sac with intracranial brain structures at the bottom; c) opened hernial sac with extracranial brain structures
and meninges (FC falx cerebri); d) intracranial brain structures (basic aspect) with cerebellum
and medulla oblongata (M). Note the spur-like cerebellar extensions embracing the brainstem
(long arrows). The cerebellar vermis is indicated by arrow heads. (Calibration bars represent
3 cm in b) and c); 2 cm in d)

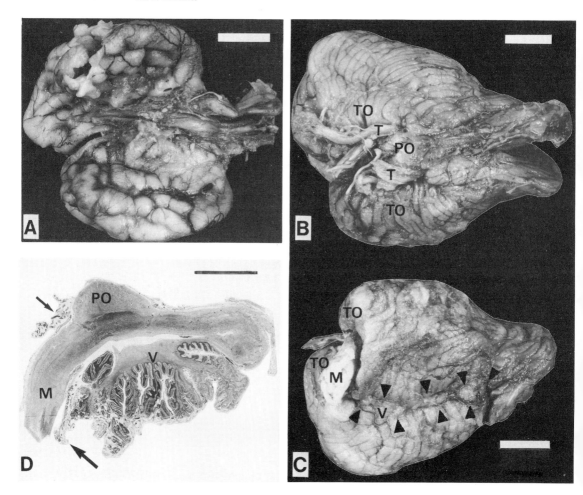

Fig. 2   a) Inferior aspect of the intracranial part of the forebrain after removing of the cerebellum. Note the smooth bowl-shaped impression with fibrous meninges and the stalk of the hernial sac; b) cranial aspect of the cerebellum. This side contacted the forebrain basis in a); c) inferior aspect of the cerebellum. The vermis (V) is indicated by arrow heads; d) microscopic slide of the cerebellum and brainstem cut in a median-sagittal plane representing their intracranial orientation: the pons is at the top and the streched vermis at the bottom. Arrows indicate the choroid plexus. M = medulla oblongata, PO = pons, T = trigeminal nerve, TO = tonsils, V = vermis. (Calibration bars represent 1 cm.)

the basal ganglia, could not be identified. Microscopically, a small nodule of poorly organized neuroectodermal tissue with neurons and glial tissue at the basis of the external brain structures and close to the opening of the stalk into the encephalocele was likely to represent rudimentary basal ganglia. These contained numerous medially and excentrically located ependymal rosettes and tubules. Both the intra- and extracranial forebrain structures exhibited servere histologic cortical disarrangement with patterns of polymicrogyria and frequent gyral fusions.

Microscopy of the cerebellum and brainstem (fig. 2d) revealed atrophic cerebellar folia in the posterior part of the stretched vermis which had been located close to the origin of the stalk of the cele. The leptomeninges covering the medulla and the pons showed sclerotic change and included heterotopic nodules of glial tissue.

Comments and conclusion

An infant delivered at the 41st week of gestation with a huge encephalocele exhibited a complete inversion of the cerebellum with the brainstem and the rhomboid fossa being located upside-down.

Unlike in the observations of Padget et al. [7] and Smith et al. [9] there was no agenesis of the cerebellar vermis. The fourth ventricle was not cystic and no communication was present with the encephalocele which contained the major parts of the forebrain. Thus, basically this malformation cannot be associated with the Dandy-Walker spectrum [1, 4, 5]. However, it shows some relations to the Arnold-Chiari spectrum [2 – 4, 8] regarding the elongation of the rhomboid fossa, the streched and irregularly formed cerebellar vermis. Furthermore the partly medial position of the choroid plexus and its downward protrusion through the foramen of Magendie and the ventral embracing of the brainstem

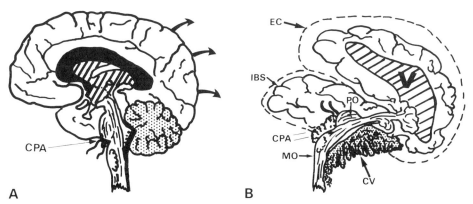

A   B

Fig. 3   Schematic drawings of the supposed developmental mechanism resulting in the upside-down position of the hindbrain. The latter is due to a dorsoflexion which occurred as a result of the extracranial displacement of the major parts of the forebrain. CPA = cerebellar pontine angle, CV = cerebellar vermis, EC = encephalocele, IBS = intracranial brain structures, MO = medulla oblongata, PO = pons, V = ventricle: a) Normal situation, b) present observation with "hindbrain upside-down".

by spur-like tonsillar extensions. In contrast to the Arnold-Chiari malformation, no downward displacement of vermal structures through the foramen magnum, or kinking of the medulla oblongata at its transition to the cervical cord was present.

The inversion of the hindbrain in the present case most likely seems to be caused by mechanical factors in conjunction with the formation of the encephalocele. This is demonstrated by the schematic drawings in figure 3. The extracranial displacement of the major parts of the forebrain has obviously resulted in a developmental retroflexion of the brainstem and the cerebellum with a bending at the cerebellopontine angle so that the pons was turned to the top and the cerebellum to the bottom, including a posterior elongation of the latter with streching of the vermis.

In five infants with occipital encephalocele, Karch et al [6] encountered cerebellar aplasia in two, while in the other three the cerebellum had been "at least partly contained within the hernial sac" and the vermis had been absent in all these cases.

The descriptions of Karch et al. [6], Padget et al. [7], Smith et al. [9] and the present observation support the view that the cerebellum and the brainstem may show a broad spectrum of malformation or morphological variation in an occipital encephalocele.

References

[1] Benda, C. E.: The Dandy-Walker syndrome or the so-called atresia of the foramen of Magendie. J. Neuropath. exp. Neurol. 13 (1954) 14 – 29.
[2] Caviness, V. S. jr: The Chiari malformations of the posterior fossa and their relation to hydrocephalus. Dev. Med. Child Neurol. 18 (1976) 103 – 116.
[3] Daniel, P., S. J. Strich: Some observations on the congenital deformity of the central nervous system known as the Arnold-Chiari malformation. J. Neuropath. exp. Neurol, 17 (1958) 255 – 266.
[4] Gardner, E., R. O'Rahiley, D. Prolo: The Dandy-Walker and Arnold-Chiari malformations. Clinical, developmental, and teratological observations. Arch. Neurol. (Chic) 32 (1975) 393 – 407.
[5] Hart, M. N., N. Malamud, W. G. Ellis: The Dandy-Walker syndrome. A clinicopathological study based on 28 cases. Neurology (Minneap.) 22 (1972) 771 – 780.
[6] Karch, S. B., H. Urich: Occipital encephalocele: a morphological study. J. Neurol. Sci, 15 (1972) 89 – 112.
[7] Padget, D. H., R. Lindenberg: Inverse cerebellum morphogentically related to Dandy-Walker and Arnold-Chiari syndromes: Bizarre malformed brain with occipital encephalocele. Johns Hopkins Med. J. 131 (1972) 228 – 246.
[8] Peach, B.: The Arnold-Chiari malformation. Arch. Neurol. (Chic.) 12 (1965) 527 – 535, 613 – 621.
[9] Smith, M. T., H. W. Huntington: Inverse cerebellum and occipital encephalocele. A dorsal fusion defect uniting the Arnold-Chiari and Dandy-Walker spectrum. Neurology (Minneap.) 27 (1977) 246 – 251.

Ocular dysraphics

R. Rochels

Introduction

Dysraphias in the more common sense means any malfusion of the neural tube. In the development of the eye the embryonic fissure of the optic cup and stalk can also fail to close. The resulting defect is traditionally called "coloboma" [13, 15]. Colobomatous malformations are consequently dysraphias and represent a wide variety of expressions from a simple notch in the pupillary region to clinical anophthalmia with orbital cyst formation [2, 4, 7]. Coloboma can be an isolated defect in an otherwise healthy person or a minor symptom of many multisymptomatic syndromes [9].

Embryology

At the 4 mm stage of development the optic vesicles pouch out of the lateral wall of the forebrain and are then invaginated along the inferior aspect of the optic cup and stalk leading to the embryonic fissure [7, 10]. At the 10 mm stage this fissure starts to fuse; this event proceeds posteriorly toward the optic disc and anteriorly towards the rim of the optic cup [9]. Any malfusion leads to eversion of the embryonic neurosensory retina over the embryonic pigment epithelium that also fails to close thus producing defects in the inner and outer layer of the optic cup and non-differentiation of the choroid along the fissure [2]. The resulting coloboma thus involves the retina as well as the choroid, whereas the sclera is not affected. Occasionally this bare sclera is covered by a bridge of atypical retina with a duplication of the neurosensory layer or rosette formation (retinal dysplasia) [8]. Typical colobomas can either lead to ectatic colobomas (staphyloma-like) or to closed cysts filling the orbit accompanied by an extreme microphthalmus [2].

Clinical manifestations

Typical *iris colobomas* are located in the inferior nasal aspect according to the site of the previous fissure; there can be a simple notch in the pupillary region, circumscribed defects in the pigment epithelium or stromal layer of the iris, or a full-thickness key-hole like defect (fig. 1). The underlying *ciliary body* can be

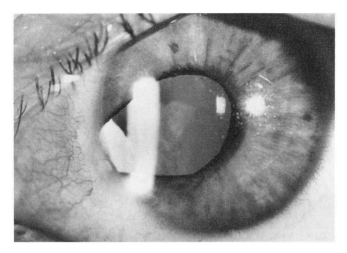

Fig. 1   Coloboma of the iris, ciliary body, zonula and lens, located typically in the nasal and inferior aspect of the (left) eye.

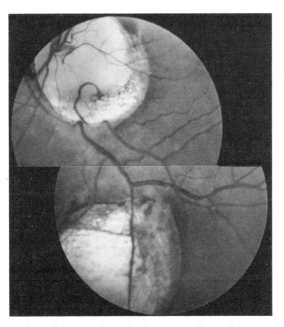

Fig. 2   Bridge-coloboma of the fundus: optic disc coloboma and retino-choroidal coloboma are separated by a bridge of dysplastic neurosensory retina.

affected; then a gap in the *zonula* as well as a small notch in the *lens* equator will be seen. Iris colobomas can be isolated or combined with *retino-choroidal colobomas*; the latter present as circumscribed white areas of bare sclera, sometimes bridged by retinal vessels or a membrane of dysplastic retina (bridge-coloboma; fig. 2). In the *posterior fundus*, colobomatous lesions can furthermore cause either outpouching of the sclera (*scleral ectasia*) or huge closed *orbital cysts* that interfere with the normal development of the globe leading to extreme microphthalmia resembling clinical anophthalmia. The *optic disc* can be colobomatous, too [1]. Minimal changes of the inferior aspect of the disc are called *spurious coloboma* of Fuchs-v. Szily, maximal variants with enlargement of the disc diameter, total cupping and abnormalities of the disc vessels are referred to as "morning glory syndrome".

All these manifestations of nonfusion of the embryonic fissure are localized inferior-nasally (typical coloboma), may be unilateral or bilateral, can interfere with the visual acuity (posterior coloboma), or be just a problem of cosmesis (iris coloboma). *Atypical colobomas* are located elsewhere in the eye; they are not related to malfusion of the embryonic fissure and do not belong to the dysraphic disorders of the eye.

Etiology

Ocular colobomas may be sporadic, autosomal dominant or recessive in inheritance and can be a part of chromosomal disorders [12] (tab. 1), or due to teratogenes such as thalidomide and perhaps LSD [9].

Table 1   Ocular colomba associated with chromosomal disorders

Trisomy	13, 18, 22
Duplication	4p, 9p, 13q, 22q
Deletion	4p, 11q, 13q, 18q
Ring	13, 18
49, XXXXX	
X-chrom.	Lenz-Syndrome, Goltz-Gorlin-Syndrome
Triploidy	

"Coloboma syndromes"

In tab. 2 all the syndromes with iridal/uveal/optic disc coloboma are listed; this variety of malformations stresses especially the fact that the period of embryonic fissure closure is a very critical one in the development of the whole body. This is seen for example in the CHARGE-association and the combination of uveal coloboma with ano-rectal defects such as anal atresia in the cat-eye-syndrome [11].

Table 2   Syndromes associated with ocular coloboma

Aicardi, Biemond I, Bietti, CHARGE-association, Goldenhar, Hennebert I, Holoprosencephaly, Laurence-Bardet-Biedl-Moon, Marfan I, Marfan-Madelung, Meckel, Peters, Reese, Rieger, Rubinstein, Stilling-Türk-Duane, Thalidomide, Ullrich-Feichtinger, Wiedemann I

Ocular symptoms in generalized dysraphic malformations

Apart from the combination of ocular coloboma and generalized birth defects, there exist ocular signs and symptoms in dysraphic malformations which are quite different from coloboma [5, 14]. *Nasofrontal encephaloceles* cause lateral displacement of the orbits with consecutive hypertelorism, ocular palsies and midfacial anomalies. *Transsphenoidal encephaloceles* affect the optic chiasm. In both of them, anomalies of the optic disc such as atrophy, pits, dysplasia or megalopapilla can be observed frequently. The more generalized *dysraphic state of Bremer* is usually associated with iridal heterochromia and Horner's trias.

Discussion

The closure of the neural tube and the embryonic optic fissure are quite comparable: the neural folds start to fuse in the region of the 4th somite; this fusion then progresses cranially to form the anterior neuroporus at day 23, and caudally to build up the posterior neuroporus at day 25, corresponding to a 4 mm stage of development [6]. The closure of the embryonic fissure starts later at about a 10 mm stage (5th week) in the midzone, then proceeding proximally and distally as already seen in the development of the neural tube. The closure in the disc is finished at the 20 mm stage (7th week); in the distal iridal region at the 65 mm stage, corresponding to about 10 weeks of gestation [3, 7, 9]. The critical period for dysraphic malformations of the neural tube is thus much earlier than that for coloboma formation; this may be one explanation for the fact that neural tube dysraphias are rarely accompanied by colobomatous eye defects. On the other hand, the sixth week of gestation, when the neural tube is already completely closed, but the embryonic fissure has just started to fuse, is a very critical point in the development of the whole body, since by this time organogenesis is nearly accomplished and histogenesis just starts [8]. Disturbances prior to that critical point thus lead to malformations affecting not only the eye but several organs at the same time. This might be another explanation for the fact that colobomatous ocular defects are more commonly associated with other non-dysraphic malformations, resulting in pathognomonic syndromes.

Conclusion

Colobomatous ocular defects can be compared with generalized dysraphic disorders not only by embryological but also by teratological findings. The different critical periods for neural tube and embryonic fissure closure explain the fact that both these dysraphias are only rarely associated. Since the embryonic fissure closes at a period sensitive for the development of the whole body, colobomas often share in the symptomatology of malformation syndromes and birth defects.

References

[1] Apple, D. J., M. F. Rabb, P. M. Walsh: Congenital anomalies of the optic disc. Surv. Ophthalmol. **27** (1982) 3 – 41.

[2] Badtke, G.: Die Mißbildungen des menschlichen Auges. In: Der Augenarzt (K. Velhagen, ed.), vol. IV, pp. 1 – 145. Thieme-Verlag, Stuttgart 1961.

[3] Duke-Elder, S. S., C. Cook: Normal and abnormal development. Part 1: Embryology. In: System of ophthalmology (S. S. Duke-Elder, ed.), vol. III, pp. 38 – 41. Kimpton, London 1963.

[4] Duke-Elder, S. S.: Anomalous closure of the embryonic cleft. In: System of ophthalmology (S. S. Duke-Elder, ed.), vol. III, part 2, pp. 456 – 488. Kimpton, London 1964.

[5] Goldhammer, Y., J. L. Smith: Optic nerve anomalies in basal encephalocele. Arch. Ophthalmol. **93** (1975) 115 – 118.

[6] Hamilton, W. J., J. D. Boyd, H. W. Mossman: Human embryology. Prenatal development of form and function. 3rd ed. Heffer and Sons, Cambridge 1966.

[7] Mann, I.: The development of the human eye. 3rd. ed. British Medical Ass., London 1964.

[8] Naumann, G. O. H.: Pathologie des Auges, Springer, Berlin – Heidelberg – New York 1980.

[9] Pagon, R. A.: Ocular coloboma. Surv. Ophthalmol. **25** (1981) 223 – 236.

[10] O'Rahilly, R.: The timing and sequence of events in the development of the human eye and ear during the embryonic period proper. Anat. Embryol. **168** (1983) 87 – 99.

[11] Rochels, R.: Anorektale Fehlbildungssyndrome mit okulärer Beteiligung. In: Anorektale Fehlbildungen (S. Hoffmann-v. Kap-herr, ed.), pp. 69 – 72. Fischer, Stuttgart – New York 1983.

[12] Rochels, R.: Chromosomale Erkrankungen mit Augenbeteiligung. Symposium der Deutschen Ophthalmologischen Gesellschaft: Ophthalmologische Genetik. Düsseldorf 1984 (in press).

[13] Szily, A. v.: Die Ontogenese der idiotypischen (erbbildlichen) Spaltbildungen des Auges, des Mikrophthalmus und der Orbitalcysten. Ztschr. ges. Anat. **74** (1924) 1 – 230.

[14] Walsh, F. B., W. F. Hoyt: Midline Craniocerebral and vertebrospinal defects. In: Clinical Neuroophthalmology (F. B. Walsh, W. F. Hoyth, eds.), 3rd. ed., vol. I, pp. 712 – 732. Williams and Wilkins, Baltimore 1969.

[15] Walther, J. (crited from S. S. Duke-Elder, 1964).

Neuropathological aspects of the syringomyelic complex

J. C. W. Kiwit, R. Schober, H. Gräfin Vitzthum, W. Wechsler

Introduction

Syringomyelia is a relatively rare disorder at a prevalence of about 8/100,000 [3] and a yearly incidence of about 0.3 to 0.4 per 100,000 [7]. The term syringomyelia includes a number of aetiologically different entities.

A considerable number of syrinx formations is of post-traumatic, post-haemato-myelic or post-infectious nature [2] and hydrodynamic effects constitute an important factor in their genesis and clinical course. Neuropathologists apply the term "secondary syringomyelia" to these lesions, which we shall not consider in this paper.

Primary forms of syringo- and hydromyelia are closely related to the dysraphic states. Some of them are easy to diagnose, while others may cause difficulties. This is particularly true of cases with tumorous changes. The purpose of our presentation is to show the possible relationship between syringomyelia, malformations and true neoplasms. We present four cases with varied morphological features: one a complex malformation syndrome, the second a case of hyperplastic or gliomatous syringomyelia, the third a congenital tumour associated with syringobulbia and the last a true malignant spinal glioma which is accompanied by syringobulbia.

Case 1

The first patient is a 39 year old male who suffered from left-sided progressive tetraspasticity since childhood. Because of a bilateral pes cavus and cerebellar symptoms Friedreich's ataxia was considered as a possible diagnosis. One month before his death he was admitted to hospital with right-sided lower cranial nerve signs, consisting of bulbar speech, an absent gag reflex and hemiatrophy of the right side of the tongue with fasciculations. A computer tomogram showed severe internal hydrocephalus internus due to a cystic space occupying lesion in the right posterior fossa, which was thought to be consistent with a cerebellar astrocytoma or an epidermoid cyst. The patient refused permission for an operation and he died.

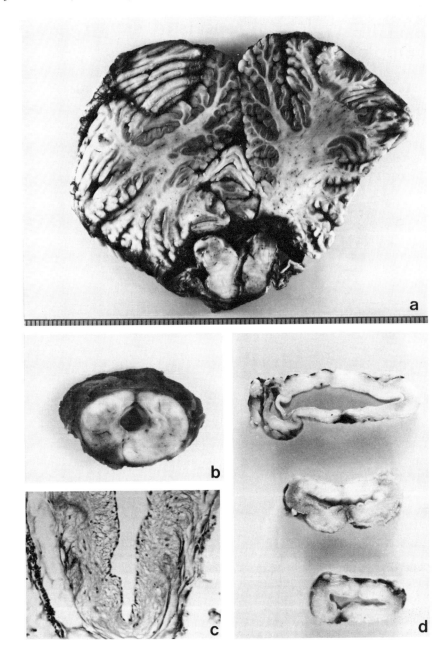

Fig. 1 a – d   Case 1: Cerebellum and upper medulla. Note slit-like syringobulbia and compression by a large cyst on the right (a). Lower medulla with hydrobulbia and subarachnoid ectopic glial tissue on the dorsal aspect (b). Wall of large glia-arachnoidal cyst with partial ependymal lining in continuity with the lateral recess of the IVth ventricle, HE (c). Hydro- and Syringomyelia of the spinal cord at the levels C4, T6 and L1 (d).

Autopsy revealed a severe scoliosis of the thoracic spine, the anticipated hydroce-phalus internus and a right sided, infratentorial membranous cyst which was filled with CSF and appeared to be a large arachnoid cyst, compressing the right cerebellar hemisphere and the right pons. The midline structures were shifted to the left (fig. 1a). Furthermore a Chiari-Type I malformation was detected with fibrotic elongated cerebellar tonsils on the dorsum of the medulla oblongata. A severe fibroglial proliferation surrounded the whole medulla which was up to 2 mm thick (fig 1b). The foramen of Luschka on the right was widely patent and led into the ependyma and a glial covered arachnoid cyst. This was considered to be a diverticulum of the IVth ventricle's right lateral recess (fig. 1c). In the medulla oblongata a round, central and partially ependymal covered syrinx was found (fig. 1b), indicating a true hydrobulbia. The cavity was occluded caudally by a fibroglial membrane at the level of the craniocervical junction.

The spinal cord was grossly deformed and flattened by a massive hydromyelia that extended down to the sacral segments (fig. 1d). Beside this hydromyelia, two lateral syringes were found in the cervical and midthoracic areas.

Case 2

A 13 year old girl suffered from progressive scoliosis and bilateral pes cavus for 7 years. 6 months before she died a slowly progressive left-sided paraparesis developed and bladder function became impaired. A CT-scan showed hydro-cephalus internus and myelography revealed an intramedullary space occupying lesion from C2 to T8. At operation a swollen yellowish spinal cord with a central syrinx was seen at the level T9, suggestive of syringomyelia. Biopsy of the syrinx wall led to the diagnosis of spongioblastoma.

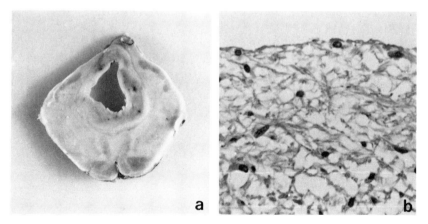

Fig. 2 a – b   Case 2: Medulla oblongata with "Gliastift" of posterior tracts surrounding central syrinx (a). Wall of syrinx with a loose meshwork of astrocytes, GFAP (b).

Autopsy showed a gross enlargement of the medulla oblongata and of the entire spinal cord. Cross sections revealed well demarcated areas in the posterior tracts with a central syrinx (fig 2a). The region was microscopically characterized by proliferation of glial cells with numerous GFAP positive fibers. The cells were spindle-shaped or spiderlike astrocytes with round regular nuclei (fig. 2b). No Rosenthal fibers or granular bodies could be detected. Vascularization was minimal. No mitotic activity could be observed. The inner wall towards the syrinx was not covered by an ependymal layer. The central canal was normal throughout the cord. At the level of the operation there was central necrosis of the cord around an inserted catheter.

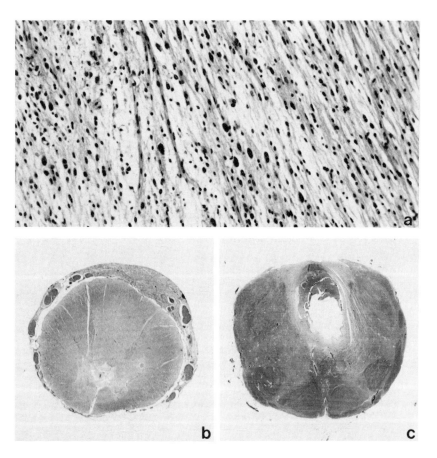

Fig. 3 a – c   Case 3: Malignant glioma of the cervical cord with small cells infiltrating along fiber tracts; sagittal section, HE (a). Extensive tumour infiltration of dorsal leptomeninges of lumbar cord, HE (b). Dorsal syringobulbia of the lower medulla, without continuity with the tumour, HE (c).

The neuropathological diagnosis in this case is difficult. Age and clinical history as well as some of the histological features may suggest a diagnosis of a so called "Stiftgliom" or a spongioblastoma (WHO-classification: pilocytic astrocytoma, grade I) with a secondary syrinx-like cavity. An alternative diagnosis in this condition could be a hyperplastic or gliomatous form of syringomyelia.

Case 3

A 34 year old woman developed acute tetraplegia and had undergone emergency laminectomy for decompression of an intramedullary space occupying lesion at the midcervical level. Due to arterial bleeding the operation was not completed and a dural patch was inserted for decompression. Intramedullary angioma was suspected, but on postoperative angiography this could not be detected.

At autopsy gross enlargement of the medulla oblongata and of the cervical cord were found with a malignant glioma with a large central necrosis in the mid-cervical area (fig. 3a). Leptomeningeal infiltration was present on the dorsal aspect of the whole spinal cord (fig. 3b). Histological features included massive proliferation of pathological vessels accompanied by perivascular pseudorosettes. The tumour was thought to be a true spinal glioblastoma by a consultant neuropathologist (L. J. Rubinstein). Cross sections of the medulla oblongata showed a large posterior syrinx (fig. 3c) surrounded by reactive gliosis with profound capillary proliferation. There was no connection between this syringob-ulbia and the malignant glioma of the cervical cord, although the tumour had spread further rostrally with marginal involvement of the lateral recessus of the IVth ventricle.

In summary, neuropathology demonstrated a syringobulbia that had been clini-cally silent together with a rapidly growing highly malignant glioma of the spinal cord.

Case 4

A twelve year old boy had suffered from extrapyramidal symptoms on the right side for more than seven years. A pseudobulbar speech and occasional swallowing cramps were noted. Neuroradiological examinations had not revealed a patho-logical process. He was admitted with severe dyspnea and he died without having regained consciousness.

On autopsy massive swelling of the medulla oblongata that extended into the upper cervical spinal cord was noted. The normal anatomical structures of the medulla oblongata had been almost completely destroyed by a large tumour infiltrating the meninges and the floor of the IVth ventricle (fig. 4a). In the area of the right olive a flat, horizontal syrinx extended from the upper medulla to

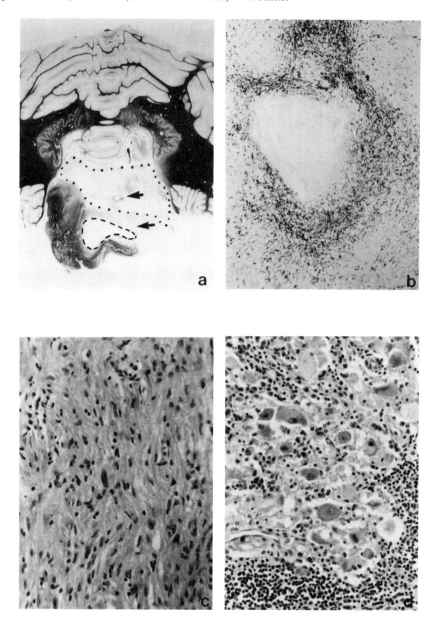

Fig. 4 a – d   Case 4: Deformity and demyelination of upper medulla oblongata by a tumour (dotted line) containing a horizontal syringobulbic cavity (dashed line, lower arrow) and smaller tumour cysts (upper arrow), Heidenhain-Wölcke (a). Smaller tumour cyst surrounded by numerous Rosenthal fibers, Heidenhain-Wölcke (b). Spongioblastic tumour component, HE (c). Gangliomatous area of tumour with extensive lymphocytic infiltration, HE (d).

the level of the cranio-cervical junction. In addition, several small tumour cysts occurred in the dorsal parts and were surrounded by numerous Rosenthal fibers (fig. 4b). Two different tumour cell populations were to be seen; there were glial cells consisting of uni- and bipolar cells characteristic of pilocytic astrocytes (fig. 4c), while in other areas the tumour consisted of neoplastic gangliocytes with an intense perivascular infiltration of lymphocytic elements (fig. 4d). The tumour had invaded the leptomeninges evoking an extensive desmoblastic reaction. Reactive changes included anterior horn degeneration with reactive gliosis in the upper cervical cord, and secondary degeneration of both pyramidal tracts.

In summary, this case represents a peculiar hamartomatous ganglioglioma of the medulla extending into the upper cervical cord. Syringobulbia was an additional morphological substrate of the long lasting clinical history of this patient. It is not clear whether the syringobulbia was a primary or a secondary one.

Discussion

Syringomyelia is a disorder of the hind-brain and the cervical and upper thoracic cord. Clinically, an intermittent or slowly progressive disease starts in the second or third decade. But it is difficult to make an accurate diagnosis in atypical cases. In none of our four cases was a clinical diagnosis established. From a neuropathological view, these cases likewise pose a number of diagnostic and nosological questions.

Several authors [11, 13, 14] have defined syringomyelia or -bulbia as a malformation related to the dysraphic states. The lesion can be associated with hyperplastic or blastomatous changes of a great heterogeneity. The extent of the maldifferentiation can vary from dorsal gliosis and gliomatous syringes to hamartomas and true tumors, such as gangliogliomas and gliomas with a different degree of malignancy. It is worth noting that in all our cases a close anatomical relationship could be detected to the dorsal midline structures. This may indicate the relationship of the syringomyelic states to the dysraphic syndromes.

In recent years the clinical entity of syringomyelia has been extensively investigated using experimental animal models [6] or new neuroradiological techniques [4, 12]. A considerable contribution to our present knowledge consists of the various hydrodynamic theories [5, 16] that emphasize the role of CSF-flow in the origin and subsequent development of the syringes. The fact that in all our cases the leptomeninges are involved might be considered as a possibly important factor regarding the pathogenesis of the syringes. However, hydrodynamic explanations cannot account for all clinical as well as morphological varieties of the disease which is often misdiagnosed and may mimic other neurological conditions.

Although two of our cases (case 1 and 2) fell in the era when CT became clinically available syringomyelia/bulbia could not be detected by neuroradiological procedures. It was not even considered in the differential diagnosis because the "classical" sign of dissociated anaesthesia was not detected. That – of course – corresponded to our neuropathological findings that the anterior commissure anterior was unaffected in all cases. One might have considered the possibility of shunting some of the above syringes if the extent of the lesion and the exact anatomical relations had been known [15].

References

[1] Banerji, N. K., J. H. D. Miller: Chiari Malformation presenting in adult life. Brain 97 (1974) 157–168.

[2] Barnett, H. J. M., J. B. Foster, P. Hudgson: Syringomyelia. Saunders Co. Ltd., London 1973.

[3] Brewis, M., D. C. Poskanzer, C. Rolland et al.: Neurological Disease in an English City. Acta Neurologica, Scandinavica 42, Supplementum 24 (1966).

[4] DeLaPaz, R. L., T. J. Brady, F. S. Buonanno et al.: Nuclear Magnetic Resonance (NMR) Imaging of Arnold-Chiari Type I Malformation with Hydromyelia. J. Comp. Ass. Tomo. 7 (1983) 126–129.

[5] Gardner, W. J., F. G. McMurry: "Non-communicating" syringomyelia: a non-existant entity. Surg. Neurol. 6 (1976) 251–256.

[6] Hall, P., M. Turner, S. Aichinger et al.: Experimental syringomelia. J. Neurosurg. 52 (1980) 812–817.

[7] Hertel, G., J. Hild, H. Mönninghoff: Geomedizinische Untersuchungen über die Verbreitung der Syringomyelie in Deutschland. Zeitschrift für Neurologie 202 (1972) 295–306.

[8] Jacob, H.: Über die Fehlentwicklung des Kleinhirns, der Brücke und des verlängerten Markes (Arnold-Chiarische Entwicklungsstörung) bei kongenitaler Hydrocephalie und Spaltbildung des Rückenmarkes. Zeitschrift für die gesamte Neurologie und Psychiatrie 164 (1939) 229–258.

[9] McComb, J. G.: Recent research into the nature of cerebrospinal fluid formation and absorption. J. Neurosurg. 59 (1983) 369–383.

[10] Oakley, J. C., G. A. Ojemann, E. C. Alvord: Posttraumatic Syringomyelia. J. Neurosurg. 55 (1981) 276–281.

[11] Ostertag, B.: Die Einzelformen der Verbildung einschließlich Syringomyelie. In: Handbuch der Speziellen Pathologischen Anatomie und Histologie (Henke, Lubarsch, eds.), Bd. XIII, Erkrankungen des Zentralen Nervensystems IV, pp 363–601. Springer Verlag, Berlin 1956.

[12] Pasto, M. E., M. D. Rifkin, J. B. Rubenstein et al.: Real-time ultrasonography of the spinal cord: intraoperative and postoperative imaging. Neuroradiology 26 (1984) 183–187.

[13] Peters, G.: Spezielle Pathologie der Krankheiten des zentralen und peripheren Nervensystems. Georg Thieme Verlag, Stuttgart 1951.

[14] Stämmler, M.: Hydromyelie, Syringomyelie und Gliose (Anatomische Untersuchungen über ihre Histogenese). Springer Verlag, Berlin 1942.

[15] Tator, C. H., K. Meguro, D. W. Rowed: Favorable results with syringosubarachnoid shunts for treatment of syringomyelia, J. Neurosurg 56 (1982) 517–523.

[16] Williams, B.: A critical appraisal of posterior fossa surgery for communicating syringomyelia. Brain 101 (1978) 223–250.

Brain cysts and dysraphism

P. C. Potthoff

Introduction

In 1981 [10] a patho-anatomical classification of brain cysts was suggested consisting of 5 categories (table 1). The number of patients with cystic cerebral lesions has increased now to 81. This material has been re-analysed to determine whether there are possible combined syndromes consisting of dysraphy and brain cysts. Three main issues are being considered:

1. Could certain combinations of dysraphy and brain cysts be established as an entity?

2. Could certain mid-line brain cysts be considered as dysraphism itself?

3. Could a dysraphic state under certain circumstances lead to secondary cyst formation within the brain?

Patient material (tab. 1)

Group 1 consists of 23 patients with cysts in the Sylvian fissure. None are associated with dysraphism but there is a male of 17 with an arterio-venous angioma of the right parietal region combined with a left Sylvian fissure cyst.

Group 2 consists of 20 patients with cysts in the hemispheres. Five of these also have occlusive hydrocephalus, including 3 with proven aqueduct stenosis. There were a pair of twins in this group, one of whom suffered from rhesus-erythro-

Table 1   Patho-anatomical topical subgroups of 81 cystic brain lesions

Brain cysts	N = 81
1. Sylvian fissure cysts	23
2. Hemisphere cysts	20
3. Midline cysts	8
(cyst. quadr. 2; III. ventricle 6)	
4. Posterior fossa cysts	11
5. Combined malformations	19
(polycystic 13; cystic plus other CNS-malf. 6)	

blastosis. There was also a child with a large parieto-occipital brain cyst in combination with a nasal encephalocele (see group 5).

Group 3 consists of 8 patients with midline cysts in the brain: these are 2 with arachnoidal cysts of the quadrigeminal cistern and the other 6 with cysts in the third ventricle. Four of these are histologically glioependymal cysts, while the other 2 are shunt-treated but no histological diagnosis is available. A one year old boy in this group has a third ventricular glio-ependymal cyst in addition to an arachnoid cyst of the right Sylvian fissure.

Group 4 consists of 11 patients with posterior fossa cysts. Two are localised in the cerebello-pontine angle; 6 in the cerebellar hemispheres; 2 in the medial vermis and in one girl with a large extension of the cerebellar midline combined with an occipital meningocele. This is the only one in this group of 11 which is combined with dysraphism, but patients with the Dandy Walker syndrome and syringobulbia are excluded in this group.

Group 5 consists of 19 patients with combined malformations. Thirteen of these have polycystic brain lesions and the other 6 brain cysts combined with other malformations consisting of: nasal encephaloceles in 2; hydrocephalus in one; polycystic malformation of the brain in another and occipital meningocele in the last 2. There are 2 patients with thoraco-lumbar myelocele, one of which is combined with a primary polycystic brain and the other with hydrocephalus plus a solitary brain cyst. Of the 13 polycystic cases there are 4 with primary polycystic brain, while the other 8 have hydrocephalus and polycystic brains, mainly due to previous ventriculitis (the so-called multiloculated hydrocephalus) [2, 9].

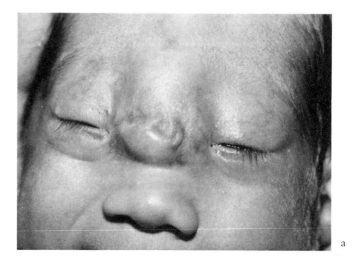

a

Fig. 1a, b   Nasal encephalocele and right temporoparieto-occipital brain cyst (L. B., female)

Different Classification

The patient material can also be divided in a different way.

Dysraphism in combination with primary cysts

This association is present in 5 patients. One of these is a child with a nasal encephalocele (figs. 1a and 1b) who is 6 years old. She had had a shunt and a frontal transcranial operation of the nasal encephalocele. The second patient in this group died at one year of age and had parieto-occipital meningocele plus a

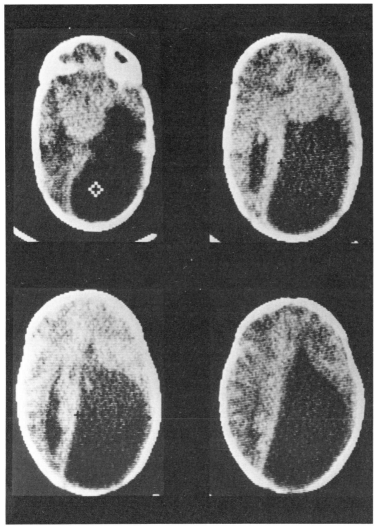

b

polycystic brain. That occurred 4 months after the shunt operation and the repair of the meningocele. A revision was followed by convulsions and pneumonia, with high fever. There was no autopsy. The third child, a girl, had a large occipital encephalocele plus a posterior fossa midline cyst. She is 7½ years of age. She had her encephalocele repaired and her hydrocephalus and the cyst treated with a combined shunt operation. Except for minimal ataxia, she has no neurological defecit. The fourth child had a lumbar myelocele and a polycystic brain. She was a permanently handicapped person who died at 6 years of age. Her myelocele was operated on and she had a cranial burrhole for multiple shunt implantation, to deal with her polycystic brain. These were followed by several revisions. The fifth patient, a girl, died at 20 months following the repair of the myelocele, shunt operation and multiple ventricular catheter revisions.

If obstructive hydrocephalus due to aqueduct stenosis or occlusion is accepted as a form of internal dysraphism, then 4 additional cases can be included in this group – 3 males and 1 female. All these children are alive and are between 5 and 11 years of age. They have minor neurological handicaps, mostly following multiple shunt operations or, in one case, following resection of a cyst, though all had hemispheric cysts.

Primary midline cysts of the brain as "inner" dysraphism

Six third-ventricle-cysts and two quadrigeminal cysts were treated. Two third-ventricle-cysts were treated by shunt operation alone and their etiology/histology was not determined. Four other third-ventricle-cysts were treated by open re-

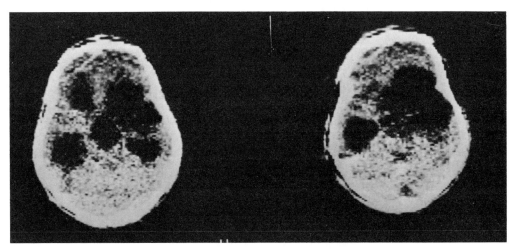

Fig. 2   Midline IIIrd ventricle glioependymal cyst – as "inner" dysraphism – in combination with Sylvian fissure arachnoidal cyst in the right side (Z. C., male)

section, only one needing an additional shunt with multiple subsequent shunt revisions. This last case (Z. C., male, fig. 2) showed a combination of a glio-ependymal cyst of the third ventricle and an arachnoidal cyst of the right Sylvian fissure. All cases with third-ventricle-cysts are doing well.

The two cases with quadrigeminal arachnoidal cysts were both subjected to open operation with histological confirmation, one case (N. M., female) was operated at the age of 39 years on the grounds of increasing headache and disturbance of concentration and memory without having developed a secondary hydrocephalus; post-operatively she has remained symptom-free except for occasional headache.

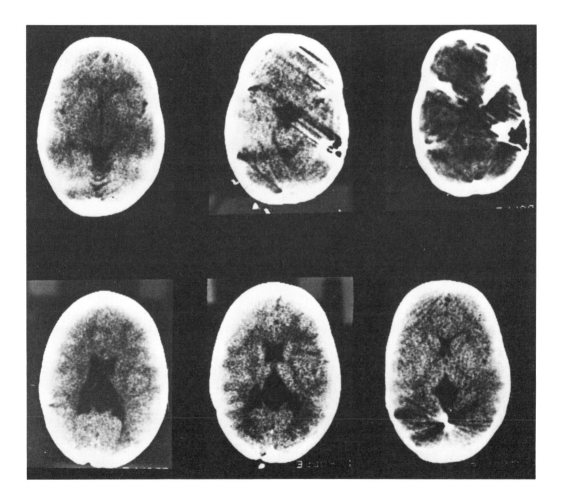

Fig. 3   Midline quadrigeminal cyst as "inner" dysraphism, combined with functional dysraphism? (K. R., male)

The second case (K. R., male, fig. 3) showed hypotonic ataxia at the age of two and additional convergent strabism at the age of four; he had his first operation at the age of four with fenestration and partial resection of his quadrigeminal cysts via occipito-supratentorial route, was slightly improved thereafter, and had a second infratentorial cyst revision and additional partial resection at the age of eight years without definite improvement; he is going to a school for intellectually disabled, and continues exhibiting hypotonic ataxia and strabism.

Dysraphism with secondary (poly-)cystic transformation of hydrocephalus

It is wellknown that hydrocephalus in spite of all therapeutic endevavour with shunting procedures may undergo polycystic transformation [9] carrying a bad prognosis. Often in these cases ventriculitis as subacute or chronic infection enhances such a deterioration. Among our own eight cases of hydrocephalus with secondary polycystic transformation were four cases combined with dysraphism: nasal encephalocele (Ö. R., male), occipital meningocele (S. S. female), thoraco-lumbar myelocele (C. K., male), aqueductal occlusion and porencephaly (H. S., female). The first child is living but severely retarded with epilepsy and hemiplegia at the age of eight, whereas the latter three children died at the age of three months, seven months, and two years and ten months respectively (for CT-documentation of polycystic transformation of hydrocephalus see [9]).

Discussion

The etiology of cystic transformation of the infant's brain is multifactorial (compare page 102 [8]). The causative factors inducing combinations of dysraphism and brain cysts remain to be determined. From our cases of brain cysts we have described three different combinations of dysraphism and brain cysts, and we suggest three entities (tab. 2).

The parallel manifestation of dysraphic lesions of the CNS on the outside (encephalocele, meningocele, myelocele) with mono- or poly-cystic brain lesions was found in five out of 81 cases. This means an incidence of 6 percent external dysraphism in patients having cystic brain lesions.

Table 2   Three suggested entities of relations of dysraphism and brain cysts

1. Dysraphism plus cysts
2. "Inner" dysraphism as cyst
3. Dysraphism followed by (poly-)cystic transformation

If, however, dysraphism is not considered only in external lesions, but if inner dys-ontogenetic lesions are also included as dysraphic, two additional forms have to be mentioned. One is the combination of occlusive hydrocephalus caused by aqueductal stenosis or occlusion and hemispheric brain cysts which we found in four additional cases.

The other, more important group is so-called "inner" dysraphism as a cyst formation in the midline of the brain reported here in six cases of third-ventricle-cysts and two cases of quadrigeminal cysts. – The reported case (fig. 3) of an arachnoidal cyst of the quadrigeminal cistern with concomitant strabism and ataxia was operated twice without major clinical improvement. This case raises an important question: Would it be possible that besides the morphological forms of external dysraphism (encephalocele or myelocele), and inner dysraphism (cysts of the cerebral midline), a type exists which might be called *"functional"* *dysraphism?* It appears feasible that – without or with minor evidence of patho-anatomical demonstration of morphological changes in the midline of the brain – a congenital faulty programme of the midline crossings might occur seldomly. This might prevent – for instance – normal development of oculo-motor functions or coordination. Thus resulting in strabism or ataxia as in the described case. The recent report of Eda et al. [5] on CT-findings in congenital occular-motor apraxia (COMA) in four cases could support this view: Besides demonstrable midline lesions as morphological "inner" dysraphism of the brain, there exist additional disturbances of midline functions in the brain stem to be considered as "functional" dysraphism.

A third relation was found for dysraphic children, namely the secondary development of polycystic transformation of hydrocephalus in the brain, as reported here in four cases. The secondary development of multiple internal cysts, "polycystic transformation" [9], has also been termed "multicystic encephalomalacia" [1], "polyporencephaly" [3], "multilocular cystic encephalopathy" [4], "multilocular encephalomalacia" [6, 7], or "multiloculated hydrocephalus" [2]. If dysraphic children are especially liable to such a secondary polycystic transformation of hydrocephalus – usually caused by subacute or chronic infection as already described by Virchow [12] – remains open. Among eight hydrocephalic children of our own collective that developed polycystic transformation of hydrocephalus, four were cases of dysraphic lesions.

Summary

A collective of 81 cystic brain lesions was analysed for relations to dysraphic lesions of the CNS. A parallel manifestation of external dysraphism with primary brain cysts in five cases (nasal encephalocele, parieto-occipito meningoceles, thoraco-lumbar myeloceles) was found, and four cases with occlusive hydroce-phalus (aqueductal stenosis/occlusion) of inner dysraphism and hemispheric brain cysts. Beside aqueductal stenosis/occlusion ("inner" dysraphism), an additional group of six third-ventricle-cysts and two quadrigeminal cysts (eight cases) were considered to be manifestation of inner dysraphism with primary midline cysts of the brain. Four more cases of dysraphic children (lumbar myeloceles, occipital meningocele, nasal encephalocele) were found to have developed a secondary polycystic transformation of their hydrocephalus. — Three dysraphic-cystic en-tities are suggested and the possibility of so-called "functional" dysraphism is discussed.

References

[1] Aicardi, I., F. Goutiers: Multicystic encephalomalacia of infants and its relation to abnormal gestation and hydroencephaly. J. of Neurol. Sciences 15 (1972) 357 – 373.

[2] Albanese, V., F. Tomasello, S. Sampaolo et al.: Multiloculated hydrocephalus. Acta Neurochir. (Wien) 69 (1983) 143.

[3] Brocher, J. E.: Polyporencephalie. Z. ges. Neurol. Psychiat. 142 (1932) 107 – 119.

[4] Crome, L.: Multilocular cystic encephalopathia of infants. J. Neurol. Neurosurg. Psychiat. 21 (1958) 146 – 152.

[5] Eda, J., S. Takashima, T. Kitahara et al.: Computed tomography in congenital ocular motor apraxia. Neuroradiology 26 (1984) 359 – 362.

[6] Kramer, W.: Multilocular encephalomalacia. J. Neurol. Neurosurg. Psychiat. 19 (1956) 209 – 216.

[7] Negrin, J.: Multilocular encephalomalacia. J. Neuropath. exp. Neurol. 11 (1952) 62 – 68.

[8] Neutatz, G.: Hirncysten und Cystenhirn. Inaug. Diss., München 1978.

[9] Potthoff, P. C.: Early and late mortality following shunt procedures in early infancy. In: Advances in Neurosurgery (W. Grothe et al., eds.), vol. 8, pp. 235 – 246. Springer, Berlin – Heidelberg 1980.

[10] Potthoff, P. C.: Evolution of brain cysts and polycystic brain. Rep. 7th World Congress Neuro-surgery, Munich, July 1981.

[11] Potthoff, P. C., R. Hemmer: The biventricular, the bilateral and the dual-unilateral shunt. Develop. Med. Child Neurol. (Suppl. 22) 12 (1970) 127 – 136.

[12] Virchow, R.: Kongenitale Encephalitis und Myelitis. Virchow's Arch. v. Path. Anat. 38 (1867) 129.

Pathogenesis and clinical aspects of congenital arachnoid cysts of the Sylvian fissure in childhood

R. Heller, J. Menzel

Introduction

Congenital arachnoid cysts belong to the space-occupying cranial processes. They were first described by Bright (1831), Starkman (1958) et al. as intra-arachnoid liquid accumulations [15]. Their size varies from the dimensions of a pea to a man's fist. The contents are mostly clear and its composition analogous to liquor, but the concentration of protein can reach a higher level. Intracranial cysts are located in most cases in relation to the basal cisterns [4, 16]. In about 50% of cases they are found in the area of the Sylvian fissure and in the insular region [4, 21].

Pathogenesis

Primary arachnoid cysts result from a defect in ontogenesis of the pia mater. In embryos of about 40 mm CR length, corresponding to the 2nd – 3rd intra-uterine month, the differentiating central nervous system is surrounded by primitive meninx, a vascularized loose tissue of mesenchymal origin. From this tissue the primitive preliminary stages of arachnoid and pia mater derive by dehiscence. This division is induced by an already pulsating choroid plexus, which ensures liquor circulation [4, 15, 19]. In the area of the spinal canal and basal cysterns the formation of free liquid space is due to a loss of leptomeningeal tissue [19], while in the region of the hemispheric rudiments only a capillary gap remains as subarachnoid space. The morphological pathogenesis of an intra-arachnoidal cyst [4, 15] is supposed to be caused by the formation of a diverticulum in the primitive external meninx in combination with a locally altered liquor circulation (fig. 1).

Besides the general formation mechanisms of congenital arachnoid cysts, great importance was attributed to the embryonic development of the insula. In the past this fact erroneously led to the hypothesis of a primary agensis of the temporal lobe [3, 10, 12, 16] – as could be demonstrated by postoperative CT controls with the proof of a complete unfolding of the temporal lobe. It has to

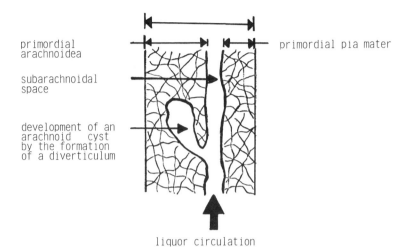

primitive meninx

primordial
arachnoidea

subarachnoidal
space

development of an
arachnoid   cyst
by the formation
of a diverticulum

primordial pia mater

liquor circulation

Fig. 1   An outline of the pathogenesis of primary arachnoid cysts during the embryonal development
of the pia mater (as modified by [4]).

a

b

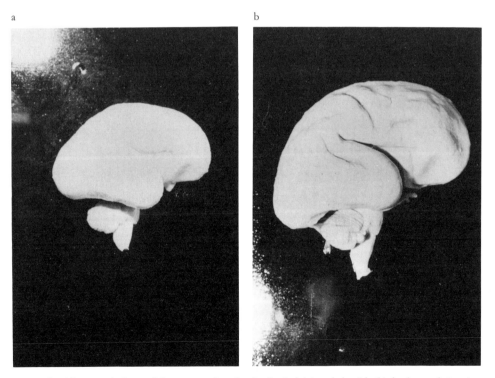

Fig. 2 a, b   The morphology of the temporal region in the 3rd (a) and the 5th (b) fetal month (text).

be considered, however, that a frequent occurrence of arachnoid cysts in the Sylvian fissure could be induced by morphological genetic aberrations.

The final morphology of the cerebral pallium is a consequence of differently growing fast processes within the 2nd and 6th fetal month [12, 19, fig. 2a and b]. In the region of the basal ganglia the growing processes fall behind, and in the 3rd month a depression is formed in a latero-basal position of the cerebral hemisphere. Later the region of the fossa lateralis remains fixed in a basal position. In its function as the future cerebral islet region, it will be covered from a frontal, parietal and temporal direction. In this connection the expanding formation of the temporal operculum is of special significance, and reaches the Sylvian fissure in the 4th fetal month. The occlusion of the fissure takes place in the 6th month. The large displacements of primitive meninx during the period of invagination into the fossa cerebri lateralis might possibly induce the development of arachnoid cysts in the islet region.

Clinical aspects

In the course of 16 months 145 intracranial tumors have been operated on in the Neurosurgical Clinic Köln – Merheim, including 15 children. Eight had arachnoid cysts. Four were in the middle cranial fossa: two of these patients were children. In one, the diagnosis was surgically confirmed. Within a period of 9 years prior to the introduction of CT scans, 3 Sylvian fissure cysts were found among 108 children with increased intracranial pressure.

Case 1

A 14-year old girl was referred to psychiatric treatment because of periodic aggression and mutism, in which she was not approachable. Neurological examination revealed unilateral mainly sensory signs on the right. EEG focal findings were ascertained in the left temporal leads. The left-sided carotid angiogram suggested a non-vascularized fronto-temporo-basal expansive process. At operation after trepanation a tight and non-pulsating dura was found. On opening it, a clear liquid spouted out under high pressure. The visible parts of the frontal and temporal lobe seemed to be hypoplastic and atrophic.

The islet-region with the ascending media-vessels on the bottom of the first-sized cavity was in a free position.

All accessible membranes were removed and a large window was created in the cisterna opto-chiasmatica. Histologically, both the visceral and the parietal membranes had the typical structure of normal arachnoid. There were no postoperative complications and all the patient's symptoms resolved.

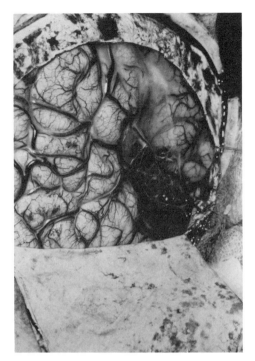

Fig. 3   Arachnoid cyst in the Sylvian fissure in a 6 year old boy – operation site.

Case 2

A 6-year old boy had been hit by a car. He became deeply unconscious and was brought to the neurosurgical clinic with a tentative diagnosis of an intracranial bleeding. Skull x-ray revealed a right-sided fracture. After 7 days the child developed a left-sided hemiparesis. Arteriography showed signs of a non-vascularized expansive process in the temporo-parietal position. There was no surgical evidence of a suspected epidural hematoma.

Opening of the tight and only slightly pulsating dura, a big cyst was found in the middle and inferior part of the Sylvian fissure (fig. 3). After removal of the external membrane a clear liquid escaped under considerably high pressure. All accessible membranes of the collapsed cyst were resected and a large communication with the basal cisterns provided. The postoperative events were protracted, but 4 months after the accident the boy was in good neurological and psychiatrical state. His school achievements were above the average level.

Case 3

A 9 months old female infant had a progressive osseous bulge at the left temporal bone. On X-ray the temporal bone proved to thinned out. Arteriography

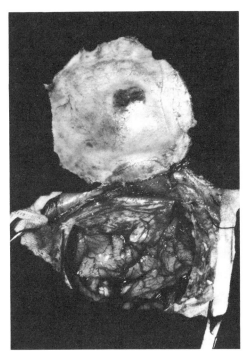

Fig. 4   Demonstration of the internal table: atrophy and perforation are caused by the pressure of an arachnoid cyst — operation site.

demonstrated the typical criteria of a big left-temporally located expansive process. During operation the temporal bone proved to be perforated by pressure atrophy in the region of the inner table. The dura was tight and in the area of the temporal lobe the cerebral convolutions had disappeared (fig. 4). After puncture a xanthochromic fluid escaped under pressure from a depth of 2 – 3 mm. A cyst was found of the size of a hen's egg. It resembled the cerebral surface and was lined from all sides with leptomeningeal membranes. Its base was in a close relation to the plexus tissue and the lateral ventricle. After the usual resection of the membranes there was sufficient drainage to the basal cisterns and to the left ventricle. Histologically the resected membranes showed the typical structure of normal arachnoid. The subsequent psycho-motor development of the child was normal.

Case 4

A 14-year old patient complained of headache for a year. This headache had appeared suddenly and caused a lack of concentration and capacity for learning.

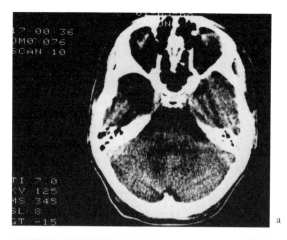

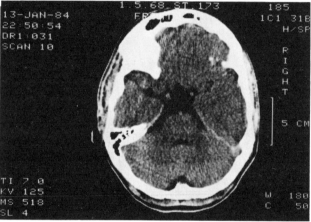

Fig. 5 a, b   Postoperative computer-tomography with the demonstration of the re-unfolding of the temporal lobe after surgical resection of a cyst in the Sylvian fissure.

Neurologically there was a slight right-sided unilateral motor deficit. Cranial computer-tomography revealed a cyst in the region of the left temporal pole (fig. 5). Selective angiography of the internal carotid artery showed the typical displacements of the middle cerebral artery in a cranial and medial direction. This was caused by a non-vascularized expansive process in a basal position. Cysto-cisternostomy was carried out. Histopathologically an arachnoidal cyst was diagnosed. The post-operative proceedings were complicated by an epidural bleeding. After its surgical removal there were no further complications. 9 months later a control-CT scan showed the complete disappearance of the cyst and the unfolding of the temporal lobe (fig. 5b). The boy is symptom-free and is making good progress in school.

Discussion

Before the CT-era arachnoid cysts were considered a rare intracranial space-occupying process. Among 700 children of the Neurosurgical University Clinic of Vienna, only 12 children had space-occupying intracerebral cysts [11]. Within 10 years Geisler and Singh found 3 arachnoid cysts in 4.000 cerebral injured children [7], and Neuhäuser [14] reported 14 within a period of 5 years. The frequency of arachnoid cysts was about 0.4 – 0.6% [3, 17] and for children about 1% [14]. The actual incidence is certainly higher. Before the introduction of cranial computer-tomography our incidence was 3% and afterwards 7%. The frequency among our patients is higher then in the above mentioned series, but it correlates very well with recent reports of Galassi et al. [6], who calculated 4.8% of all intracranial tumors.

Clinically these cysts can cause various unspecific symptoms, such as dull headache and other symptoms of brain pressure, either organic or even more psychomotor but also focal and generalized attacks. Less frequently, sensory or motor hemisyndroms and eye-muscle- or optic disturbances may occur. Some temporal arachnoid cysts remain without symptoms, even if these are of considerable size, and are merely radiological findings [1, 2, 20].

Skull X-rays demonstrate bulging and thinned out temporal bone, an extension of middle cranial fossa and an elevation of the small wing of sphenoid. The computer-tomography reveals an area of the density of CSF in the temporal region, without marginal enhancement. The coronal and sagittal reconstructions demonstrate a topographical relation to the Sylvian fissure and give the impression of a polydimensional extension of the cyst (fig. 6a and b). A reciprocal relation was found between the communication of the cyst with the subarachnoidal space and the extension of the cyst [6]. A transition from one type into the other remains hypothetical, but a possible tendency of rapid growth could be proved by sequential examinations [1, 8, 18, 22].

The prolonged latency of clinical symptoms without any particular event seems remarkable. This could possible be explained by a progressive expansion of the cysts.

Typical complications are either the development of subdural hematoma (fig. 7) or intracystic bleedings after minor injuries [3, 5, 9, 13, 18]. A primary manifestation of arachnoid cysts of the Sylvian fissure following head injury without haemorrhagic component is rarely described [5, 12]. With reference to the studies of Galassi et al. [6] obstruction of the CSF dynamics is pathogenetic to be considered between the contents of a cyst and the subarachnoid space, due to the obstruction of cerebral pathways, caused by the traumatic cerebral edema.

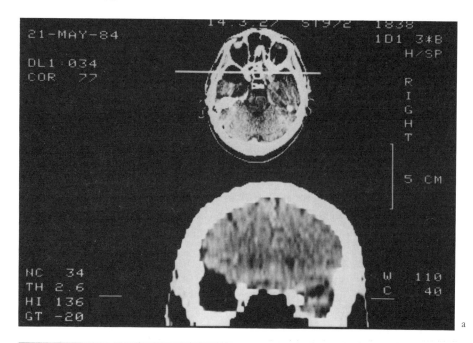

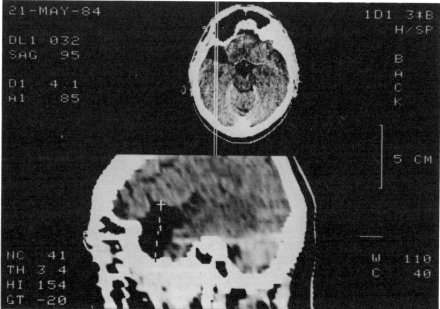

Fig. 6 a, b   Coronal (a) and sagittal (b) reconstruction of an arachnoid cyst of the left Sylvian fissure.
A spatial impression of the cystic extension.

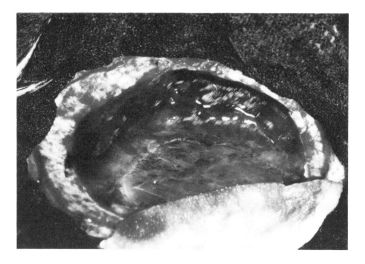

Fig. 7 Operation site of a subdural haematoma as the primary manifestation of an arachnoid cyst of the Sylvian fissure.

Arachnoid cysts must be differentiated from porencephaly and cysts of epithelial or ependymal origin. Ependymal cysts mostly derive from embryonic dispersed parts of the neural tube, whereas porencephaly communicates with the ventricular system or the subarachnoid space. Most frequently ependymal cysts are located in an intracerebral position. In case of a topographic relation to the subarachnoid space, the differentiation from an arachnoid cyst can only be established by histology.

Cysts of the Sylvian fissure have to be removed. In children all approachable membranes must be removed. Cystocisternostomy should be preferred to shunting. This technique avoids shunt dependence and its complications. It is possible to eliminate the potential postoperative haemorrhagic complications by coagulating the vessels in the outer cyst membrane [10].

Summary

Congenital cystic lesions of the arachnoid and of the Sylvian fissure, and the insular region are considered to be the consequence of aberrant embryonal development. Four examples have been presented and discussed.

References

[1] Anderson, F. M., B. H. Landing: Cerebral arachnoid cysts in infants. J. Pediatrics **64** (1966) 88–96.

[2] Anderson, F. M., H. D. Segall, W. L. Caton: Use of computerized tomography scanning in supratentorial arachnoid cysts. J. Neurosurg. **50** (1979) 333–338.

[3] Auer, L. M., B. Gallhofer, G. Ladurner et al.: Diagnosis and treatment of middle fossa arachnoid cysts and subdural hematomas. J. Neurosurg. **54** (1981) 366–369.

[4] Brackett, C. E., S. S. Rengachary: Arachnoid Cysts. In: Neurological Surgery (J. R. Youmans, ed.), pp. 1436–1446. W. B. Saunders Comp., Philadelphia – London – Toronto – Mexico City – Sydney – Tokyo 1982.

[5] Galassi, E., G. Piazza, G. Gaist et al.: Arachnoid Cysts of the Middle Cranial Fossa: A Clinical and Radiological Study of 25 Cases Treated Surgically. Surg. Neurol. **14** (1980) 211–219.

[6] Galassi, E., F. Tognetti, G. Gaist et al.: CT Scan and Metrizamide CT Cisternography in Arachnoid Cysts of the Middle Cranial Fossa: Classification and Pathophysiological Aspects. Surg. Neurol. **17** (1982) 363–369.

[7] Geisler, E., M. Singh: Arachnoidalcysten bei Kindern. Kinderärztl. Prax. **35** (1967) 411ff.

[8] Geissinger, J. D., W. C. Kohler, B. W. Robinson: Arachnoid cysts of the middle cranial fossa: Surgical considerations. Surg. Neurol. **10** (1978) 27–33.

[9] Kadowaki, H., M. Ide, E. Takara et al.: A case of Arachnoid Cyst Associated with Chronic Subdural Hematoma. No Shinkei Geka **11** (1983) 431–436.

[10] Karvounis, P. C., J. C. Chiu, K. Parsa et al.: Agenesis of Temporal Lobe and Arachnoid Cyst. N. Y. St. J. Med. **70** (1970) 2349–2353.

[11] Koos, W. T., M. H. Miller: Intracranial tumours of infants and children. Thieme-Verlag, Stuttgart 1971.

[12] Markakis, E., R. Heyer, L. Stöppler et al.: Agenesis of the Perisylvian Region (Temporal Lobe Agenesis): Neurological Symptoms and Therapy. Adv. Neurosurg. **5** (1978) 297–305.

[13] Nabeshi, S., Y. Makita, M. Motomochi et al.: Three Cases of Arachnoid Cysts Associated with Chronic Subdural Hematoma. No To Shinkei **34** (1982) 173–178.

[14] Neuhäuser, G.: Zerebrale Arachnoidalzysten bei Kindern. Fortschr. Med. **90** (1972) 66–70.

[15] Rengachary, S. S., I. Watanabe, C. E. Brackett: Pathogenesis of Intracranial Cysts. Surg. Neurol. **9** (1978) 139–144.

[16] Robinson, R. G.: The Temporal Lobe Agenesis Syndrome. Brain **87** (1964) 87–106.

[17] Robinson, R. G.: Congenital Cysts of the Brain: Arachnoid Malformations. Prog. Neurol. Surg. **4** (1971) 133–174.

[18] Smith, R. A., W. A. Smith: Arachnoid Cysts of the Middle Cranial Fossa. Surg. Neurol. **5** (1976) 246–252.

[19] Stark, D.: Embryologie, 3. Aufl. Georg Thieme-Verlag, Stuttgart 1975.

[20] Starkman, S. P., T. C. Brown, E. A. Linell: Cerebral Arachnoid Cysts. J. Neuropath. Exp. Neurol. **17** (1958) 484–500.

[21] Vigouroux, R. P., M. Choux, C. Baurand: Les Kystes arachnoidiens congénitaux. Neurochirurgia **9** (1966) 169–187.

[22] Williams, B., A. N. Gutkelch: Why do central arachnoid pouches expand? J. Neurol. Neurosurg. Psych. **37** (1974) 1085–1092.

II Epidemiology, antenatal diagnostics and prevention of dysraphias

The distribution of anencephalus and spina bifida in Germany

M. Koch

New development of the last years concerning spina bifida and anencephalus (neural tube defects) have interested investigators for epidemiologic data of these malformations again. Now there exist reliable methods for the prenatal diagnosis-skilled ultrasound, measurement of alphafetoprotein and acetylcholinesterase in amniotic fluid and screening procedures of alphafetoprotein in maternal serum [6, 7]. In the last years some investigators started methods of primary prevention by vitamin supplements before conception and during pregnancy [11, 20]. On the other hand there exist more improved surgical methods and follow-up clinics for the handicapped survivors.

It is well known that a considerable variation in the prevalence of neural tube defects (NTD) exists at birth and in different populations.

In Great Britain the prevalence at birth for this group of malformations is higher than in countries of Continental Europe and North America while the malformation is very rare in Black and Asian people.

In the FRG official statistics of population surveys for malformations in live-born children are published by the Statistisches Bundesamt Wiesbaden [21]; but it is estimated that only 10% of the malformed newborns are reported, making the figures too low and unrepresentative. In the FRG therefore we have to rely on different local investigations to be able to follow the epidemiological trend of NTD.

Several studies on the prevalence at birth of NTD are available for this country. The comparison of the figures from various studies is difficult because their methods are different. The material of most series was collected retrospectively and based on birth records of maternity hospitals. In contrast to community surveys, hospital series may overestimate the prevalence. Figures collected during the last years show the results of prospective studies as the data of screening programs for maternal serum alphafetoprotein became available [7, 10, 16].

Most important for the interpretation of the percentages rates of NTD given in the literature is the question whether stillbirths are included in the series. The frequency of NTD is calculated to be ten times higher in embryos and fetuses than in neonates [2, 15]. Studies considering live births only will therefore have a lower prevalence at birth than those which include stillbirths as well.

Only studies for which the mode of selection was evident were reviewed and a selection of these data are presented in this paper and summarized in table 1 and 2 [9].

Table 1   Prevalence rates of NTD per 1000 births in Germany (Retrospective Studies)

Authors	Area	Time period	SB	A
Eichmann und Gesenius [5]	Berlin	1935 – 1939	0.96	0.85
		1945 – 1949	2.4	2.55
Winter und Pätz [22]	Berlin	1951 – 1956	0.96	1.05
Lenz [13]	Hamburg	1935 – 1939	2.05	1.07
		1945 – 1949	0.96	0.95
		1960 – 1963	–	0.5
Canzler et al. [1]	Leipzig	1946 – 1950	–	2.05
		1961 – 1965	–	0.53
Karkut [8]	Berlin (FRG)	1971 – 1982	0.81	0.43

Table 2   Prevalence rates of NTD per 1000 births in Germany (Prospective studies)

Authors	Area	Time period	SB	A
Michaelis [16]	FRG	1964 – 1972	1.1	0.8
Fuhrmann und Weitzel [7]	FRG	1980 – 1982	0.53	0.55
Körner und Horn [10]	GDR	1981 – 1982	0.68	0.78

The largest retrospective study of the prevalence of NTD at birth for a specific region in Germany was reported by Eichmann und Gesenius [5] and followed up by Winter and Pätz [22] for Berlin. These authors found an increasing prevalence during and shortly after the Second World War, reaching a pick after the Second World War. A significant heterogeneity among the data could be demonstrated by the chi-square test.

In a follow-up study, Winter and Pätz [22] reported a decreasing frequency but the low percentages observed before the Second World War were not reached again. The overall rate at this time was about 2‰ in Berlin. In 1971 Karkut [8] started another retrospective study in Berlin, these rates for NTD were lower again, especially for anencephalus.

An epidemic increase of anencephaly was also noted by Canzler et al. [1] in the area of Leipzig, here the high plateau continued until 1955, when a decrease to levels comparable to those found by Lenz [13] in Hamburg occured.

Concerning the cited figures of Lenz [13] it is remarkable that he reported high rates already *before* the Second World War but no increase after the war. The figures for Hamburg decreased slowly and constantly over the years and at the end of the survey the occurrence of anencephalus had fallen to 0.5‰ comparable to the new data presented by Karkut [8].

Figures of the last decade were presented by new prospective studies. The prospective study of pregnancy and child development of the Deutsche For-schungsgemeinschaft [16] showed relatively high rates when compared to those studies by Fuhrmann and Weitzel [9] and Körner and Horn [10]. The differences among these figures might include a certain selection for the prenatal screening studies and also considerable random fluctuation in smaller surveys like these. As mentioned above the figures of the official notification system for congenital malformations in the FRG [21] are much too low and not representative; the register gives figures for spina bifida – 0.2‰ and for anencephalus – 0.06‰.

In conclusion it can be confirmed that the prevalence rates for NTD show an increase during and shortly after the war and a decline in the last two decades. From the reviewed data it can be assumed that the decrease was more obvious for anencephalus than for spina bifida. It can be confirmed that Germany – the FRG as well as the GDR – belongs to the countries having a low prevalence for NTD at birth like other Continental European countries and North America.

The current prevalence of NTD at birth can be estimated for Germany to be about 1.0 – 1.5‰ with about an even distribution to anencephalus and spina bifida.

An apparent decline of the prevalence rates of NTD first observed in Germany is also reported from Great Britain and other European countries, Australia, and the USA [3, 4, 12, 14]. Larger declines were seen in regions with high incidence and were more marked for anencephalus than for spina bifida [8, 14].

A reasonable explanation for the falling rates cannot be stated. The falling birth rates, prenatal diagnostic, the considerable number of early terminated pregnancies are only responsible for a small portion of the decline, and none of the factors are sufficient to explain the early decline in Germany.

Poor nutrition and other socio-economic factors concerning the mothers during and after the war do not seem to account for the decreased rates. For example in the area of Hamburg an increase was not recorded at this time. It has also to be considered that at present other congenital malformations are not decreasing neither in Germany nor in other countries.

References

[1] Canzler, E., G. Funk, L. Schlegel: Mißbildungshäufigkeit an der Universitätsfrauenklinik Leipzig in den Jahren 1941 bis 1965. I. Mitteilung: Mißbildungshäufigkeit unter besonderer Berücksichtigung der Gestosen. Zentralbl. Gynäkol. **26** (1969) 833 – 847.

[2] Creasy, M. R., E. D. Alberman: Congenital malformations of the central nervous system in spontaneous abortions. J. Med. Genet. **13** (1976) 9 – 16.

[3] Czeizel, A., C. Révész: Major malformations of the nervous system in Hungary. Br. J. Prev. Soc. Med. **24** (1970) 205 – 210.

[4] Danks, D. M., J. L. Halliday: Incidence of neural tube defects in Victoria, Australia. Lancet **I** (1983) 65.

[5] Eichmann, E., H. Gesenius: Mißgeburtenzunahme in Berlin und Umgebung in den Nachkriegsjahren. Arch. Gynecol. **181** (1952) 168 – 184.

[6] Ferguson-Smith, M. A.: The reduction of anencephalic and spina bifida births by maternal serum alphafetoprotein screening. Brit. Med. Bull. **39** (1983) 365 – 372.

[7] Fuhrmann, W., H. K. Weitzel: Maternal serum alpha-fetoprotein screening for neural tube defects. Hum. Genet. **69** (1985) 47 – 61.

[8] Karkut, G.: Personal communication (1983).

[9] Koch, M., W. Fuhrmann: Epidemiology of neural tube defects in Germany. Hum. Genet. **68** (1984) 97 – 103.

[10] Körner, H., A. Horn: Pränatale Diagnostik von Neuralrohrdefekten als Massenscreening. Vortrag auf der 18. Tagung der Gesellschaft für Anthropologie und Humangenetik, Münster 1983.

[11] Laurence, K. M.: Primary prevention of neural tube defects by dietary improvement and folic acid supplementation. In: Spina bifida – neural tube defects (D. Voth, P. Glees, eds.), pp. 107. Walter de Gruyter, Berlin – New York 1986.

[12] Le Merrer, M., M. L. Briard, F. Demenais et al.: Etude épidémiologique et génétique du spina bifida. Arch. Fr. Pediatr. **37** (1980) 521 – 525.

[13] Lenz, W.: Epidemiologie von Mißbildungen. Padiatr. Padol. **1** (1965) 38 – 50.

[14] Lorber, J.: Spina bifida – a vanishing nightmare? In: Spina bifida – neural tube defects (D. Voth, P. Glees, eds.), pp. 3. Walter de Gruyter, Berlin – New York 1986.

[15] Mac Henry, J. C. R. M., N. C. Nevin, J. D. Merrett: Comparison of central nervous system malformations in spontaneous abortions in Northern Ireland and South-east England. Brit. Med. J. **1** (1979) 1395 – 1397.

[16] Michaelis, H.: Personal communication about the data of the prospective study of pregnancy and child development. In part published in Koller, S.: Risikofaktoren in der Schwangerschaft. Auswertung von 7870 Schwangerschaften der prospektiven Untersuchungsreihe "Schwangerschaftsverlauf und Kindesentwicklung" der Deutschen Forschungsgemeinschaft. Springer Verlag Berlin, Heidelberg – New York – Tokyo 1983.

[17] Nevin, N. C., W. P. Johnston: A family study of spina bifida and anencephalus in Belfast, Northern Ireland (1964 to 1968). J. Med. Genet. **17** (1980) 203 – 211.

[18] Owens, J. R., F. Harris, E. McAllister et al.: 19-year incidence of neural tube defects in area under constant surveillance. Lancet **I** (1981) 1032 – 1035.

[19] Romijn, J. A., P. E. Treffers: Anencephaly in the Netherlands: A remarkable decline. Lancet **I** (1983) 64 – 65.

[20] Seller, M. J., N. C. Nevin: Periconceptional vitamin supplementation and the prevention of neural tube defects in south-east England and Northern Ireland. J. Med. Genet. **21** (1984) 325 – 330.

[21] Statistisches Bundesamt Wiesbaden: Todesursachen der Gestorbenen, Fehlbildungen bei Geborenen. Schriftenreihe des Bundesminsteriums für Jugend, Familie und Gesundheit, 77. Verlag W. Kohlhammer, Stuttgart – Berlin – Köln – Mainz 1980.

[22] Winter, G. F., A. Pätz: Die Mißbildungshäufigkeit in Berlin und Umgebung in den Jahren 1950 – 1956. Arch. Gynecol. **190** (1958) 404 – 418.

Primary prevention of neural tube defects by dietary improvement and folic acid supplementation*

K. M. Laurence

Introduction

Family studies suggest that neural tube defects (NTD) like most of the other common malformations, have a multifactorial aetiology: early embryonic development of a polygenically susceptible fetus is interfered with by environmental trigger influences [1], setting off the defect. As little can be done to modify the genetic component, any primary prevention would be dependent on identifying the environmental triggers, which then might either be eliminated from the environment or avoided.

Nutrition has been suspected as an aetiological factor for NTD for some time because in the British Isles with its high incidence, those regions that seem to be more deprived such as the Irish Republic, Northern Ireland, South Wales, North West of England and the South West of Scotland, have the highest incidence [2]. In these area, and elsewhere, social class IV and V families have a much higher incidence than those of social class I and II [3 – 5]. Seasonal variations, with a higher incidence amongst winter and spring conceptions when fresh foods are less plentiful and more expensive have also been reported [3]. Secular trends have been noted in the past but these have usually been difficult to interpret. The sharp rise in the incidence of NTD in Boston during the depression years and in a number of German cities immediately after the Second World War, have been attributed to the poor maternal nutrition prevailing at the time [6, 7]. However, in the last decade there has been a dramatic fall in the incidence of NTD in the United Kingdom, especially in high incidence regions [8 – 10] and social class and seasonal variations have become less pronounced [3]; changes which may be due to improvement in the general standard of maternal nutrition.

Although the effect of poor maternal nutrition on the developing embryo may be due to a number of vitamin deficiencies acting together to interfere with the closure of the neural tube, it seemed to be more likely, on experimental,

---

* This paper is based partly on a presentation given on the 1st International Meeting on Cleft lip and Palate, Birmingham July 1983.

embryological, epidemiological and clinical grounds, that the main cause, in the British Isles at least, might be a folate lack for the developing embryo [11]. NTD can be induced in the rat by exposing developing embryos to a variety of teratogens, amongst them anti-folic acid agents [12]. In the rat about the 9th day after fertilisation, the time when its neural tube is being formed and when the chorio-allantoic placenta begins to develop, the embryonic heart starts to perfuse it and the pace of development and energy requirement increases significantly [13]. There are also considerable changes in the metabolic processes and the embryo's folate requirements increase steeply [14, 15]. It might therefore be supposed that should insufficient folate be present in the substrate of the developing embryo, the neural crests may fail to meet properly, or having met may dehisce again leading to NTD. Clinically, any deficiency must act before the 28th day following fertilisation, as this is the stage by which the neural tube completes closure in man.

It has been found that both serum and red cell folate levels are lower in women who are taking an unsatisfactory diet and also that women from social class III, IV and V both non-pregnant and during the first trimester of pregnancy, tend to have low levels of both serum and red cell folate. Such levels seem to be particularly low in the first trimester of those pregnancies which end in NTD [16, 17]. Finally, there is the small human experience with Aminopterin, at one time used as an abortifacient precipitating NTD, leading to malformation including NTD [18]. To elucidate the possible role of poor maternal diet and of folic acid lack in the genesis of NTD, a prospective preconception dietary counselling and folic acid supplementation study was undertaken in women at increased risk for NTD in South Wales.

NTD dietary and folic acid supplementation studies

Patients and methods

902 women resident in South Wales, who had previously had a pregnancy with an NTD, were visited in their homes by two experienced medically qualified field workers between 1969 and 1974. 415 who were not already pregnant, not on folate therapy and who had not decided against having further children, were enrolled into the dietary study. They were interrogated about their usual diet at the time of the field worker's visit (the inter-pregnancy diet) and enquiries were made about the diet during the first trimester of their previous pregnancies, both those that ended in an NTD (index pregnancies) and those which had a normal outcome (other pregnancies).

A simple diet sheet was used that provided a general pattern for meals, together with a checklist which included protein rich foods, diary products, vegetables and fruits, brown and white bread, confectionery and soft drinks. It was designed to reveal especially any deficiency in the consumption of foods containing folic acid. Diets were classified as good, fair or poor. Good diets were those comprising of a large variety of foods, particularly meats, eggs, milk, green vegetables and fruit with a relatively low consumption of confectionery and soft drinks. Such diets would be expected to provide generous intakes of all the nutrients including folic acid and dietary fibre. Poor diets were monotonous, restricted in variety with very low intakes of animal foods (including milk) and fruits and vegetables and an over-dependence on convenience foods and high in refined carbohydrates and fat. The poor diets were also associated with irregular meal patterns and a high consumption of confectionery. Fair diets were intermediate between these extremes. Classification was carried out after the study was completed by an independent research worker who was unaware of the outcome of the preg-nancies. Blood samples for serum and red cell folic acid and B_{12} estimation were taken after the interview.

The women in the western half of the project area were counselled to improve their diets and to stop smoking not later than the time that contraceptive precautions were stopped. Those in the eastern area were not specifically coun-selled. Previous epidemiological studies had shown there to be no demographic or social differences between the 2 areas, nor did there seem to be any differences in the dietary habits of the women [2, 3, 19].

These women were also invited to participate in a double blind randomised controlled trial of folate treatment without promise of reduction in the risk recurrence. Those who agreed were randomised to either taking 4 mg of folic acid per day from the time that contraceptive measures were dispensed with, or to taking placebo, and were instructed to continue until the end of the first trimester of the pregnancy. Neither the patient nor research staff knew to which the former had been assigned until the end of the trial.

All the women were requested to notify pregnancy to the field workers as soon as possible, but in any case not later than 9 weeks after the last menstrual period, when they were revisited as quickly as possible to make enquiries about the quality of the diet in the pregnancy so far, any illness, nausea, vomiting and medicines used. A further blood sample was taken for folate and B_{12} estimation. They were revisited in mid-trimester and immediately after the end of the pregnancy.

As pregnant women are known to not necessarily take the medicines prescribed for them, we planned to use the serum folate concentration as a screening test for compliance for those assigned to taking folate, reasoning that any woman with a serum folate of less than 10 mg/l was not receiving folic acid supplementation. However, a judgement as to compliance was not made until after the conclusion of the trial when the biochemical results were to be analysed.

Results of the dietary study

There was a significant relationship between the quality of the diet as judged for this study and the mean levels of both serum and red cell folate but not of B_{12} (tab. 1). Of the 174 women who joined the prospective study and achieved pregnancy, 25% were on a poor diet and only 14% on a good diet in the inter-pregnancy period. However, over 50% of these women reported a poor diet in the first trimester of their pregnancy that ended in a NTD, though rather less (30%) seemed to be on a poor diet in their previous pregnancies that had a normal outcome (tab. 2).

Table 1   NTD dietary study: Women with a previous fetal neural tube defect. Quality of inter-pregnancy diet and mean concentration of serum folate red blood cell folate and serum D_{12}

| Quality of diet | Subjects | | Mean serum folate | RBC folate | Serum B_{12} μg/l |
	n	%	μ/l	μg/l of red cells	
Good	65	16	8.9	295	283
Fair	197	47	5.4	236	272
Poor	149	36	4.9	197	285*
Not know	4	1	—	—	—
All women	415	100	5.9	238	277

* Two sera with concentrations of B_{12} over 1000 μg/l excluded as subjects were likely to have been on B_{12} treatment.

Table 2   NTD dietary study: Quality of previous diet

| | n | Quality if diet (percentage of cases) | | |
		Good	Fair	Poor
Inter pregnancy	174	14	61	25
Index pregnancy	174	10	37	53
Other pregnancy	123	19	51	30

The 174 women reported 186 pregnancies during the period of the study (1969 – 1974), 12 of them reporting two. There were 103 women reporting 109 pregnancies who received dietary counselling prior to their pregnancy and 71 women with 77 pregnancies who did not. Seventy-one percent of the counselled women significantly improved the quality of the diet in time for the pregnancy, whereas in the uncounselled the diet remained essentially unchanged (tabs. 3 and 4). There were 3 recurrences amongst the 109 pregnancies of the counselled women (approximately half the expected number) and 5 (the expected number) amongst

Table 3   NTD dietary study: Effect of counselling for project pregnancies

	n	Quality of diet (percentage of cases)		
		Good	Fair	Poor
Counselled	109	37	45	18
Uncounselled	77	17	51	32

Table 4   NTD diety study: Change of diet in project pregnancy compared with index pregnancy

	n	Quality of diet percentage of cases		
		improved	no change	deteriorated
Counselled	109	71	27	2
Uncounselled	77	12	82	6

Table 5   NTD dietary study: Outcome of project pregnancies (number of pregnancies)

	Quality of diet								
	Counselled				Uncounselled				
	Good	Fair	Poor	Total	Good	Fair	Poor	Total	Totals
Normal outcome	40	46	10	96	13	39	12	64	160
Recurrences	–	–	3	3	–	–	5	5	8
Miscarriages	–	3	7	10	–	–	8	8	18
Totals	40	49	20	109	13	39	25	77	186

the 77 pregnancies in the women who received no counselling, a difference which, though of interest, is not statistically significant. What is, however, highly significant ($p < 0.001$) is that all the recurrences occurred in the 45 pregnancies where the women remained on a poor diet; the 141 pregnancies where the women were on a fair or good diet had none (tab. 5).

Results of folate supplementation trial

Of the 123 pregnancies reported to us that met with the criteria for inclusion in the folic acid supplementation study, 60 were in the folate group and 63 were randomised to placebo (fig. 1). There was no test for compliance in taking placebo tablets but of the 60 women randomised to folate, 15 were, by the criteria, regarded as being non-compliers. We were however surprised to find one woman

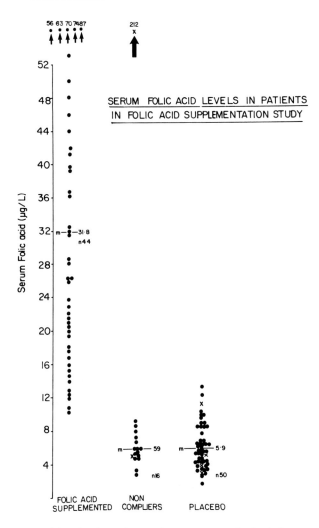

Fig. 1   Serum folate levels in the supplementation study divided into groups according to whether the patients were on folic acid supplementation or placebo, or whether they were non compliers. All but one of those regarded to have been non-compliers had serum folate levels below 10 mg/l. (x denotes patients with a recurrence.)

in the folate tablet group with a serum folate level of 212 mg/l and a rather low red cell folate (tab. 6). It was thought that this might possibly have been a laboratory error and she was retained as a folate complier. She had a miscarriage of an anencephalic fetus at 12 weeks of pregnancy. In 1980 at the time of the publicity following the publication of another vitamin supplementation trial [20], she volunteered that she had not taken the tablets during early pregnancy but when she realised that the field worker would take a sample of blood on revisiting

Table 6   NTD folic acid supplementation trial: Recurrence of neural tube defects

| Case | Treatment | Diet | Wk. | Blood estimations | | | | Outcome | | |
				Serum folate	Red cell folate	B_{12}	Delivery	Lesion	Gestation Mths.
A	F.NC	Poor	7	212.0	259	112	MC	AN	3
B	F.NC	Poor	8	4.8	155	167	LB	SB	9
C	PL	Poor	6	3.7	226	89	LD	SB	8
D	PL	Poor	7	11.0	275	210	MC	AN	4
E	PL	Poor	8	5.0	380	217	LD	SB	9
F	PL	Poor	7	2.9	76	371	T	AN	5

Estimations in µg/l; F.NC = Folate non complier; PL = Placebo; LB = Live birth; MC = Miscarriage; AN = Anencephalic; SB = Spina bifida cystica.

at 7 weeks gestation, she took a large number on the evening before the visit. She had not been supplemented during the teratogenic period and was therefore a non-complier.

There were 4 recurrences out of 63 pregnancies in the placebo group and 2 recurrences out of the 60 pregnancies in the folate prescribed group. This is a 50% reduction in the recurrence which is not significant with such small numbers. However, both the recurrences amongst the folate prescribed group were in non-compliers and so all 6 recurrences occurred in the 79 unsupplemented pregnancies and none in the 44 supplemented (tab. 7), which is significant by Fisher's exact test ($p = 0.04$). The data therefore suggests that there is a biological effect of taking folate which could be demonstrated even though in practice it was difficult to ensure that women took the tablets. The specific effect of taking folate has, however, to be separated from the more general effect of diet. There were no recurrences amongst the 91 pregnancies who received a good or fair diet, but there were 6 recurrences amongst the 32 pregnancies receiving a poor diet (tab. 8) ($p < 0.001$, Fisher's exact test). Within this high risk group of women, however, there were no recurrences in the 10 who had taken folate supplementation but 6 in the 22 who had a poor diet and had not been supplemented ($p = 0.004$, Fisher's exact test) [21].

Table 7   NTD folic acid supplementation trial: Outcome of pregnancy by treatment group

| | Folate supplementation | | Placebo | All cases |
	Compliers	Non-compliers		
Normal fetus	44	14	59	117
NTD	0	2	4	6
All outcomes	44	16	63	123

Table 8   NTD folic acid supplementation trial: Outcome of pregnancy by quality of diet and by folate supplementation

| | Outcome | | | | |
| Diet | Received folate | | Did not receive folate | | All cases |
	Normal	NTD	Normal	NTD	
Good	18	0	25	0	43
Fair	16	0	32	0	48
Poor	10	0	16	6	32
All cases	44	0	73	6	123

Discussion

The NTD Dietary and Supplementation study has demonstrated that even then a considerable number of women of reproductive age are asked to help in the evaluation of a treatment, it is difficult to collect sizeable numbers of prospectively studied pregnancies with reasonable compliance with the study protocol especially when no promise of beneficial effect are made. This is even so when the women concerned are kept under constant review by caring experienced field workers. To obtain adequate numbers for a statistically significant effect, an enormous number of women at increased risk for having a child with malformation will need to be ascertained, the more so when that effect may not be a complete prevention of recurrence. Such studies will therefore need to involve several centres if they are to be completed within a reasonable time span.

As a trial of methodology of a double blind randomised placebo controlled trial of folic acid supplementation for the prevention of NTD recurrences, the South Wales study must be regarded as having been a failure, with its non-significant results because of the high rate of non-compliance. However by combining the non-compliers with those assigned to placebo, all patients who had not been supplemented with folic acid, it seemed to be a successful test of the biological effect of taking a pharmacological daily dose of folic acid (about 10 times the usually recommended dose).

The supplementation study suggests that folic acid unavailability for the embryo during the first few weeks of development is an important factor in the aetiology of NTD in South Wales, and probably in the British Isles in general and possibly elsewhere in the world as well. However, it does not exclude the possibility that other deficiencies or some abnormality of folic acid metabolism, which can be swamped by a pharmacological dose of folic acid, may not also play a part. In addition NTD also has other aetiologies and aetiological triggers, most of which have not yet been identified.

Table 9   Outcome of pregnancies supplemented with Pregnavite Forte F[®]

	Supplemented	Unsupplemented
Number of pregnancies*	459	529
Infants with NTD	3	24
Miscarriages not examined	30	19
Normal outcome	429	510
Recurrences	0.7%	4.7%

* Including 15 twin pairs (5 suppl., 10 unsuppl.),
  (After Smithells et al. [29]).

Folic acid lack for the fetus does not necessarily imply a lack of foods containing the folic acid in the diet [11, 21]. Much of the folic acid in food may be destroyed in storage, in processing (canning) or in the preparation of meals. Lack of dietary zinc may interfere with folic acid absorption from the gut [22] and on the analogy with absorption of zinc, folic acid absorption could be inhibited by excessive amounts of refined carbohydrates and fats in the diet [23, 24]. Folic acid metabolism does appear to be deranged in some women on oral contraceptives [25] and a greater proportion of women who have just had a child with an NTD show evidence of folic acid metabolism abnormality, than do women with a normal outcome [26]. The study also suggests that in the apparently highly successful supplementation trial of Smithells and his colleagues [20, 27, 28] who used Pregnavite Forte[®]*, it is likely that it was the folic acid which was the major, if not the only active ingredient [11, 21].

Contrary to what has been suggested [29, 30] the evidence is not yet sufficiently strong for widespread introduction of preconceptional supplementation with folic acid, or for that matter, Pregnavite Forte F, with promise of success for women at increased risk for NTD, let alone on a population basis. The South Wales study was not only of small numbers but has been criticised because of the way that the non-compliers of folic acid treatment have been combined with those on placebo [31]. The compliers and the non-compliers undoubtedly differ from each other and this may well have introduced some bias. The Smithells supplementation study [20, 27, 28] which suggested that Pregnavite Forte F is highly effective in reducing the recurrence risk is also open to serious criticism [32 − 34], not because of inadequate numbers (tab. 9) but because of their choice of controls who consisted of those women who where already pregnant when ascertained or who for one reason or another were not supplemented or did not want

---

* Daily intake in 3 tablets per day: vit. A 4000 iu, vit. D$_2$ 400 iu, vit. B$_1$ 1.5 mg, vit B$_6$ 1 mg, nicotinamide 15 mg, vit C 40 mg, dried ferrous sulphate 252 mg, calcium phosphate 480 mg, folic acid 0.36 mg.

supplementation. Supplemented women certainly differed from the unsupplemented by having more social class I, II and non-manual III and in that more
did not have a miscarriage in their preceding pregnancy, both factors known to
be associated with a lower risk for NTD [31, 35, 36]. Because of these differences
and probably other more suitable ones the "self-selected" controls are far from
ideal [34]. The British Medical Research Council's multicentre placebo-controlled
trial to test out 4 mg per day of folic acid alone and a vitamin preparation akin
to Pregnavite Forte, with and without 4 mg of folic acid, against a placebo, on
up to 2,000 adequately prospectively studied pregnancies is therefore to be
welcomed despite the objections and criticisms on ethical and other grounds,
that this trial has attracted [37, 38]. However provided that potential volunteers
are given a full and honest explanation and there is no direct or indirect pressure
for them to participate there can be no real ethical objection to the trial.

If the MRC trial confirms the promising results of the 2 trials so far carried out
then supplementation for planned high-risk pregnancies should become part of
normal "care". If it also shows that suplementation with a pharmacological dose
of folic acid on its own is as effective as with a relatively expensive multivitamin
preparation which contains a relatively small dose of folic acid and some items
of uncertain value, then it may be possible to offer it more widely. It might be
possible not only to prevent the relatively few cases that recur in women with
an obstetric or a family history but to supplement all planned pregnancies
whether at increased risk or not and thereby make a real impact on the incidence
of NTD in the British Isles and perhaps elsewhere as well. Folic acid on its own
seems to be safe in childbearing women, to be without unpleasant side effects
(even in pharmacological amounts) and is sufficiently cheap to be considered
as an addition to staple items of the diet and thereby perhaps prevent NTD
in the many unplanned pregnancies which tend in any case to be the ones
more at risk [39].

As a good diet seems to be an important factor in the reduction of neural tube
defect, dietary education needs to be given early to our potential mothers and
should be part of the schools' curriculum. Good genetic counselling for high risk
women should include dietary counselling which must be given before pregnancy
is begun with the aim of making sure that she is on a good diet. She should also
be offered preconceptional supplementation with 4 – 5 mgm of folic acid per day.
This has to be given at least from the first day of the monthly cycle during which
the pregnancy is to be started and preferably longer if it is to have any chance
of being effective and it should be continued until the end of the first trimester.
In the last two years 47 women who were supplemented with folic acid alone
have had normal outcomes, 2 have had miscarriages and there have been no
outcomes with a neural tube defect. In a further 8, the pregnancy is still continuing
but prenatal diagnostic tests have not demonstrated an NTD. Unfortunately,

many women at risk for neural tube defect attend for advice (and generally for prenatal diagnosis) only after the pregnancy has been started, thus severely limiting their options [40].

References

[1] Carter, C. O.: Multifactorial inheritance revisited. In: Congenital Malformations (F. R. Fraser, V. A. McKusick, eds.), pp. 227–237. Exerpta Medica, Amsterdam 1969.

[2] Laurence, K. M., C. O. Carter, P. A. David: The central nervous system malformations in South Wales: I incidence, local variations and geographical factors. Brit. J. Prev. Soc. Med. **22** (1968a) 146–160.

[3] Laurence, K. M., C. O. Carter, P. A. David: The major central nervous system malformations in South Wales: II pregnancy factors, seasonal variations and social class effects. Brit. J. Prev. Soc. Med. **22** (1968b) 212–222.

[4] Nevin, N. C.: Recurrence risk of neural tube defects. Lancet I (1980) 1301–1302.

[5] Record, R. G., T. McKeown: Congenital malformations of the central nervous system I; a survey of 930 cases. Br. J. Prev. Soc. Med. **3** (1949) 183–219.

[6] MacMahon, B., S. Yen: Unrecognised epidemic of anencephaly and spina bifida. Lancet II (1971) 260–261.

[7] Wynn, M., A. Wynn: In: Prevention of Handicap and the Health of Women, pp. 26–42. Routledge Kegan Paul, London 1979.

[8] Bradshaw, J., J. Weale, J. Weatherall: Congenital Malformation of the Central Nervous System. Population Trends **19** (1980) 13–18.

[9] Laurence, K. M.: Spina Bifida and anencephaly in South Wales. In: Genetic and Population Studies in Wales (P. S. Harper, E. Sunderland, eds.). Universitiy of Wales Press, Cardiff 1984 (in press).

[10] Nevin, N. C.: Neural Tube Defects. Lancet II (1981) 1290–1291.

[11] Laurence, K. M., H. Campbell, N. James: The role of improvement in the maternal diet and preconceptional folic acid supplementation in the prevention of neural tube defects. In: Prevention of spina bifida and other neural defects (J. Dobbing, ed.), pp. 85–125. Academic Press, London 1983.

[12] Elwood, J. M., J. H. Elwood: Epidemiology of Anencephaly and Spina Bifida, p. 23. Oxford University Press, Oxford University Press, 1980.

[13] Beck, F.: Personal Communication, 1983.

[14] Sheppard, T. H., T. Tanimura, M. A. Robkin: Energy metabolism in early mammalian embryos. Dev. Bio. Suppl. **4** (1970) 42–58.

[15] Tanimura, T., T. H. Sheppard: Glucose metabolism by rat embryos in vitro. Proc. Soc. Ex Biol. Med. **135** (1970) 51–54.

[16] Smithells, R. W., C. Ankers, M. E. Carver et al.: Maternal nutrition in early pregnancy. Br. J. Nutr. **38** (1977) 497–506.

[17] Smithells, R. W., S. Sheppard, C. J. Schorah: Nutritional deficiencies and neural tube defects. Arch. Dis. Childh. **51** (1976) 944–950.

[18] Thiersch, K. B.: Therapeutic abortions with folic acid antagonist, 4-amino pteroyglutamic acid (4-amino PGA) administered by oral route. Am J. Obstet. Gynecol. **63** (1952) 1298–1304.

[19] Richards, I. D. G., C. R. Lowe: Incidence of congenital malformations in South Wales 1964–1966. Brit. J. Prev. Soc. Med. **25** (1971) 59–64.

[20] Smithells, R. W., S. Sheppard, C. J. Schorah et al.: Apparent prevention of neural tube defects by periconceptional vitamin supplementation. Lancet I (1980) 339–340.

[21] Laurence, K. M., N. James, M. Miller et al.: Double-blind randomised controlled trial of folate treatment before conception to prevent recurrences of neural tube defects. Brit. Med. J. **282** (1981) 1509 – 1511.

[22] Tanimura, T., B. Shane, M. T. Boer et al.: Absorption of mono- and polyglutamyl folates in zinc depleted man. Am. J. Clin. Nutr. **31** (1978) 194 – 1987.

[23] Brenner, I., C. F. Mills: Absorption, transport and tissue storage of essential trace elements. Phil. Trans. Roy. Soc. London B **294** (1981) 75.

[24] Elmes, M. E.: Zinc absorption and metabolism. In: Paediatric Nutrition (J. A. Hodge, ed.), pp. 170 – 179. Pitmans Medical Publications, Thunbridge Wells 1983.

[25] Shojonia, A. M., E. J. Hornaby: Oral contraceptives and folate absorption. J. Clin. Lab. Med. **82** (1973) 869 – 875.

[26] Hibbard, E. D., R. W. Smithells: Folic acid metabolism and human embryopathy. Lancet **I** (1965) 1254.

[27] Smithells, R. W., S. Sheppard, C. J. Schorah et al.: Apparent prevention of neural tube defects by periconceptional vitamin supplementation. Arch. Dis. Child **56** (1981) 911 – 918.

[28] Laurence, K. M., N. James, M. Miller et al.: Increased risk of recurrence of neural tube defects to mothers on poor diets and the possible benefits of dietary counselling. Brit. Med. J. **281** (1980) 1544.

[29] Smithells, R. W., N. C. Nevin, M. J. Sellar et al.: Further experience with vitamin supplementation for prevention of neural tube defect recurrences. Lancet **I** (1983) 1027 – 1031.

[30] Edwards, J. H.: Vitamins to Prevent neural tube defects. Lancet **I** (1982) 1458 – 1459.

[31] Lorber, J.: Vitamins to Prevent neural tube defects. Lancet **II** (1982) 1458 – 1459.

[32] Stone, D. H.: Possible prevention of neural tube defects by preconceptional vitamin supplementation. Lancet **I** (1980) 647 – 648.

[33] Wald, N.: Possible prevention of neural tube defects by vitamin supplementation. In: Prevention of spina bifida and other neutral tube defects (J. Dobbing, ed.), pp. 231 – 239.

[34] Wald, N. J., P. E. Polani: Neural tube defects and vitamins: the need for a randomised clinical trial. Brit. J. Obst. Gynae. **91** (1984) 516 – 523.

[35] Cuckle, H. S.: Recurrence risk of neural tube defects following a miscarriage. Prenatal Diagn. **3** (1983) 287 – 289.

[36] Edwards, J. H.: Congenital malformations of the central nervous system in Scotland. Br. J. Prev. Soc. Med. **12** (1958) 115 – 130.

[37] Nature. Spina Bifida: controversy continues (comments). Nature **300** (1982) 396 – 397.

[38] Lancet: Vitamins to prevent neural tube defects (Leading Article) Lancet **II** (1982) 1255 – 1256.

[39] Laurence, K. M.: Neural tube defects: a two-prolonged approach to primary prevention. Paediatrics **70** (1982) 648 – 651.

[40] Carter, J., K. M. Laurence: Genetic Counselling for neural tube defect in high risk couples during pregnancy: is this the optimum time to attend? Biology and Society (in press).

Periconceptional vitamin prophylaxe — ethical and other problems

J. Lorber

Introduction

Neural tube defects (NTD) (spina bifida, encephalocele and anencephaly) were the commonest congenital malformation until recently. The prognosis for the overwhelming majority of the babies was devastating in spite great advances in the treatment of spina bifida. Those women who already had at least one baby with neural tube defect were at substantially greater risk of having recurrences than women in the general population. It is, therefore, clear that attempts should be made to prevent these conditions. This can only be undertaken if the cause, or causes, of NTDs is at least partly known.

It is generally considered that the causes of NTDs are multifactorial. These include genetic background plus adverse environmental circumstances, such as poverty and poor nutrition [1]. There may be other factors which are at present unknown. There are as yet no known means to manipulate the genetic background but it is possible to improve the environment which could lead to a reduction in NTDs.

There is some evidence that a poor and unbalanced diet may contribute to the risk of having NTD babies [1]. The evidence is partly epidemiological in as much as NTDs are commoner in the women in lower socio-economic classes who are more often on an inadequate or unbalanced diet. NTD births are also commoner when whole communities live under very unfavourable circumstances such as during wars or economic depressions. Further, there is some evidence that women who had a baby with neural tube defect sometimes have minor vitamin deficiencies which could be shown, in at least some, by the demonstration of low serum or red cell levels of either folic acid, vitamin B complex or vitamin A [8]. It is not known, however, whether such minor deficiencies are constant or are merely random observations.

Against the dietary theory are the observations that a large majority of the babies in the world are born to grossly underprivileged and underfed mothers, yet the overwhelming majority of their babies do not have NTD. Further, none of the women in Western societies who had a baby with NTD suffered from clinically evident vitamin deficiency and many with low serum vitamin levels produced normal babies and vice versa. There are also plenty of women in social classes 1 and 2 on a splendid, well-balanced diet who have babies with NTD.

Another major difficulty in accepting that diet plays a major role is the observations on twins. Even like-sexed twins are rarely concordant for NTD [5]. It is difficult to understand how and why vitamins would protect only one of two twins. The observation on twins is also a major defect in understanding the genetic background of these conditions.

Previous trials on vitamin supplementation

Nevertheless the theory of vitamin deficiency led to 2 clinical trials to test this hypothesis on women who had a high risk of recurrence because they already had at least one child with NTD. The risk of recurrence for this group was approximately 5% [9, 10].

These trials produced partial evidence that supplementary vitamins are of value, but because of faults in the protocols of the trials or other reasons, their conclusions are not scientifically acceptable. Consequently, further trials appeared to be necessary and justified. The problem is to find a protocol which is ethically acceptable to a sufficient number of women and doctors, so that a conclusive result would be achieved in a reasonable time.

The trial by Smithells and his team [9] was not randomised because the ethical committees to whom the plan was submitted did not agree that high risk women should be deprived of periconceptional vitamin supplementation because it appeared promising and harmless, although at that time it was not known whether vitamins could be of benefit. Further, it was not normal practice to give extra vitamins to pre-pregnant women.

Consequently, high risk women who came for advice at least 28 days before planning a pregnancy and who agreed to take part in the trial were given Pregnavite Forte F®. It is known that these women did not conceive for at least 28 days after starting to take Pregnavite Forte F®. This was the "fully supplemented" group.

There was another group of women who also attended for the same reason who were prescribed Pregnavite Forte F®, but they were either already pregnant and did not know it, or they conceived within 28 days of starting to take the tablets. This was a "partially supplemented" group.

The third and last group were women who were not supplemented, either because they were unwilling to take the tablets or they were already known to be pregnant at their first visit to the clinic.

The recurrence rate of NTDs was:

- 0.7% (3 out of 454) in the fully supplemented group;
- none out of 114 in the partially supplemented group and
- 4.6% (24 out of 519) in the unsupplemented group, as would be expected.

These results indicated the apparently high protective value of Pregnavite Forte F® but, interestingly, the partially supplemented women, though fewer in number, did at least as well as the fully supplemented. This poses the question whether it is necessary to give vitamins prior to conception.

This trial has been criticised [11] on the grounds that as it was not properly randomised and that there was a disproportionately high ratio of women in social classes 1 and 2 in the fully supplemented group. The reverse applied to the unsupplemented group. It was suggested that women in social classes 1 and 2 may have a lower recurrence risk than women in social classes 3 to 5 and that this made the conclusions that vitamin supplementation is of benefit, open to doubt. Analysis of Smithells' data, in my opinion, successfully counters this argument because in socal classes 1 and 2 there was a 3.9% recurrence rate in the 102 unsupplemented and nil in the 143 who were fully supplemented. In contrast, in social classes 3 to 5 there were 4.8% recurrences in the 417 unsupplemented but only 1% in the 311 fully supplemented women. Consequently, the recurrence rate was only a little lower in women in social classes 1 and 2 compared to those in social classes 3 to 5. The risk without supplementation remained high in all classes. These results suggested a major advance in the true prevention of neural tube defects.

Laurence et al. [2] conducted a randomised, controlled trial on high risk women. One group were treated with folic acid alone in approximately 10 times the dose as in Pregnavite Forte F®. The second group were untreated controls. Unfortunately, too few women were enrolled and many did not adhere to the protocol, so, although the findings were encouraging, no proof emerged that folic acid would reduce the risk of recurrences.

The possibility and aims of further trials

The trials which had been completed did not command universal acceptance that periconceptional vitamin supplementation is of value. Nor did the trials produce evidence of which vitamin or vitamin combinations are essential. It is possible that folic acid is the essential vitamin.

Further trials could elucidate many of the outstanding problems. As things are, it would not be feasible to recommend that all women of childbearing age should take periconceptional vitamins. Nor would it be possible to organise such a public health measure. Yet, restricting periconceptional vitamin supplementation only to high-risk women would only result in a minimal reduction of the total NTDs in the community because only some 5% of NTD babies are born to high-risk mothers, not all of whom could be reached for vitamin supplementation.

Concurrently with the progress of the trials already completed and also after their conclusion there has been a substantial reduction in the incidence of NTDs independant of antenatal diagnosis and therapeutic terminations of pregnancy [4]. These heartening epidemiological facts had to be considered prior to planning a new trial on high-risk women because the number of women potentially eligible to take part is rapidly decreasing. This may make the recruitment of women to the trial very difficult and it would be impossible to recruit enough women to reach statistically valid conclusions within a reasonable time.

The results achieved in Smithells' trials make the planning of new trial(s) even more difficult from the ethical point of view. If it was considered by some ethical committees that it was unethical to deprive women of vitamin supplementation at a time when their potential value was unknown. Would many ethical committees approve a new trial which included untreated controls when the results of supplementations were apparently so successful?

This was the background before the Medical Research Council Committee which was set up to investigate these problems.

The trend of decrease in NTD prevalence must have been already obvious when new trials were being planned and maybe for this reason the MRC needed and succeeded in obtaining co-operation of workers in a few countries abroad, such as Australia, Israel and Hungary. The ethical considerations mentioned certainly also applied to Australia but not to Hungary. In Hungary Pregnavite Forte F® or folic acid are not available to high-risk pregnant women. Consequently, taking part in this trial would ensure that at least some Hungarian women could benefit if the vitamins were of protective value. Nevertheless, the enrollment of women abroad is still unlikely to boost the numbers sufficiently for a statistical conclusion.

The MRC trial

The problem of numbers and time

In spite of the difficulties, a Committee of the Medical Research Council decided to carry out new trials. The Committee consists of top class, highly respected experts from the relevant fields of medicine. After prolonged considerations extending over 2 years, it was decided to start the trial in December 1982. There were to be 4 groups to which women would be randomly allocated. Neither the women nor their doctors would know what preparation was prescribed. The women, however, were given a printed sheet of information to answer their potential questions and to ensure that they are fully informed before giving their agreement for inclusion. This information for patients could be considered biased in favour of joining the trial and some of the statements in it are, at least, contentious [6].

The MRC planned to recruit 2000 women, approximately 500 per group, and the trial was to run for 5 years. The practical problems of recruiting such numbers and of completing the trial in time were likely to be very difficult, if not impossible, because many major units and doctors and many mothers would not agree to take part in the trial. The numbers potentially available would be further and progressively reduced because of the rapidly declining rate of prevalence of neural tube defects. In any case, it is probable that much larger numbers than 2000 would be needed to reach statistically valid conclusions [3]. The MRC trial, therefore, could be considered unethical on the grounds that it was unlikely to be completed in a reasonable time and unlikely to lead to definite conclusions. As it is by June 1984 only 132 patients were recruited, only 18 became pregnant and only a single baby was born [7].

The use of untreated controls

It is difficult to accept that it is ethical to include untreated controls after the conclusion of Smithells' trials. The benefit of the doubt must be given to parents at high risk. Vitamins could be considered at least for this group, even if their value is not considered to be totally proven and even if it is not known which of the vitamins, if any, in Pregnavite Forte F® is effective or essential. They are all harmless.

In the MRC trial [11] 25% of women receive only minerals, as a placebo, and so remain unprotected. It is this 25% which caused much public concern but, in truth, more than 25% are unprotected and the participants are being misled by this figure. This is because it is considered, at least by some, that the essential protective vitamin is folic acid. For this reason, 25% of the women in the trial receive folic acid alone. Consequently, if this theory is incorrect, then those receiving folic acid alone will remain unprotected or only partially protected. If the folic acid theory is correct, then the third group of 25% who receive multivitamins without folic acid remain unprotected. This makes the total unprotected at least 50%. If a combination of vitamins, including folic acid and other vitamins, is necessary then more than 50% of the participants remain unprotected or incompletely protected and the proportion of unprotected could be as high as 75%.

All these calculations are based on the assumption that at least some of the vitamins are of value. If this is not the case then the whole argument falls to the ground. The MRC trial will not show whether this is the case or not, because they will have far fewer women in the Pregnavite Forte F® group than was available to Smithells and his colleagues. So whatever will be the outcome in this group, it is unlikely to contribute to the available information because the numbers will be so small.

What appears certain is that, if the vitamins are of value, then the only truly protected groups could be those receiving Pregnavite Forte F® or folic acid alone, or 50% of the participants.

It is also questionable whether all the women who were willing to enrol in the trial will keep to the protocol. As they do not know to which group they belong, and as most of them do know that Pregnavite Forte F® or vitamins in general could at least be beneficial, the chances are that they will buy the vitamins for themselves from the chemist or eat high vitamin-containing foods. They could also get a prescription for Pregnavite Forte F® or folic acid from their family doctor to benefit their potential offspring. There is no way in which the MRC can check what the women really do, nor can they check whether they take the prescribed tablets, even if they do occasional periodic blood levels. The results, therefore, will be unreliable even if the desired number were to take part.

In other words, the trial is also unethical because it is impossible to ensure that the women taking part will, in fact, adhere to the protocol.

In the context of the need for vitamins and a good diet, the MRC leaflet to mothers is self-contradictory, misleading and biased to benefit the trial rather than the participants. In this leaflet there is a hypothetical question "Will I need to change my diet if I enter the study?" The answer given is "No. There is no need for any special diet.". Yet, the hypothesis is that a poor, unbalanced diet contributes to the conception of NTDs. Consequently, the ethical answer to the question must be "Yes. You must take the best possible diet, including vitamins.". If, however, the women did that, the trial would collapse.

Conclusion

In conclusion, it is unlikely that the MRC trial will produce an answer to the questions on the value of periconceptional vitamin supplementation, above and beyond what is already known.

It is difficult to think of a better, properly controlled and ethical trial than the one the MRC have decided to use, but reasons have been put forward why their trial is unlikely to advance our knowledge and why it could be considered unethical in practice.

References

[1] Laurence, K. M., et al.: Increased risk of recurrence of neural tube defects to mothers on poor diets and the possible benefits of dietary counselling. Br. Med. J. **281** (1980) 1542 – 1544.

[2] Laurence, K. M., et al.: Double-blind randomised controlled trial of folate treatment before conception to prevent recurrence of neural tube defects. Br. Med. J. **282** (1981) 1509 – 1511.

[3] Lorber, J.: Vitamins to prevent neural tube defects. Lancet II (1982) 1458.

[4] Lorber, J.: Spina bifida — a vanishing nightmare? In: Spina bifida — neural tube defects (D. Voth, P. Glees, eds.), pp. 3. Walter de Gruyter, Berlin – New York 1986.

[5] Lorber, J., S. C. Rogers: Spina bifida cystica and anencephalus in twins. Zeitschrift für Kinderchirurgie **22** (1977) 565 – 571.

[6] Medical Research Council: Vitamin study information for patients. April (1983).

[7] Medical Research Council: Vitamin study report of meeting of 4th June 1984. Lancet I (1984) 1308.

[8] Smithells, R. W., et al.: Vitamin deficiencies and neural tube defects. Archives of Disease in Childhood **51** (1976) 944 – 950.

[9] Smithells, R. W., et al.: Apparent prevention of neural tube defects by periconceptional vitamin supplementation. Archives of Disease in Childhood **56** (1981) 911 – 918.

[10] Smithells, R. W., et al.: Further experience of vitamin supplementation for prevention of neural tube defect recurrences. Lancet I (1983) 1027 – 1031.

[11] Wald, N. J., P. E. Polani: Neural tube defects and vitamins: the need for a randomised clinical trial. Br. J. Obstet. Gynaecol. **91** (1984) 516 – 523.

Anencephalus and spina bifida in Germany, the risk of recurrence

M. Koch

Despite extensive research into the etiology of anencephalus and spina bifida (neural tube defects) the cause remains unknown, but genetic and environmental factors are thought to contribute to their manifestation [23].

Since the mode of inheritance and the role of exogenous factors are not understood practical counselling depends on empirical risk data. Recurrence risk data of neural tube defects (NTD) in sibs of affected individuals are needed for genetic counselling, for decision on prenatal diagnosis and for the planning of preventive measures.

Different data have been reported from various populations and the risk in sibs is always higher than the risk of newborns in the general population. In the high risk population of Great Britain with a prevalence at birth of 3 – 9‰ [1, 16, 17] the recurrence risk in sibs ranges between 3.2 – 9% [16, 17]. In lower risk populations like in Continental Europe and North America with a prevalence at birth of about 1 – 2‰ [14, 15, 25] the recurrence risk in sibs is about 2 – 3‰ [4, 13, 14].

The prevalence at birth for NTD in the population of the FRG is estimated to range between 1 – 1.5‰ nowadays [9]. The FRG belongs to the low prevalence areas and the risk in sibs of affected children should be in the range of the lower risk populations.

Risk data for the counselling of families with one affected NTD-child for the population in the FRG derived from a family study in the Bundesland of Hessen and surrounding areas.

In this study altogether 240 families were interrogated and by a structured interview informations of epidemiological interest were collected. Ten mothers with two affected NTD children were investigated. None of the mothers had a history of three or more affected pregnancies. Thus the risk among sibs with one affected NTD-child could be calculated to 2.6% [10].

The 240 mothers had 13 stillborn children (3.45%) without reporting of having NTD and they had 79 miscarriages (17.3%) thus 20.2% of all pregnancies ended with a fetal loss. Gynaecologists usually estimate the miscarriage risk about

Table 1   Prevalence rates for NTD in different populations

		after one affected child (%)	general population (‰)
Belfast	[16, 24]	4.2	6.52
South Wales	[1]	5.2	7.6
London	[2, 22]	3.2	2.95
France	[13]	1.9	1.02
FRG	[9, 10]	2.6	1.0 – 1.5
GDR	[11, 19, 27]	2.9, 5.04	1.46
Poland	[20, 21]	3.4	0.93
Switzerland	[15]	2.9	0.95
Canada	[14]	2.4	1.55
USA	[4, 25]	3.0	1.11

10 – 15% in the general population. The stillbirth rate is said to be 1% by official population statistics [26].

The presented data for the recurrence risk of NTD are in good agreement with the results of other studies of Continental Europe – including data of the GDR – and North America. A selection of those data in comparison to the British figures is presented in table 1.

In the meantime British investigators published data about recurrence rates after periconceptional vitamin supplementation [12]. Seller and Nevin [24] presented comparative data and found a 3.6 fold reduction after vitamin supplementation for Northern Ireland and a less than 2.0 fold reduction in South-east England. Thus, the effect is less in the lower than in the higher prevalence population. This fits in with the hypothesis that in low prevalence areas the environmental factors are of less importance than in high prevalence areas. Therefore it might not be reasonable to start a vitamin supplementation for prevention of neural tube defects in low prevalence populations like in Continental Europe.

For genetic counselling of neural tube defects in the FRG it can be assumed:

The prevalence in sibs of one affected child with isolated spina bifida, encephalocele or anencephalus is about 2.6%.

The prevalence in half sibs of one affected child is 3.1% in the cited study; the high figure might be due to the small number of ascertained cases. Thus it seems reasonable to use those figures of other low prevalence areas: 1 – 2% [2].

Data for the recurrence risk in sibs after two affected children could not be established by the study. According to other low prevalence populations a risk of 5% might be given in genetic counselling [14].

Risk figures for offsprings of affected parents are only available from smaller studies. According to the combined data of Carter and Tünte [3, 28] the suggested risk is about 3%.

Different risks have been assumed and calculated for special situations in families with several close relatives affected, for those rare cases with suggestive evidence of monogenic inheritance [8, 27] and for those in which NTD is a part of a special syndrome or a chromosome anomaly.

A special and difficult question for genetic counselling are those schisis-type abnormalities [6] or midline defects [18] where NTD is associated with other malformations and/or occurs with different cleft-anomalies in one family [7].

References

[1] Carter, C. O., P. A. David, K. M. Laurence: A family study of major central nervous system malformations in South Wales. J. Med. Genet. 5 (1968) 81 – 106.

[2] Carter, C. O., K. Evans: Spina bifida and anencephalus in Greater London. J. Med. Genet. 10 (1973) 209 – 234.

[3] Carter, C. O., K. Evans: Children of adult survivors with spina bifida cystica. Lancet II (1973) 924 – 926.

[4] Cowchock, S., E. Ainbender, G. Prescott, et al.: The recurrence risk for neural tube defects in the United States: A collaborative study. Am. J. Med. Genet. 5 (1980) 309 – 314.

[5] Creasy, M. R., E. D. Alberman: Congenital malformations of the central nervous system in spontaneous abortions. J. Med. Genet. 13 (1976) 9 – 16.

[6] Czeizel, A.: Schisis-association. Am. J. Med. Genet. 10 (1981) 25 – 35.

[7] Fraser, F. C., A. Czeizel, C. Hanson: Increased frequency of neural tube defects in sibs of children with other malformations. Lancet II (1982) 144 – 145.

[8] Fuhrmann, W., W. Seeger, R. Böhm: Apparently monogenic inheritance of anencephaly and spina bifida in a kindred. Hum. Genet. 13 (1971) 241 – 243.

[9] Koch, M., W. Fuhrmann: Epidemiology of neural tube defects in Germany. Hum. Genet. 68 (1984) 97 – 103.

[10] Koch, M., W. Fuhrmann: Sibs of probands with neural tube defects – a study in the FRG. Hum. Genet. (in press 1985).

[11] Körner, H., A. Horn: Pränatale Diagnostic als Massenscreening. Vortrag auf der 18. Tagung der Gesellschaft für Anthropologie und Humangenetik, Münster 1983.

[12] Laurence, K. M.: Primary prevention of neural tube defects by dietary improvement and folic acid supplementation. In: Spina bifida – neural tube defects (D. Voth, P. Glees, eds.), pp. 107. Walter de Gruyter, Berlin – New York 1986.

[13] Le Merrer, M., M. L. Briard, F. Demenais, et al.: Etude épidémiologique et génétique du spina bifida. Arch. Fr. Pediatr. 37 (1980) 521 – 525.

[14] McBridge, M. L.: Sib risk of anencephaly and spina bifida in British Columbia. Am. J. Med. Genet. 3 (1979) 377 – 387.

[15] Moser, H., H. P. Böss, C. H. Neuenschwander: Epidemiologie der offenen Neuralrohrmissbildungen in der Schweiz. Vortrag auf der 4. Tagung der Arbeitsgemeinschaft Klinische Genetik der Gesellschaft für Anthropologie und Humangenetik, 1984.

[16] Nevin, N. C.: Neural tube defects. Lancet II (1981) 1290 – 1291.

[17] Nevin, N. C., W. P. Johnston: A family study of spina bifida and anencephalus in Belfast, Northern Ireland (1964 to 1968). J. Med. Genet. **17** (1980) 203 – 211.

[18] Opitz, J. M., E. F. Gilbert: Editorial comment: CNS anomalies and the midline as a "developmental field". Am. J. Med. Genet. **12** (1982) 443 – 455.

[19] Pelz, L., J. M. Hille: Familiäres Vorkommen dorsaler Schlußstörungen des Neuralrohres. Kinderärztl. Praxis **45** (1977) 219 – 225.

[20] Pietrzyk, J. J., J. Grochwoski, B. Kanska: CNS malformations in the Krakow region I. Birth prevalence and seasonal incidence during 1979 – 1981. Am. J. Med. Genet. **14** (1983) 181 – 188.

[21] Pietrzyk, J. J.: Neural tube malformations: complex segregations analysis and recurrence risk. Am. J. Med. Genet. **7** (1980) 293 – 300.

[22] Seller, M. J.: Recurrence risks for neural tube defects in a genetic counselling clinic population. J. Med. Genet. **18** (1981) 245 – 248.

[23] Seller, M. J.: The cause of neural tube defects: some experiments and a hypothesis. J. Med. Genet. **20** (1983) 164 – 168.

[24] Seller, M. J., N. C. Nevin: Periconceptional vitamin supplementation and the prevention of neural tube defects in South-east England and Northern Ireland. J. Med. Genet. **21** (1984) 325 – 330.

[25] Sever, L. E., M. Sanders, R. Monsen: An epidemiologic study of neural tube defects in Los Angeles Country. I. Prevalence at birth based on multiple sources of case ascertainment. Teratology **25** (1982) 315 – 321.

[26] Statistisches Jahrbuch der Bundesrepublik Deutschland, Fachserie 1, Reihe 2, Bevölkerungsbewegung (1980 – 1982).

[27] Theile, H., G. J. Hermsdorf: Familienuntersuchungen bei Neuralrohrdefekten. Dt. Gesundh. Wesen **39** (1984) 1857 – 1861.

[28] Tünte, W.: Fortpflanzungsfähigkeit, Heiratshäufigkeit und Zahl und Beschaffenheit der Nachkommen bei Patienten mit Spina bifida aperta. Humangenetik **13** (1971) 43 – 48.

Relevance of biochemical parameters in the prenatal diagnosis of dysraphic malformations

G. Hoffmann, R. Wellstein, E. Merz, B. Manz, R. Kreienberg, K. Pollow

Children with dysraphic malformations are a great medical as well as social problem. Approximately half of these children die within first 24 hours post partum. Among the survivors, 75% suffer from severe physical handicaps and another 20% from retardation, which can be more or less severe [10].

The most relevant biochemical parameters in prenatal diagnostic of dysraphic malformations are α-1-fetoprotein and, more recently, acetylcholinesterase. Determination of 5-hydroxy-indole acetic acid and of ferritin are of minor importance, due to less reliability. Since 1972, when Brock and Sutcliffe [2] showed that elevated levels of α-1-fetoprotein in amniotic fluid are coincident with open neural tube defects of the fetus, this parameter gained increasing importance in prenatal diagnosis.

Alpha-fetoprotein (AFP)

AFP is a fetal glycoprotein with a molecular weight of about 70.000. It is synthesized in the fetal liver, in the yolk sac and, to a minor extent, in the gastrointestinal tract. It reaches the amniotic fluid via the fetal urine and passes across the amnion to the maternal blood (fig. 1). A significant decrease in concentrations between these three compartments (fetal serum: 10^6 IU/ml, amniotic fluid: $10^3 - 10^4$ IU/ml, maternal serum: 10^2 IU/ml) can be demonstrated [6, 17, 20]. The amniotic fluid AFP level is diminished by the fetus' swallowing and digesting some of the fluid. Therefore increasing levels of AFP can be found in cases of gastrointestinal atresias. In fetal blood, AFP is about 200 times more concentrated, compared to the amniotic fluid. Fetal bleeding necessarily leads to an elevation of AFP level in the amniotic fluid. In the fetal spinal fluid, high levels of AFP are detectable. The presence of open neural tube defects facilitates the passage of AFP from the fetal spinal fluid to the amniotic fluid, and in this case, an increase of AFP levels can be detected not only in the amniotic fluid itself, but also in the maternal blood. In cases of congenital nephrosis, an increased excretion of AFP is demonstrable as well as increased amniotic fluid AFP concentrations. Additionally, contact between the amniotic fluid com-

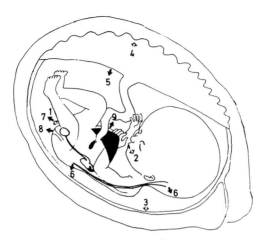

Fig. 1   AFP-synthesis and transfer to the amniotic fluid (Weitzel et al., 1979 [18]). AFP-synthesis in
the fetal liver and yolk sac. Ways of AFP-transfer to the amniotic fluid:

Physiological transfer	*Pathological transfer*
1. fetal urine	5. fetal bleeding
2. oral ingestion	6. neural tube defect
3. amniomaternal transfer	7. renal loss
4. transplacental transfer?	8. meconium
	9. omphalocele

partment and the content of a hernia, as seen for example in cases of ventral defects, leads to elevation of the AFP level.

AFP levels are measured by means of radioimmunoassay or enzyme-linked immunosorbent assay [19].

AFP in amniotic fluid

Physiologically, a marked increase of the AFP level in amniotic fluid is demonstrable in early pregnancy, with a maximum of approximately 20.000 ng/ml found in the 13th to 24th week of gestation (fig. 2). Between the 15th to 24th week of gestation, which is the most interesting time for prenatal diagnostic, AFP levels decrease significantly, so that the values determined can only be evaluated correctly with respect to exact knowledge of duration of pregnancy. No accurate discrimination exists between normal or pathologically elevated AFP levels. Therefore, it is absolutely important to estimate limiting values, with regard to the week of gestation, that neither false positive AFP levels during a normal pregnancy nor false negative AFP levels due to open neural tube defects can be found. Extensive studies have revealed a 2.5-fold of the median as a useful level. Values above have to be considered pathological [6, 17, 20]. The accuracy of

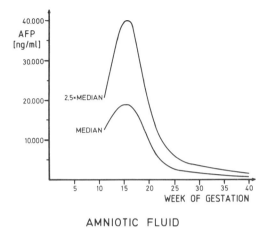

AMNIOTIC FLUID

Fig. 2   Amniotic fluid AFP-level during gestation.

elevated amniotic fluid AFP levels for detection of open neural tube defects is about 90 – 98% [9, 13]. While evaluating AFP levels, one has to consider also the a priori risk. If amniocentesis has been because of a known increased risk, there is more of a probability that the fetus has a neural tube defect, compared to a pregnancy with an unobtrusive case history, where a similar AFP level has been found.

Elevated AFP levels (tab. 1) can be found in various other malformations, intrauterine fetal death, tendency to abortion, "fetal distress"-syndrome, rhesus incompatibility, but also in multiple pregnancy. False positive values can also be obtained in case of inaccurate determination of the gestation week and in case of blood-contaminated amniotic fluid [5, 20]. Therefore, it has to be emphasized that in case of elevated amniotic fluid AFP level, further investigations (e.q. ultrasound) have to be performed to exclude reasons other than fetal malformations.

Table 1   Differential diagnosis of elevated amniotic fluid AFP-levels

Anencephalus	Intrauterine fetal death
Spina bifida	Tendency to abortion
Meckel's syndrome	"fetal distress" syndrome
Coccygeal teratoma	Rhesus incompatibility
Atresia of esophagus or duodenum	Multiple pregnancy
Omphalocele	
Congenital nephrosis	Wrong estimation of the week of gestation
Trisomy	
Turner's syndrome	Contamination by fetal bleeding

AFP in maternal serum

From the 7th week of gestation, a marked increase in AFP levels can be seen in the maternal serum, with a maximum of approximately 250 ng/ml at the 32nd – 34th week (fig. 3). A maximum of 2,5-fold the median is a useful criterium of elevated AFP levels in the maternal serum, too [17]. The determination of AFP in maternal serum is about 80% accurate for open neural tube defects [11]. There is a relationship between AFP levels determined in serum and in amniotic fluid, but no strict correlation. Sometimes, the parallel determination of AFP in both of these is of additional diagnostic importance. If the maternal blood level is elevated, a slightly increased amniotic fluid AFP level has to be considered as being more serious. On the other hand, a slightly elevated amniotic fluid level is explainable by the presence of fetal blood, if the maternal blood shows normal range levels [17].

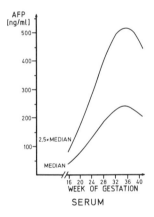

Fig. 3   Maternal serum AFP-level during gestation.

If serum AFP levels are found to be elevated, consideration should also be given to maternal diseases such as hepatoma, hepatocellular carcinoma or carcinoma of the ovaries. In order to prevent misinterpretations, it should be stressed again that exact knowledge of gestation duration is prerequisite for the evaluation of amniotic fluid or serum AFP levels.

Figure 4 shows our normal range values for AFP in amniotic fluid and in maternal serum as well as all pathological levels, found in 1.213 pregnancies screened throughout 1983 and 1984. The coincidence of elevated levels in serum and in amniotic fluid is obvious. One case studied was a trisomy 18. Unfortunately, from the patient no amniotic fluid sample was available.

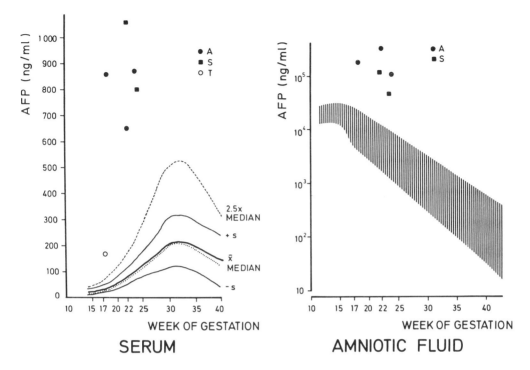

Fig. 4   Determination of AFP in maternal serum and amniotic fluid: Normal range and pathological values found in our own investigations (n = 1.213). A = anencephaly; S = spina bifida aperta; T = trisomy 18.

Acetylcholinesterase (AChE)

The most useful and predictive parameter besides AFP is the determination of acetylcholinesterase in the amniotic fluid [14]. Quantification can be performed by a photometric assay combined with inhibition of AChE-activity [4, 15]. However, the slightest blood contamination of the sample can induce false positive results. Therefore, the method of choice is presently a qualitative analysis using agar gel electrophoresis [15, 16]. An essential advantage of this method is, that the evaluation of this assay is independent of exact knowledge of the week of gestation.

The results of gel electrophoresis of two normal and eight pathological amniotic fluid samples are shown on figure 5. Besides a cholinesterase, appearing in all amniotic fluid samples, in those cases with an open neural tube defect, a second enzyme (acetylcholinesterase) is demonstrable. This AChE is characterized by a different electrophoretic mobility. Measuring this activity, it has to be selectively

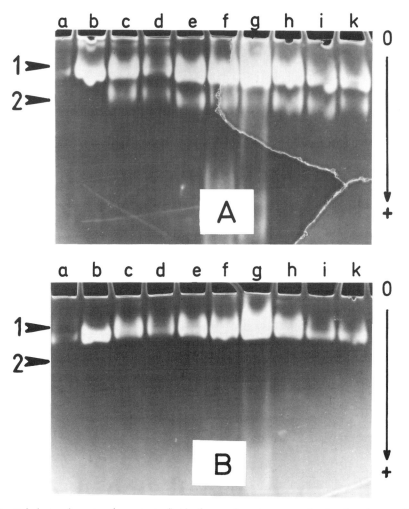

Fig. 5   Gel-electrophoresis of amniotic fluids from selected pregnancies in the absence (A) and
presence (B) of the specific AChE inhibitor (BW 284 C 51).
1 → slow migrating first band of cholinesterase
2 → additional fast moving second band of AChE
a, b: normal pregancy   i: anencephalus
c – h: open spina bifida   k: amniotic bands syndrome

inhibited by addition of a specific AChE inhibitor (BW 284 C 51) in a parallel
experimental setup.

In a collaborative study [12] qualitative analyses of AChE-activity were performed
on all amniotic fluid samples, in which AFP was positive (tab. 2). A positive
AChE-result was found in the case of anencephalus in 99.6%, in presence of
spina bifida in 99.4%. Also in malformations with no neural tube defect positive

AChE were found at a high percentage. However, in no case of congenital nephrosis were positive AChE demonstrable. This provides an interesting possibility for differential diagnosis.

On the other hand, false positive amniotic fluid AChE results are only seen in about 6% of samples with confirmed pathological AFP levels, when no malfor-

Table 2   Numbers of pregnancy (n = 1.099) with positive amniotic fluid AFP results and proportions with positive Ge-AChE results according to the outcome of pregnancy (Report of Collaborative AChE Study [12])

Outcome of pregnancy	No. of pregnancies	Positive AChE result No.	(%)
Neural tube defect			
Anencephaly	478	476	(99,6%)
Open spina bifida	335	333	(99,4%)
No neural tube defect			
Exomphalos*	63	47	(75%)
Congenital nephrosis	11	0	(0%)
Other serious malformation**	14	7	(50%)
Miscarriage	73	34	(47%)
Without serious malformation or miscarriage	125	8	(6%)

 * Including 3 cases of gastroschisis.
** 4 with Turner's syndrome (all with positive AChE); 3 with teratoma (1 with positive AChE); 1 with trisomy E; 1 with trisomy 13; 1 with trisomy 18 (positive AChE); 1 with Potter's syndrome; 1 with kidney agenesis; 1 with hypoplasia of heart and lung (positive AChE); 1 with multiple abnormalities.

Table 3   Summary of the amniotic fluid AChE and AFP results in 83 pregnancies studied [1]

Outcome of pregnancy	Amniotic fluid AFP*	No. of pregnancies	Gel AChE result
Anencephaly	positive	8	all positive
Open spina bifida	positive	8	all positive
	negative	*1 (1,2%)*	*positive*
Exomphalos	positive	3	all positive
	negative	3	1 positive
			2 negative
Unaffected	*positive*	*4 (4,8%)*	*all negative*
	negative	56	all negative

* A positive amniotic fluid AFP was defined an being ⩾ 5,0 standard deviations above the mean.

Table 4   Amniotic fluid AFP and AChE results according to the outcome of pregnancy in 738
pregnancies prospectively studied (own investigation 1983/84)

Outcome of pregnancy	Amniotic fluid AFP*	No. of pregnancies	Gel AChE result
Anencephalic	positive	1	positive
Open spina bifida	all positive	6	all positive
Amniotic bands syndrome	positive	1	positive
Unaffected	all negative	723	all negative
	borderline	7	all negative
	after reamniocentesis of 5 cases negative	5	all negative

* positive ⩾ 3-fold median; borderline ⩾ 2,5-fold < 3-fold median.

mation is detectable. So AChE in considered to be a more specific and sensitive indicator for neural tube defects as AFP.

Barlow, Cuckle and Wald [1] showed in a prospective study with 83 pregnancies that in no case of open neural tube defect a false-positive AChE-result was found, whereas AFP determinations showed false-negative results in 1.2%. No false-positive AChE results were found in contrast to 4.8% for AFP (tab. 3).

Our own investigations of 738 pregnancies within 1983 – 1984 confirm these result. Borderline AFP levels in 7 cases with values between 2,5 – 3-fold of the median were AChE negative. On 5 of these patients was a second amniocentesis performed resulting finally in normal AFP levels (tab. 4).

Screening of dysraphic malformations

Recently there is increasing interest in biochemical screening parameters during the $16^{th} - 18^{th}$ week of gestation. The fact, that only 5 – 10% of fetuses with dysraphic malformations are born in families with obtrusive history but more than 90% of these children remain undetected prenatally, justifies an intensified screening.

Determination of amniotic fluid parameters is not useful in terms of large scale screening due to possible complications during amniocentesis. As mentioned above, maternal serum contains elevated AFP levels in case of a fetus with an open neural tube defect. This would be a possible parameter for a general screening. Pathologically elevated AFP levels in maternal serum can be found with an accuracy of about 90% in case of anencephalus and 80% in case of spina bifida aperta [11].

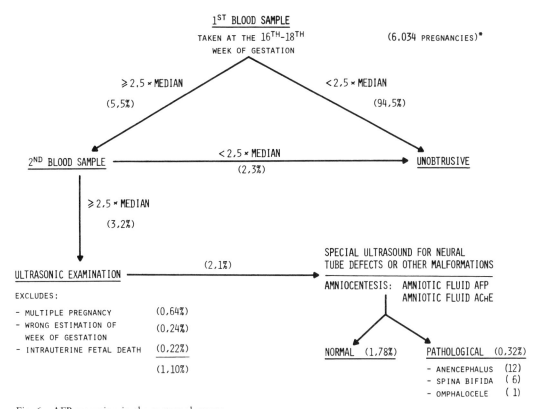

Fig. 6   AFP-screening in the maternal serum.
            *The values (...) are taken from the investigations performed by Brock [3].

The following schedule (fig. 6) has been applied with success for AFP screening. A first maternal serum AFP determination takes place within the 16th – 18th week of gestation. If the level is found to be more than 2,5-fold above the median, additional examinations should be performed. If the repeated AFP determination confirms the pathologically elevated value, the following situations have to be excluded by ultrasonic investigations: wrong estimation of gestational period, multiple pregnancy, or intrauterine fetal death. The final diagnosis of open neural tube defects or other malformations can be proofed by increased amniotic fluid AFP levels or a significant AChE value.

By means of such screening examinations in England open neural tube defects were detected in 3% of all pregnancies. In his study of 6.034 pregnancies Brock [3] found elevated AFP levels in 5.5% after the first examination, 3.2% remained pathological after the second control. Careful ultrasonic investigation showed other reasons than malformation in 1.1%. Of the remaining 2.1%, further diagnosis was performed by amniocentesis. 1.78% showed normal range AFP levels. Among the remaining 0.32% with pathologically elevated AFP were 12 fetuses with anencephalus. 6 with spina bifida aperta and one with an ompha- locele (fig. 6). The value of a predictive test has to be — at least to some extent — related to expenditure and usefulness. The exposed schedule for a screening has been applied with success, especially in areas with a high incidence of such malformations. This is proven by examinations in Great Britain, but there are also positive evaluations reported from the USA, Canada and other countries with a similar incidence as in Germany [6—8, 11, 19].

The success of prenatal diagnostic is not only restricted to the finding of fetal malformation, but lies also in their exclusion, especially in risk patients.

References

[1] Barlow, R. D., H. S. Cuckle, N. J. Wald: A simple method for amniotic fluid gel-acetylcholin- esterase determination, suitable for routine use in the antenatal diagnosis of open neural tube defects. Clin. Chim. Acta **123** (1982) 137—142.

[2] Brock, D. J. H., R. G. Sutcliffe: Alpha-fetoprotein in the antenatal diagnosis of anencephaly and spina bifida. Lancet **II** (1972) 197—199.

[3] Brock, D. J. H.: Screening for neural tube defects. In: Towards the prevention of fetal malforma- tions (J. B. Scrimgeour, ed.), pp. 37—46. Edinburgh University Press, Edinburgh 1978.

[4] Chubb, I. W., P. M. Pilowsky, H. J. Springell et al.: Acetylcholinesterase in human amniotic fluid: an index of fetal neural development? Lancet **I** (1979) 688—690.

[5] Cremer, M., W. Schmidt, T. Voigtländer et al.: Pränatale Diagnostik bei erhöhter Alpha- Fetoprotein-Konzentration im Fruchtwasser. Z. Geburtsh. u. Perinat. **185** (1981) 299—304.

[6] Fuhrmann, W.: Die Alpha-Fetoproteinbestimmung in der pränatalen Diagnostik und Vorsorge. Diagn. Intensivther. **16** (1983) 1—7.

[7] Grob, P. J.: Pränatales α-Fetoprotein-Screening für Neuralleistendefekte. Schweiz. med. Wschr. **108** (1978) 1302—1307.

[8] Kjessler, B., S. G. O. Johansson: Alpha fetoprotein (AFP) in early pregnancy. Acta Obstet. Gynecol. Scand. (Suppl.) **69** (1977) 50—53.

[9] Kleijer, W. J., H. W. A. de Bruijn, N. J. Leschot: Amniotic fluid alpha fetoprotein levels and the prenatal diagnosis of neural tube defects: a collaborative study of 2.180 pregnancies in the Netherlands. Br. J. Obstet. Gynaecol. **85** (1978) 512—517.

[10] Ramzin, M. S.: Physikalische Diagnostik in der Geburtshilfe: Biochemische Diagnostik. In: Gynäkologie und Geburtshilfe, vol. II/1, Schwangerschaft und Geburt (O. Käser, V. Friedberg, K. G. Ober, K. Thomson, J. Zander, eds.), pp. 6.72—6.82. Georg Thieme Verlag, Stuttgart—New York 1981.

[11] Report of UK Collaborative Study on alpha-fetoprotein in relation to neural tube defects: Maternal serum alpha-fetoprotein measurement in antenatal screening for anencephaly and spina bifida in early pregnancy. Lancet **I** (1977) 1323—1332.

[12] Report of the Collaborative Acetylcholinesterase Study: Amniotic fluid acetylcholinesterase electrophoresis as a secondary test in the diagnosis of anencephaly and open spina bifida in early pregnancy. Lancet **II** (1981) 321—324.

[13] Second report of the UK Collaborative Study on alpha-fetoprotein in relation to neural tube defects: Amniotic fluid alpha-fetoprotein measurement in antenatal diagnosis of anencephaly and open spina bifida in early pregnancy. Lancet **II** (1979) 651—662.

[14] Smith, A. F.: Amniotic fluid acetylcholinesterase assay and the antenatal detection of neural tube defects. Clin. Chim. Acta **123** (1982) 1 – 9.

[15] Smith, A. D., N. J. Wald, H. S. Cuckle et al.: Amniotic-fluid acetylcholinesterase as a possible diagnostic test for neural tube defects in early pregnancy. Lancet **I** (1979) 685 – 688.

[16] Voigtländer, T., W. Friedl, M. Cremer et al.: Quantitative and qualitative assay of amniotic-fluid acetylcholinesterase in the prenatal diagnosis of neural tube defects. Hum. Genet. **59** (1891) 227 – 231.

[17] Wald, N. J., H. S. Cuckle: Pränatale Diagnostik von Neuralrohr-Defekten. Laboratoriumsblätter **31** (1981) 27 – 41.

[18] Weitzel, H., K. Schumann, H. Rehder et al.: Prenatal diagnosis of neural tube defects by AFP analysis. In: Prenatal diagnosis (J. D. Murken, S. Stengel-Rutkowski, E. Schwinger, eds.), pp. 94 – 98. Enke Verlag, Stuttgart 1979.

[19] Weitzel, H. K., F. Dati, G. Grenner: α-Fetoprotein-Bestimmung in der Schwangerschaft mittels Enzymimmunoassay. Laboratoriumsblätter **32** (1982) 136 – 150.

[20] Weitzel, H.: Alpha-fetoprotein in der Geburtshilfe. Gynäkologe **16** (1983) 148 – 154.

Ultrasound in the prenatal diagnosis of dysraphic malformations of the head

W. Goldhofer

With high-resolution ultrasound equipment (Combison 202, real-time, Kretz 3.5 MHz) it is now possible to diagnose certain fetal anomalies, in some cases even before the 20th week of gestation. With ultrasound, the obstetrician has a non-invasive method by which he can routinely diagnose serious diseases and malformations of the fetus early in the course of pregnancy. The basis for this is the experience gained from the widespread use of ultrasound in Germany. In 1980 Germany became the first country of the world to demand the routine performance of two ultrasound examinations during the course of normal pregnancy. The fact that 90% of all fetal malformations occur without alterations in the genetic code or without a previous history of birth defects, underlines the importance of ultrasound as a screening method for the detection of fetal malformations.

With a frequency of 1:2000 deliveries, *anencephalus* represents the most serious dysraphic malformation of the head [6, 7, 9]. At the same time it is the malformation diagnosed most easily – and most frequently – by ultrasound. The prognosis of the malformation is poor, resulting in death within a few hours post partum.

Normally, the fetal skull is first detectable by ultrasound in the 13th or 14th week of gestation. In anencephalus the first sonographic sign is that a normal presentation of the fetal head is not obtained. The final diagnosis of anencephalus is made if the typical spherical outline of the fetal head is replaced by an irregular mass without intracranial structures [1, 2, 5, 7, 10, 11] (fig. 1). Because of the missing cranial vault, the eyes are protruded (so-called frog-eyes) and can be seen very often by ultrasound (fig. 2). In most cases the rest of the body demonstrates normal development. On the sonographic picture, the normal structure of the body together with the irregular mass of the fetal skull give the fetus a torpedo-like appearance (fig. 2). The malformation is sometimes accompanied by a defective closure of the spine (spina bifida) in the cervical region which is then called craniorachischisis (fig. 3). Anencephaly is often associated with polyhydramnion and hectic movements of the fetus. The diagnosis is difficult to make before the 13th week of gestation, but should not be missed after the 16th week [4, 7]. Ultrasound is the only procedure necessary for the final

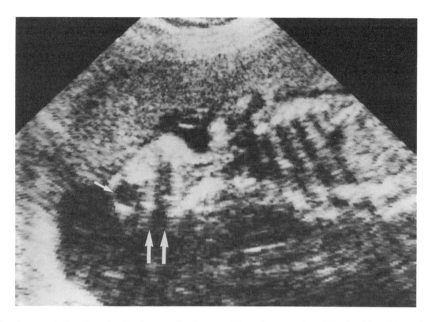

Fig. 1   Anencephalus. Longitudinal scan of a fetus at 27 weeks gestation. The fetal head is replaced by an irregular mass without intracranial structures (↑↑). Eye (↑).

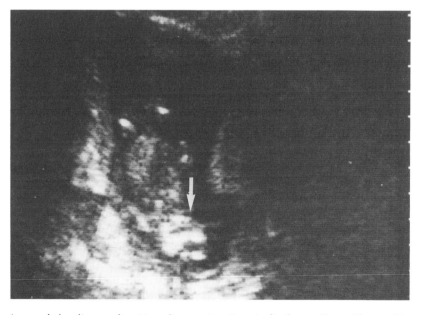

Fig. 2   Anencephalus diagnosed at 14 weeks gestation. Longitudinal scan. Face with eyes (↓).

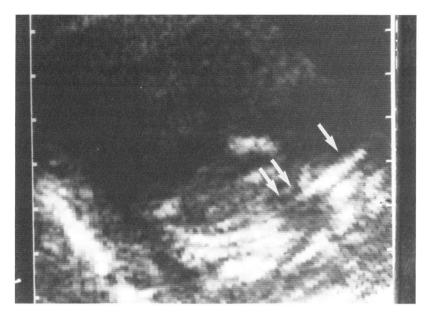

Fig. 3   Craniorachischisis. Longitudinal scan (spine) of the same fetus as fig. 2 with anencephaly (↓) and spina bifida in the cervical region (↓↓). The lower spine was normal.

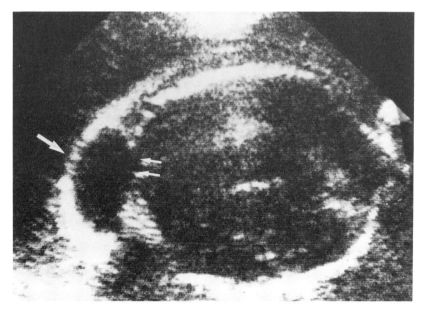

Fig. 4   Encephalocele. Transverse section of the fetal head at 35 weeks gestation. Cystic bulge beside the fetal cranium (↑) with a defect in the normally rounded outline of the occipital region (⇐).

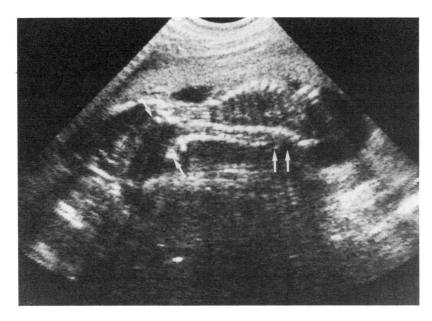

Fig. 5a   Arnold-Chiari malformation. Longitudinal scan of a fetus at 20 weeks gestation. Wide foramen magnum (↕) with lumbosacral myelomeningocele (↑↑).

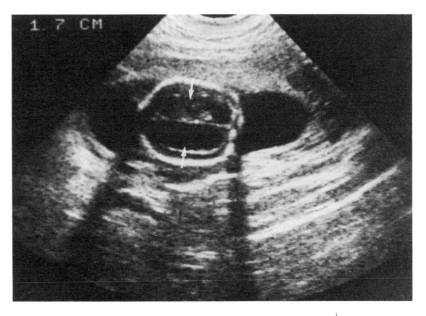

Fig. 5b   The same fetus as fig. 5a. Hydrocephalus. Dilated lateral ventricles (↕).

diagnosis of anencephalus. Confirmatory x-ray have been abandoned because ultrasound has proved extremely accurate and x-ray pictures before the 20th week of gestation are not sufficiently reliable.

The maternal serum Alpha-Fetoprotein levels are often elevated and usually increased in the amniotic fluid. Because the risk of having another anencephalic fetus increases 4% after one child with anencephalus and 10% after two, the early sonographic control of succeeding pregnancies is extremely important.

Two other rare dysraphic malformations of the head are the encephalocele and the Arnold-Chiari malformation.

The *encephalocele* is a cystic expansion of meninges and brain tissue outside the cranium, possibly covered by normal or atrophic skin. The most common site is the occipital region, but it may be located in the frontal, parietal, orbital or nasal part of the fetal skull. Ultrasonically encephaloceles are recognized by a cystic bulge beside the fetal cranium and/or a defect in the normally rounded outline of the head [2, 6, 8, 9, 10] (fig. 4).

The *Arnold-Chiari malformation* represents a combined malformation characterized by a displacement of parts of the cerebellum, fourth ventricle, pons and medulla oblongata into the spinal canal, usually always associated with hydrocephalus and myelomeningocele [3]. The most common sonographic finding is the simultaneous diagnosis of hydrocephalus and myelomeningocele. The final diagnosis of Arnold-Chiari malformation can be made, if, in addition, a wide foramen magnum and a striking enlargement of the spinal canal in the cranio-cervical region (figs. 5a and 5b) are present.

In summary, sonography has proven to be of essential importance in the prenatal diagnosis of fetal head malformations. The prerequisites, however, are high-resolution ultrasound equipment and wide experience in normal fetal sonoanatomy and fetal malformations.

References

[1] Bernaschek, G., Ch. Dadak, A. Kratochwil: Frühzeitige Diagnose fetaler Mißbildungen durch Ultraschall. Geburtsh. u. Frauenheilk. 40 (1980) 868 – 875.
[2] Campbell, S.: Early prenatal diagnosis of fetal abnormality by ultrasound B-scanning. In: Prenatal diagnosis (J. D. Murken, S. Stengel-Rutkowski, E. Schwinger, eds.), pp. 155 – 171. Proceedings of the 3rd European Conference of Prenatal Diagnosis of Genetic Disorders. Enke Verlag, Stuttgart 1979.
[3] Gardner, W. J.: The dysraphic states from syringomyelia to anencephaly. Excerpta medica, Amsterdam 1975.
[4] Hansmann, M.: Sonar in prenatal diagnosis. In: Prenatal diagnosis (J. D. Murken, S. Stengel-Rutkowski, E. Schwinger, eds.), pp. 155 – 171. Proceedings of the 3rd European Conference of Prenatal Diagnosis of Genetic Disorders. Enke Verlag, Stuttgart 1979.

[5] Hobbins, J. C., P. Grannum, R. Berkowitz et al.: Ultrasound in the diagnosis of congenital anomalies. Amer. J. Obstet. Gynec. **134** (1979) 331–345.

[6] Holländer, H.-J.: Die Ultraschalldiagnostik in der Schwangerschaft, 3rd ed. Urban & Schwarzenberg, München–Wien–Baltimore 1984.

[7] Kurjak, A., P. Kirkinen, V. Latin et al.: Diagnosis and assessment of fetal malformation and abnormalities by ultrasound. J. Perinat. Med. **8** (1980) 219–235.

[8] Miskin, M., N. L. Rudd, M. R. Dische et al.: Prenatal ultrasonic diagnosis of occipital encephalocele. Amer. J. Obstet. Gynec. **130** (1978) 585–587.

[9] Ramzin, M. S.: Mißbildungsdiagnostik im Rahmen der Schwangerenvorsorge. Swiss. Med. **4**, Nr. 6a (1982) 77–81.

[10] Schlensker, K.-H.: Atlas der Ultraschalldiagnostik in Geburtshilfe und Gynäkologie. Thieme Verlag, Stuttgart–New York 1984.

[11] Winter, R.: Die Diagnose angeborener fetaler Mißbildungen mittels Ultraschall. Ultraschall **2** (1981) 235–243.

Diagnostic ultrasound in children with meningomyelocele-hydrocephalus and Arnold-Chiari-malformation

K. H. Deeg, W. Dick, D. Wenzel

Introduction

According to the relevant literature 80–90% of all children suffering from meningomyelocele caused by an Arnold-Chiari-syndrome (ACS) develop eventually a progressive shunt dependent hydrocephalus [12–14, 17, 18]. A few years ago the ACS could only be detected by computed tomography (CT) [12, 13, 18] or invasive diagnostic procedures such as pneumencephalography [14] and ventriculography [8, 14, 17].

The development of high resolution sector scanners allows the sonographic examination of the infant's brain, using the anterior fontanelle as an acoustic window [1, 4, 6, 11, 16]. Comparative investigations using computed tomography and sonography showed such a good correlation between the two methods, that an indication for CT in babies is hardly necessary [11, 16].

Patients and investigating methods

22 newborn infants (11 boys and 11 girls) suffering from meningomyeloceles were examined on the day of birth and from then on twice a week using a mechanical sector scanner. In all the children sagittal, parasagittal and coronal sections were performed and the ventricular system was measured in defined places for early recognition of ventricular dilation. The examinations were carried out using a RA-1 sonographic system (Frequency 3.5 MHz; sector 60° and 100°) and an ATL Mark 600 (Frequency 3.5 MHz, 5 MHz and 7 MHz; sector 90°).

Results (Tables 1, 2, 3)

The initial ultrasound examination on the day of birth yielded a normal ventricular system in only three children (14%). The remaining 19 children (86%) displayed varying degrees of ventricular dilation: 12 children (55%) already

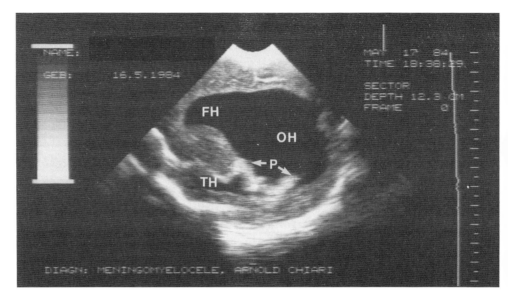

Fig. 1   Parasagittal section of the dilated lateral ventricle: Extensive hydrocephalus with dilation of the occipital horn (OH) and frontal horn (FH). Temporal horn (TH) normal in size: Prominent plexus chorioideus (P) floating freely in the ventricular lumen.

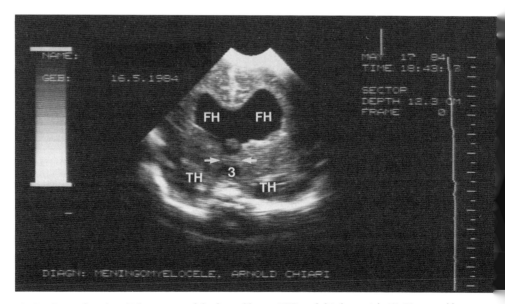

Fig. 2   Coronal section: Enlargement of the frontal horns (FH) and third ventricle (3). Temporal horns (TH) normal in size. Enlarged massa intermedia (arrows) and absent septum pellucidum.

had a massive hydrocephalus; the remaining 7 children (32%) displayed slight ventricular dilatation. The hydrocephalus always began with the dilatation of the *occipital horns* (fig. 1), followed by the enlargement of the *frontal horns* (figs. 1 and 2). Even in cases of massive hydrocephalus the *temporal horns* were normal in size or only slightly dilated (figs. 1 and 2), as opposed to forms of hydrocephalus of different origin such as the posthemorrhagic hydrocephalus, where all parts of the ventricular system are enlarged [4, 5]. The highest degree of dilatation could always be detected in the area of the occipital horn or the atrium (fig. 1), where the brain mantle had often narrowed to a few millimeters (fig. 1). For this reason the brain mantle in the area of the occipital horns is a sensitive indicator of progressive ventricular dilatation, especially in the first few days after birth, and is well suited for short-term controls. However, in the case of a very pronounced hydrocephalus, where the brain mantle over the occipital horns is only a few millimeters thick, measurements taken in the area of the frontal horns are better suited for the further controls.

The *third ventricle* was usually of normal width or at the most slightly dilated (fig. 3). All children with ACS displayed a ventral and caudal displacement of the dysplastic third ventricle (fig. 3), which showed atypical and enlarged recesses (fig. 3). In 41% of the cases a prominent recessus pinealis could be detected. None of the children had a dilated *aqaeduct of Sylvius*. In most instances the aqueduct also displayed ventral and caudal displacement and an angulation after leaving the third ventricle.

The *fourth ventricle* could not be detected by sonography in the case of 4 children (18%) due to its displacement in the foramen magnum. The remaining 18 children

Table 1   Sonographic characteristics of hydrocephalus in children with meningomyeloceles (n = 22)

Normal ventricular system at birth	3	(14%)
Ventricular enlargement at birth	19	(86%)
− moderate enlargement at birth	7	(32%)
− severe enlargement at birth	12	(55%)
Progressive hydrocephalus	18	(82%)
Dilatation of the lateral ventricles	20	(91%)
− dilatation of the occipital horns	20	(91%)
− dilatation of the frontal horns	19	(86%)
− dilatation of the temporal horns	3	(14%)
Third ventricle: Dilated	4	(18%)
Displaced ventrally and caudally	18	(82%)
Prominent pineal recess	8	(41%)
Fourth ventricle: Elongated and displaced caudally	18	(82%)
Not visible	4	(18%)
Cerebellum: Displaced caudally	18	(82%)
Hypoplastic or dysplastic	18	(82%)

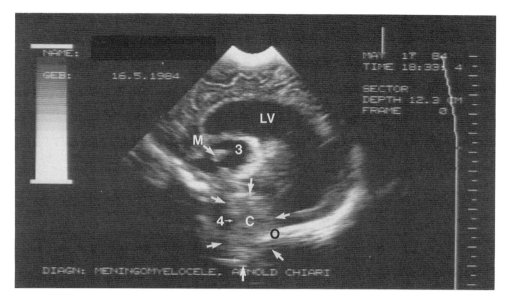

Fig. 3   Sagittal section of midline structures: Arnold-Chiari-malformation. Caudally displaced third
ventricle (3), fourth ventricle (4) and cerebellum (C). Dysplastic third ventricle and cerebellum
(arrows) impressed by the os occipitale (0). Thick massa intermedia (M). LV = lateral
ventricle.

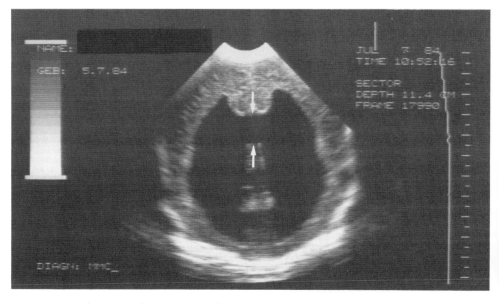

Fig. 4   Semiaxial section: Absent septum pellucidum (arrows). Symmetrical dilatation of the lateral
ventricles.

(82%) displayed an elongated fourth ventricle with caudal displacement and a sagittal flattening (fig. 3).

The *cisterna magna,* which can normally be detected by sonography in 90% of all children, could not be seen in any child suffering from ACS due to the caudal displacement of the cerebellum (fig. 3).

The hydrocephalus of children suffering from meningomyelocele is caused by the *Arnold-Chiari malformation,* characterized pathologically and anatomically by the caudal displacement of the cerebellum and brainstem, seen by sonography in 18 children (82%) (fig. 3). In 82% of the children the *cerebellum* was dysplastic or hypoplastic and impressed caudally by the os occipitale (fig. 3). In rare instances (4 children) the cerebellum was displaced into the foramen magnum. Whereas the cerebellum, brainstem, fourth ventricle and the cisterna magna can normally be clearly shown by gray scale ultrasonography only on obscure image of the above structures could be obtained in the case of ACS (fig. 3).

Table 2   Sonographic characteristics of Arnold-Chiari-malformation

Cerebellum	Displaced caudally Hypoplastic or dysplastic
Fourth ventricle	Displaced caudally and flattend sagittally
Cisterna magna	Not visible
Third ventricle	Displaced caudally and ventrally Dysplastic with atypical recesses
Lateral ventricles	Dilated occipital and frontal horns Temporal horns normal in size
Associated malformations of the brain	Enlarged massa intermedia Absent septum pellucidum Prominent plexus chorioideus Agenesia of the corpus callosum

Table 3   Associated malformations of the brain in children with myelomeningoceles (n = 22)

Large massa intermedia	12	(55%)
Prominent plexus chorioideus	11	(50%)
Absent septum pellucidum	8	(36%)
Fenestrated septum pellucidum	2	(9%)
Agenesia of the corpus callosum	1	(5%)

Malformations of the central nervous system (tab. 3) associated with ACS were thickening of the *massa intermedia,* found in 12 children (55%) (figs. 2 and 3), an *agenesia of the corpus callosum* (1 child), a *missing* (8 children) or *fenestrated* (2 children) *septum pellucidum* and a *prominent plexus chorioideus* (11 children).

The *plexus chorioideus* was thickened in 50% of all children floating freely in the ventricular lumen (fig. 1). Although a prominent choroid plexus floating freely in the lateral ventricles is not pathognomic for ACS, it is often in association with ACS.

Further associated malformations of the central nervous system were an *absent septum pellucidum* in 9 children (36%) or a *fenestration* of it in 2 children (9%) (figs. 2 and 4). Using sonography it could not be determined whether this was a case of agenesia or a secondary tearing of the septum pellucidum in the course of progressive ventricular dilation. In some children an intact septum pellucidum could be detected at birth, but absent at later ultrasound checks as the enlargement of the ventricular system had advanced.

Discussion

Our sonographic findings are in good agreement (tabs. 1–3) with the results of ventriculography [8, 14, 18], pneumencephalography (14) and computertomography [12, 13, 18], especially regarding the Arnold-Chiari-syndrome and hydrocephalus of varying degrees [8, 12, 13, 14, 18]. Progressive ventricular dilatation was found in 86% of our patients in accordance to the frequency of 80–90% reported in literature [10, 12, 13, 17, 18].

Associated malformations of the brain (tab. 3), seen by other authors too [8, 12–14, 17, 18], were also present in more than 50% of our patients.

The sonographic findings at birth and further echographic controls of children with myelomeningoceles throw light on the pathogenesis of ACS and progressive hydrocephalus: 55% of all children displayed severe hydrocephalus and ACS already at birth. The enlargement of the ventricular system could be an expression of a primary CNS-malformation as already discussed by Chiari himself and later on by other authors too [3, 9]. On the other hand some children had a normal ventricular system (3 children) or only slight ventricular enlargement (7 children) at birth, but progressive hydrocephalus could be shown in 18 children postnatally. This indicates that other factors may play an important role in the pathogenesis such as disturbances of cerebrospinal fluid (CSF) circulation near the foramina Luschkae or the basal cisterns [10, 17]. Ventriculographic and cisternographic studies of Yamada [17] demonstrated a total obstruction of the CSF-pathways from the fourth ventricle to the subarachnoidal space in 15% and a partial obstruction in 54%. The obstruction in this region is caused by a displacement of the vermis towards the fourth ventricle [17]. McCoy [10] saw disturbances in the CSF pathways in the basal cisterns e.g. in the cisterna ambiens; Masters [9] considers that a deficiency in the CSF resorption is due to subarachnoidal fibrovascular attachments. The literature relevant to morphology and pathogenesis of hydrocephalus due to malformations of the fossa posterior is discussed by Schmidt [13].

Based on the dynamic ventricular changes in hydrocephalus caused by an ACS in children with myelomeningocele [6] and on our own results reported above, we postulate, that a prenatal imbalance in CSF circulation may cause a severe ventricular dilatation. These prenatal intracerebral CSF imbalances can disturb the development of the brain and help to explain the associated brain malformations found in more than a half of our patients. A prenatally increased intracranial CSF pressure appears to be a pathogenetic factor in associated malformations. This is in good agreement with our findings of a normal septum pellucidum at the beginning of progressive ventricular dilatation, the septum disappears during further controls, mimicking an agenesia of the septum pellucidum at a later stage. The increased CSF-pressure on periventricular structures may be due to several defects in the midline structures of the brain especially during the stage of fast brain development in the fifth to sixth fetal month.

The finding of a prominent choroid plexus in half of our children and especially in the patients with the severest forms of hydrocephalus deserves special attention. The enlargement of a plexus showing hypervascularisation and hyperproduction of CSF may play an important role in CSF imbalance of production and resorption and thus contribute to the development of a dynamic hydrocephalus. Obstruction of CSF-circulation cannot be the sole cause of the hydrocephalus in myelomeningoceles, for in one child, a primary ventricular enlargement had totally reversed afterwards. In two other children the ventricular system remained normal throughout repeated controls during the first year of life. But as a rule (in 19 of 22 children) disturbances in CSF dynamics may well play the major role in the pathogenesis of hydrocephalus in ACS prenatally and postnatally. An obstruction of the CSF-pathways near the fourth ventricle and the outlet to the basal cisterns, can be a primary cause while a less important reason is an overproduction of CSF from the enlarged plexus combined with a decreased CSF-resorption in the subarachnoidal space, resulting in a "reduced communicated" hydrocephalus in Arnold-Chiari-syndrome.

The scope of the diagnostic information of high resolution ultrasonography approximately equals that of neuroradiology, sonography in addition does have a number of significant advantages: it can be performed without using ionizing radiation or contrast media and requires neither sedation or anaesthesia nor transport of the child. Bedside examination can be carried out, even in the case of seriously ill newborn infants without interrupting vital therapeutic measures. As ultrasound examination does not require ionizing radiation, it can be performed repeatedly and is especially suited for short-term checks.

Conclusion

Using the anterior fontanelle as an acoustic window, two-dimensional echoencephalography is able to detect Arnold-Chiari-syndrome, a developing hydrocephalus and associated malformations of the central nervous system. Invasive diagnostic procedures, such as ventriculography and pneumencephalography are no longer indicated for the diagnosis of ACS. The use of computed tomography should be limited in view of ionizing radiation.

Using sonography it is possible to obtain useful information, already at birth, concerning ventricular dilatation or the risk of a developing hydrocephalus. If, at birth, no indications of an ACS are present and the ventricular system is normal in size, only a slight probability of a progressive hydrocephalus exists. The detection of an ACS requires many ultrasound checks, to be able to detect a progressive hydrocephalus at an early stage and to provide an appropriate therapy. Furthermore, sonography is well suited for controls after shunt implantation, allowing shunt insufficiency and shunt complications to be detected at an early stage. After closure of the fontanelles computer tomography is the first choice for further diagnostic investigations.

References

[1] Bejar, R., V. Curbelo, R. W. Coen et al.: Diagnosis and follow-up of intraventricular and intracerebral hemorrhages by ultrasound studies of infant's brain through the fontanelles and sutures. Pediatrics 66 (1980) 661–673.
[2] Bliesener, J. A.: Die Sonographie der Arnold-Chiarischen Mißbildung. Monatsschr. Kinderheilkd. 131 (1983) 688.
[3] Caviness, V. jr.: The Chiari malformations of the posterior fossa and their relation to hydrocephalus. Dev. Med. Child. Neurol. 18 (1976) 103–116.
[4] Deeg, K. H., W. Dick, V. Spitzer et al.: Sonografische Verlaufskontrolle der fortschreitenden Ventrikelerweiterung beim posthämorrhagischen Hydrocephalus. In: Hydrocephalus im Kindesalter (D. Voth, P. Gutjahr, P. Glees, eds.), pp. 143–149. Enke Verlag, Stuttgart 1983.
[5] Deeg, K. H., K. Richter, K. Steh: Diagnose und Verlauf von Hirnblutungen im Säuglingsalter mit Hilfe der Sonografie. Pädiatr. Pädol. 19 (1984) 25–34.
[6] Dick, W., K. H. Deeg, D. Wenzel et al.: Dynamik der Ventrikelveränderungen im prä- und postoperativen Verlauf beim angeborenen Hydrocephalus. Entscheidungshilfen für Ventilrevision? In: Hydrocephalus im Kindesalter (D. Voth, P. Gutjahr, P. Glees, eds.), pp. 220–224. Enke Verlag, Stuttgart 1983.

[7] Gardner, W. J.: Hydrodynamic factors in Dandy-Walker and Arnold-Chiari malformations. Childs Brain 3 (1977) 200–212.

[8] Kellermann, K., J. A. Bliesener, J. M. Kyambi: Positive ventriculography using water-soluble contrast media in infants with myelomeningocele and hydrocephalus. Neuropädiatrie 9 (1978) 49–58.

[9] Masters, C. L.: Pathogenesis of the Arnold-Chiari malformation: The significance of hydrocephalus and aqueduct stenosis. J. Neuropath. Exp. Neurol. 37 (1978) 56–74.

[10] McCoy, W. T., D. A. Simpson, R. F. Carter: cerebral malformation complicating spina bifida. Clin. Radiol. 18 (1976) 176–182.

[11] Morgan, C. L., W. S. Trought, S. J. Rothman et al.: Comparison of gray-scale ultrasonography and computed tomography in the evaluation of macrocrania in infants. Radiology 132 (1979) 119–123.

[12] Naidich, T. P.: Cranial CT signs of the Chiari II malformation. J. Neuroradiol. 8 (1981) 207–227.

[13] Naidich, T. P., R. M. Pudlowski, J. B. Naidich: Computed tomographic signs of the Chiari II malformation. Ventricles and cisterns. Radiology 134 (1980) 657–663.

[14] Raimondi, A. J.: Pediatric neuroradiology, pp. 295–343. Sounders, Philadelphia 1972.

[15] Schmitt, H. P.: Der Hydrocephalus bei Mißbildungen der hinteren Schädelgrube im Umfelde des dysraphischen Formenkreises. In: Hydrocephalus im Kindesalter (D. Voth, P. Gutjahr, P. Glees, eds.), pp. 79–88. Enke Verlag, Stuttgart 1983.

[16] Skolnick, M. L., A. E. Rosenbaum, T. Matzuk et al.: Detection of dilated cerebral ventricles in infants: A correlative study between ultrasound and computed tomography. Radiology 131 (1979) 447–451.

[17] Yamada, H., S. Nakamura, Y. Tanaka et al.: Ventriculography and cisternography with water-soluble contrast media in infants with myelomeningocele. Radiology 143 (1982) 75–83.

[18] Zimmermann, R. D., D. Breckbill, M. W. Dennis et al.: Cranial CT findings in patients with meningomyelocele. AJR 132 (1979) 629–632.

Prenatal diagnosis of neural tube defects by ultrasound

E. Merz

In spite of the introduction of an ultrasound screening program during pregnancy, neural tube defects are rarely discovered during a routine ultrasound examination. The first accurate ultrasound scanning is usually performed after a raised maternal serum-AFP-level or an elevated amniotic fluid-AFP-level or in patients with a familial risk of neural tube defects.

With a modern realtime ultrasound equipment of high resolution not only gross neural tube defects are demonstrable but also small defects such as spina bifida occulta. The examination has to be carried out at an appropriate gestational age by an experienced investigator provided there is enough amniotic fluid and the fetus is in a normal position.

The optimal period for the prenatal diagnosis of neural tube defects (NTD) is between 16 and 22 weeks' gestation. The fetal spine can be visualised along its full length on a single longitudinal scan, and it is early enough for terminating the pregnancy if there is a large spinal defect.

Reduced quantity of amniotic fluid (oligohydramnios) can complicate the prenatal sonographic diagnosis, as the fetal back is mostly adjacent to the uterine wall covering the neural tube defect. Especially in an occiput posterior position the spine defect can be covered up by a limb bone in front of the fetal body. Even when a normal quantity of amniotic fluid is present the diagnosis can be difficult in a low lesion in the lumbo-sacral area or if the fetus is in a breech presentation deep in the pelvis. For the diagnosis of a NTD it is important that the fetal spine can be visualised in its full length and without superposition of other structures.

The sonographic visualisation of the fetal spine is possible as early as 14 weeks menstrual age, a more detailed examination should be delayed until 16 weeks' gestation. The normal spine in the longitudinal axis can be identified as a pair of continuously interrupted parallel lines which are confluent in the sacral area (fig. 1). In the transverse scan the fetal spine shows a closed ring structure with a dorsal shadowing. In case of a NTD distinct changes can be found according to the kind of the defect and the position of the fetus. In case the fetus is in a dorso-lateral position, the *spina bifida aperta* shows diverging walls at the level of the defect (fig. 2); if the fetus is in a dorso-anterior position, the skin defect

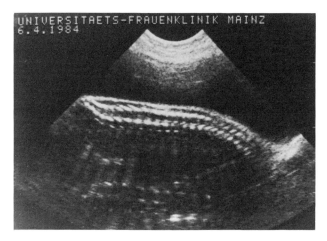

Fig. 1   Normal fetal spine in the longitudinal axis (24 weeks' gestation).

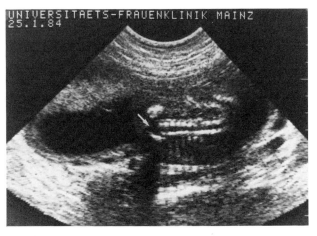

Fig. 2   Spina bifida aperta in the lumbo-sacral area (↘). Dorso-lateral position of the fetus (18 weeks' gestation).

can also be shown by the interruption of the fetal surface (fig. 3). In the transverse section instead of the normal ring structure of the spine a dorsal open U- or V-shaped canal is found. Occasionaly a spina bifida can be simulated by the dorsal shadowing of the fetal ilium wing if the fetus is in a lateral position. As this, however, is only a superimposition effect, the supposed defect can no longer be printed out after a change in fetal position.

In case the defect is a *spina bifida occulta*, a longitudinal section shows a local diverging of the spinal walls, but in contrast to the spina bifida aperta no defect

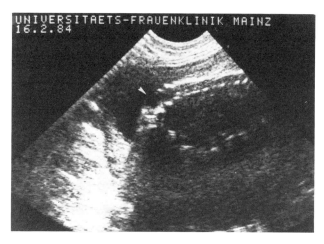

Fig. 3   Spina bifida aperta in the lumbo-sacral area (↘). Dorso-anterior position of the fetus (23 weeks' gestation).

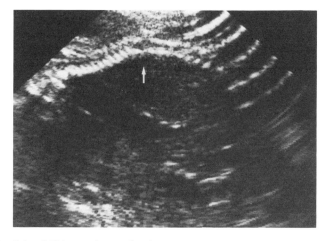

Fig. 4   Spina bifida occulta in the thoracic area. Local diverging of the spinal walls (↑) without defect of the fetal surface (24 weeks' gestation).

of the fetal surface is seen in the dorso-anterior position of the fetus (fig. 4). In these cases where a *meningocele* or *myelomeningocele* in addition to the spine defect is present, a round or oval well defined cystic mass is found behind the spine defect. In the meningocele no echoes are shown from the interior of the cyst, whereas in the myelomeningocele singular string-like echoes can be visualised (fig. 5). In the transverse section the direct course of the nerves passing through the spine defect to the border of the cyst can be seen.

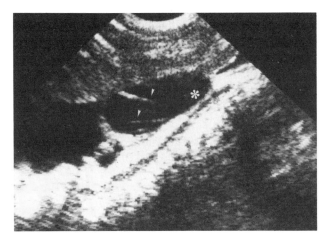

Fig. 5   Spina bifida with myelomeningocele in the lumbo-sacral area (38 weeks' gestation).
* Defect of the spinal wall. ↙ String-like echoes within the cystic mass behind the spinal defect.

In cases of reduced amniotic fluid, without optimal position of the fetus, the spina bifida cystica can be mistaken for an area of amniotic fluid or for a placental cyst. Longer observation however shows a synchronous movement of the cystic mass with fetal movements. Regarding the growth pattern in fetuses having spina bifida, a reduced growth of the fetal head is often found. Wald et al. [3] found in 20 fetuses with spina bifida that the mean bi-parietal diameter was 16% less than that of unaffected fetuses. Hansmann [2] also observed in spina bifida cases to start with a microcephalic growth pattern, which was compensated by the later development of hydrocephaly. Each observation of a reduced growth pattern of the fetal head in early pregnancy should call for a control of the fetal spine for a possible defect.

For the prognosis of the affected fetus not only the position of the defect is important but also the malformations which are associated with the NTD. Sonographic diagnosis should not only be limited to the proof of a spinal defect, but must result in an exact sonographic search for further malformations such as hydrocephaly, anencephaly, club-foot, cleft lip and palate or eventeration.

Intrauterine fetal limb movement was studied in the hope to determine whether ultrasound examination could reveal early evidence of paralysis, but it appears that for this no clear prognosis is a yet possible. Campbell [1] found in 2 cases having major lesions, limb movements, which were apparently normal. In our observations of 2 fetuses an apparently normal limb movement could also be seen, but the children showed post partum a partial paralysis of the lower limbs.

We conclude that in exact sonographic examination spina bifida can be prenatally detected or ruled out, whereas in the routine ultrasound examination a spinal defect is often overlooked. For these reasons an AFP estimation should be made at least from the maternal serum. If the AFP-level is raised an accurate ultrasound examination can then be performed in order to detect the size and position of the spinal defect. However the accuracy of the ultrasound examination depends greatly on the experience of the investigator, a sufficient amount of amniotic fluid and a normal position of the fetus. Small defects in the lumbo-sacral area can remain undetected, especially if there is a breech presentation deep in the pelvis.

References

[1] Campbell, S.: Early prenatal diagnosis of neural tube defects by ultrasound. Clin. Obst. Gynecol. **20** (1977) 351 – 359.
[2] Hansmann, M.: Nachweis und Ausschluß fetaler Entwicklungsstörungen mittels Ultraschallscreening und gezielter Untersuchung – ein Mehrstufenkonzept. Ultraschall **2** (1981) 206 – 220.
[3] Wald, N., H. Cuckle, J. Boreham et al.: Small biparietal diameter of fetuses with spina bifida: implications for antenatal screening. Brit. J. Obstet. Gynaecol. **87** (1980) 219 – 221.

Midtrimester prenatal diagnosis of neural tube defects following amniocentesis and selective termination of pregnancy in South Wales 1973 – 1983*

K. M. Laurence, J. O. Dew, C. Dyer

Introduction

Prenatal diagnosis of neural tube defect (NTD) in midtrimester, by means of amniocentesis followed by amniotic alphafetoprotein (AFP) estimation and other biochemical tests and then selective termination of pregnancies shown to be of an abnormal fetus, has become an essential part of the management of the pregnancy at increased risk of NTD [1]. Sophisticated ultrasonography (USS) for the detection of NTD (anencephaly as well as spina bifida) is increasingly used not only in high risk pregnancies but as a screening procedure. Any suspicious USS findings should be followed by a diagnostic amniocentesis as should any abnormal serum AFP levels in pregnancy NTD screening programmes [2, 3]. Between 1973, when prenatal diagnosis for NTD in midtrimester first became available in South Wales, and the end of 1981, over 3,800 amniocenteses have been carried out for NTD indications alone. This paper is concerned with the outcome of these pregnancies and the findings in some of the terminated fetuses.

Materials and methods (tab. 1)

3,849 amniotic fluids, on pregnancies either known to be at increased risk for NTD, with a suspicious USS finding or a raised serum AFP result in an NTD screening programme [4, 5] nearly all from amniocenteses carried out at the University Hospital of Wales were sent for AFP estimation. Up to the beginning of 1978, in addition to having the AFP measured, all fluids also had amnion cell culture carried out for chromosome analysis. However, from that time onwards this was done only on those fluids from pregnancies where there was a definite "chromosome indication" or where the woman was aged 30 years or over. Since

---

* Based in part on a paper published in Prenatal Diagnosis [9].

the beginning of 1979 fluids from problem cases (blood contaminated fluids, those from gestations of 19 weeks or more, and those with equivocal, borderline raised or with frankly abnormally raised AFP levels) also had a gel-electrophoresis for iso-enzymes of acetyl cholinesterase [6 – 8] carried out before any offer of a termination of pregnancy was made.

Nearly all the fetuses terminated as a result of the amniocentesis programme were sent for detailed pathological examination and where relevant or possible, for chromosome analysis as well. However, as the terminations had mostly been carried out with extra-amniotic prostaglandin some of the fetuses were quite macerated precluding chromosomal analysis or a detailed examination of the brain. All continuing pregnancies have been followed up to term and any fetal abnormalities present have been recorded.

Results

Outcome of pregnancies terminated for fetal malformation

The largest group, the 1,411 pregnancies that came to amniocentesis because the normality of the fetus was called to question following a raised maternal serum AFP level led to the termination of 144 fetuses with an NTD, 70 with anencephalus, 74 with "open" spina bifida and four with encephalocele (tab. 1). Two of the four encephaloceles had Meckel-Gruber's syndrome (Dysencephalia splanchnocystica) with what appears to have been "closed" and quite small encephaloceles.

The second most common indication for amniocentesis was where the pregnancy was known to be at increased risk for NTD because the mother had previously had a pregnancy with an NTD fetus or occasionally because the father has had a child with an NTD in a previous marriage/liaison. Monitoring the 1294 such pregnancies led to the termination of 29 fetuses with an NTD (17 with

Table 1   Amniocenteses for NTD indications 1973 – 1983 and termination of pregnancy

Indications	No	Malformations terminated					
		An	SBC	En	Exomp	Chrom	Other
Previous NTD	1294	17	11	1	–	3	1
FH of NTD	938	4	1	–	2	3	2
Parent with NTD	62	–	–	–	–	–	–
Raised serum AFP	1411	70	74	4	13	3	2
Other indications	144	17	2	–	–	1	1
Totals	3849	108	88	5	15	10	6

anencephalus, 11 with "open" spina bifida and one with encephalocele), two with Down's syndrome and a normal looking fetus with a dubious chromosome anomaly mosaicism which had probably arisen spontaneously in the amnion cell culture [9]. The parents of this "mosaic" elected to have what was really an unwanted pregnancy terminated as they could not be assured absolutely of the fetal normality. Another pregnancy was terminated because of possible rubella embryopathy.

No fetal abnormalities were found in the 62 pregnancies monitored because one parent him or herself had spina bifida, most frequently of the "complicated" spina bifida occulta variety [10].

In one of these the amniotic AFP was elevated while the other was associated with a normal amniotic AFP level but suspicious USS led to a positive fetoscopic diagnosis. The other two cases of encephalocele were associated with an elevated amniotic AFP level one of whom also had a very abnormal USS. In addition, four pregnancies of fetuses with exomphalos and 9 with gastroschisis, three with chromosome abnormalities were terminated. The latter three were a severely phenotypically abnormal true hermaphrodite with a 46XX/46XY chromosome constitution. Two pregnancies of a normal fetus were also terminated and two phenotypically normal fetuses, a female with 47XXX and a male with 48XXXY. (see below).

The 144 amniocenteses carried out for "other indications" included history of hydrocephalus without SBC, mental retardation or microcephaly and those where there was a suspicious finding on routine antenatal USS. 19 pregnancies with an NTD (17 anencephalus and 2 open spina bifida), one with a chromosome abnormality (Trisomy 18) and one with a bone dysplasia (lethal type of osteogenesis imperfecta) were terminated.

Malformations missed or indentified but not terminated

Six NTD's were identified but the pregnancies were deliberately not terminated. Three couples, having had an "open" NTD identified changed their minds about having a termination carried out. Three twin pregnancies, where only one co-twin was shown to have an NTD were allowed to go to term with the delivery of one normal surviving child in each case. In addition one pregnancy diagnosed to be of an NTD ("open" spina bifida) miscarried spontaneously before the planned termination could be carried out.

"Closed" NTD's remained undetected as did cases of hydrocephalus unassociated with spina bifida. All these might possibly have been identified by careful high precision USS. One case of Down's syndrome was born to a mother of 32 where amnion cell culture and chromosome analysis was mistakenly omitted.

There were 4 pregnancies where the amniotic fluid contained only a marginally elevated amount of AFP where the pregnancy was not terminated, including one where the obstetrician made this decision against the advice of the other clinicians involved. All these pregnancies ended about term in newborn infants, three of them with large "open" lesions, none of whom survived beyond 3 months. The fourth resulted in an infant with a quite small "open" sacral spina bifida who is surviving with no hydrocephalus but incontinence and relatively little limb paralysis. All the women concerned had their amniocentesis before 1979 and now in all of them the pregnancy would probably have been offered termination as on retrospective testing of the amniotic fluid a second acetyl cholinesterase band was [11] seen on gel-electrophoresis.

False positive AFP results and termination of pregnancies with a normal fetus

There were two false positive amniotic AFP results. In one an amniotic AFP level of 72 mg/l in a clear amniotic fluid taken at 16 weeks from a high risk woman who had a normal USS led to a termination of an apparently normal fetus. Congenital nephrosis was excluded by electromicroscopy of the kidneys. In the other the mother concerned had a stillborn NTD following her first pregnancy. She had an amniocentesis and AFP estimation carried out elsewhere in the next pregnancy. Because the AFP level was considerably elevated the pregnancy was terminated, but the fetus was reported as entirely normal. In her third pregnancy, an amniocentesis at 20 weeks again yielded amniotic fluid with an elevated AFP level (43 mg/l). This time the parents elected not to have a termination and a "normal" infant was born at term who had abnormalities of one external ear and who then developed normally. These were true false positives where no explanantion for the raised AFP level has been found. In neither of these cases tested before 1979 was a gel-electrophoresis carried out. Examined retrospectively neither amniotic fluids contained isoenzymes of acetylcholinesterase [12].

One pregnancy of a normal fetus was terminated in spite of contrary advice. The woman concerned, with no history of NTD had a greatly elevated serum AFP level at 16 weeks. Two amniocenteses yielded clear amniotic fluid containing raised AFP levels but with normal gel acetylcholinesterase electrophoresis results. In spite of repeated high precision USS with normal appearances the parents were too worried about the normality of the fetus to continue with the pregnancy.

Findings in anencephalic fetuses terminated

Those fetuses with anencephaly only tended to have a relatively normal body form and few other defects. Those that had spinal rachischisis or spina bifida in addition, often had other abnormalities and malformations such as leg abnormal-

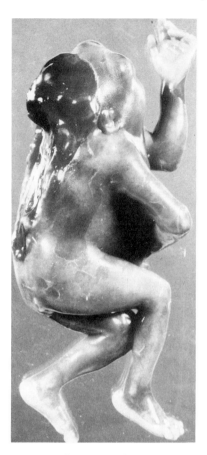

Fig. 1   A 19 week fetus with a florid anencephalus and spinal rachischisis.

ities, exomphalos, cleft palate, pulmonary hypoplasia and horseshoe kidney. In both groups the central nervous system lesions tended to be more florid than those seen at term (fig. 1), with better organised and preserved central nervous system tissue in which areas reminiscent of cerebral cortex, cerebellum and choroid plexus could be recognised. Presumably much of this tissue normally degenerates between mid-trimester and term. An anterior pituitary could usually be found. The suprarenal glands at this stage of development were relatively larger than in anencephalics delivered nearer term.

Findings in spina bifida fetuses terminated

Eighty eight spina bifida fetuses were referred for pathological examination. Those fetuses terminated because of a raised maternal serum AFP led to the detection of the abnormality, tended to be of greater gestational age than those

Table 2   Spina bifida fetuses — gestation at termination

Gestation	Reason for amniocentesis Raised serum AFP	Previous NTD FH of NTD
16	–	1
17	9	3
18	14	2
19	10	3
20	22	2
21	9	–
22	6	–
22	6	1
Total	76	12

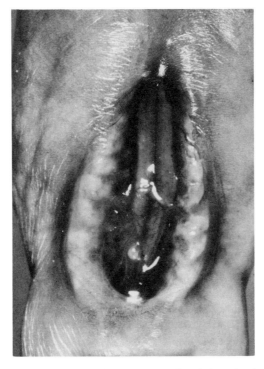

Fig. 2   A 20 week fetus with a large open florid dorso-lumbar spina bifida.

detected in women who were at increased risk because of a positive obstetric or family history (tab. 2). For a maternal serum AFP to be as informative as possible, blood for the test is not normally taken until 16 or 17 weeks [13]. By the time the AFP level is found to be raised, an amniocentesis is organised, the amniotic

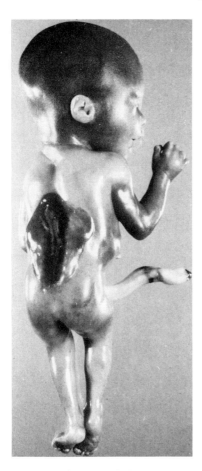

Fig. 3   A 20 week fetus with hydrocephalus and a large open dorso-lumbar spina bifida. The head
is somewhat unusual in that it is enlarged and shows the typical hydrocephalic shape.

AFP level is found to be elevated the termination is often not carried out until the
19th or 20th week. In a high risk pregnancy, on the other hand, an amniocentesis is
generally timed for the 15th or 16th week of gestation [14].

Due to the extra-amniotic prostaglandin technique used for many of the terminations, maceration was too advanced in 11 fetuses for the degree of hydrocephalus
or the severity of the Arnold-Chiari or both to be assessed properly. In mid-
trimester fetuses, the "open" spinal lesion also tends to be rather more florid
than that seen in infants born at or near term (fig. 2). In the better preserved
fetuses, the neural plaque was often covered with an ependyma-like layer of cells
and contained a fair number of neurons, sometimes organised into recognisable
centres. In the majority of the fetuses the head appeared normal in size and
shape, but in some it was obviously enlarged with a characteristic disproportion-

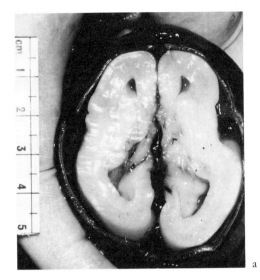 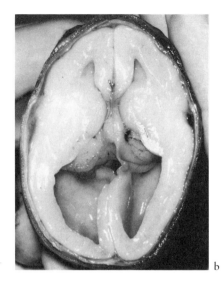

Fig. 4a and b   The transected head of a normal 20 week fetus (terminated for social reasons) showing that the ventricular system is more than a "potential space" (a). The transected head of a 20 week fetus with spina bifida. Hydrocephalus is well established and of + + degree by our classification. The dilatation is most severe in the occipital horns and the cerebral mantle is considerably reduced (b).

ately large vault and frontal bossing (fig. 3). In all but 8 of the 86 fetuses (fig. 8) in which ventricular size could be assessed, hydrocephalus was already present though this was only mild in 14. Ventricular dilatation affecting the lateral and third ventricles symmetrically was marked in 26 and severe in a further 13 and usually most pronounced in the posterior horns (figs. 4a and b). The severity of the ACM which could be assessed in 78 fetuses (fig. 8) was present to some degree in all but 9 and was quite pronounced in 35 (fig. 5). The more severely dilated ventricles tended to be associated with a more pronounced ACM but there were notable exceptions (fig. 6). The degree of hydrocephalus as well as the severity of the ACM bore some relation to the level of the spinal lesion and with some exceptions, both tended to be less marked in association with the lower spinal defects (figs. 7a and b), and both were entirely absent in four with sacral lesions.

There seemed to be no obvious relationship between the total size of the spinal lesion or of the area of the neural plaque and the AFP content of the amniotic fluid, even when allowances were made for the gestation at which both the amniocentesis and the termination had been carried out. There also seemed to be no obvious relationship between the degree of hydrocephalus and the level of amniotic AFP. In about one fifth of the fetuses (16 cases) spina bifida and any associated hydrocephalus and ACM were the only malformations or deformities

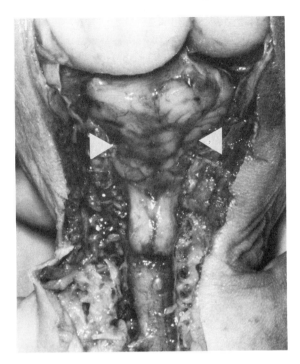

Fig. 5   The dissected posterior fossa of a 20 week fetus showing a well-developed Arnold-Chiari malformation. The arrows indicate the level of the foramen magnum.

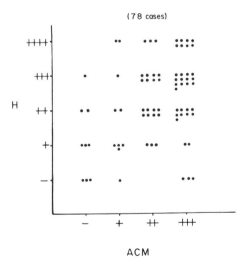

Fig. 6   Mid-trimester spina bifida fetuses. The relationship between the degree of hydrocephalus (H) and the severity of the Arnold-Chiari malformation (ACM).

detected. Many of the remainder showed club foot often bilateral, kyphosis or scoliosis. Most of the extracranial internal malformations were confined to the urinary tract with horseshoe kidney, agenesis of the kidney and polycystic kidney being found most frequently (tab. 3). Four fetuses showed abnormalities of other systems; two had severe hyperplasia of both lungs, one ano-rectal agenesis and another had a cleft palate.

Table 3   Spina bifida fetuses (58 cases) associated abnormalities (other than ACM or hydrocephalus)

Scoliosis	5
Kyphosis	25
Unilateral TEV	15
Bilateral TEV	23
Polycystic kidney	2
Absent kidney (unilat)	2
Absent kidney (bilat)	3
Horseshoe kidney	5
Hydronephrosis	1
Hypoplastic lungs	2
Imperforate anus	1
Single umbilical artery	2
Cleft palate	1
No obvious malformations	16

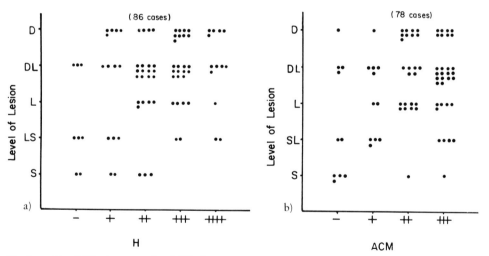

Fig. 7a and b   Mid-trimester spina bifida fetuses.
a) Relationship between the level of the spinal lesion and the degree of hydrocephalus (H). LD = dorso-lumbar; DS = dorso-lumbal-sacral; L = lumbar; LS = lumbo-sacral; S = sacral. (In one the degree of hydrocephalus could not be assessed.)
b) The relationship between the level of the spinal lesion and the severity of the ACM.

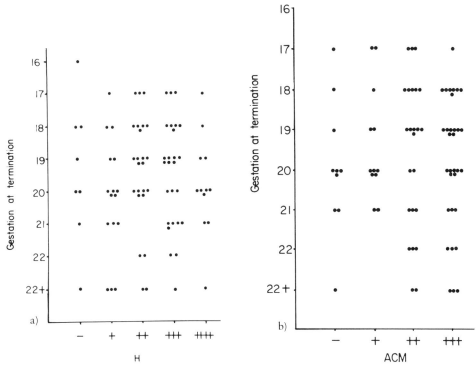

Fig. 8a and b   The relationship between gestation at termination and the degree of hydrocephalus (H) in the 87 fetuses and the degree of the Arnold-Chiari malformation (ACM) in the 78 fetuses in which an assessment was possible.

Other fetuses terminated

The cases of encephalocele and the normal fetuses have already been referred to. The two "rubella" fetuses were also normal and no virus was recovered. The cases of Down's syndrome looked remarkably normal at termination, showing few characteristic facial features or single palmar creases [15]. For this reason alone the diagnosis must be confirmed from the terminated fetus. The amniotic AFP level was of no help in distinguishing between the pregnancies of fetuses with the relatively operable exomphalos and the fetuses with the more serious gastroschisis. The cases of gastroschisis did not show the degree of secondary pathology usually seen in such infants born at term.

Discussion

Prenatal diagnosis of NTD using amniotic AFP levels is a quite reliable investigation in the hands of experienced and careful clinicians [16, 17]. The chance of equivocal AFP levels being obtained at between 15 and 19 weeks gestation is small and false positive results, which are tragic if they lead to the mistaken termination of a normal fetus, are relatively uncommon, but they are reckoned to occur without explanation once in 500 amniotic fluids [18, 19]. In this series the incidence of the latter was only about 1 in 2000 amniocenteses [20]. However, neither the difficulties with equivocal AFP levels, nor with mistaken terminations of normal fetuses need occur if repeat high precision USS and gel-electrophoresis for iso-enzymes of acetylcholinesterase are routinely carried out following all equivocal or borderline raised and obviously raised amniotic AFP results before an offer of termination of pregnancy is made. Though an invasive procedure, the risk of amniocentesis precipitating sequential miscarriage, fetal death or damage is generally less than 1% [21].

In any antenatal diagnosis programme all abortuses should be examined by the laboratory associated with the prenatal diagnostic service and all pregnancies followed up, only in this way can a check be kept on the efficiency of the service [22]. Malformations and abnormalities identified antenatally must be confirmed from the fetus, something that is especially important with chromosome anomalies and biochemical disorders. The amniotic AFP level is quite unhelpful in distinguishing between the smaller and possibly less serious 'open' spinal abnormalities from the large spinal inoperable lesions, but only the 'open' from the "closed" [23, 24]. To some extent, anencephaly can be separated from spina bifida, the former often being associated with very high AFP levels only rarely seen with the latter.

In our cases, as in those of others [25, 26], the pattern of hydrocephalus and ACM in the mid-trimester fetus is remarkably similar to that seen in the full term neonate with spina bifida with a proportion of sacral lesions escaping one or both [27, 28]. Both the hydrocephalus and the ACM are well established by 16 weeks and also do not seem to increase in severity with increasing gestation between 16 and 23 weeks. These findings suggest even if the technical problems are overcome, that any attempts at intrauterine treatment of the hydrocephalus are likely to have poor results as the hydrocephalus is already well established by 16 weeks. They also mean that information as to the causation and sequence of events therefore have to be obtained from fetuses of shorter gestation than 16 weeks.

Referral for amniocentesis for NTD indications have risen very greatly with greater public and professional familiarity with this investigation; referrals are likely to rise further in the immediate future. However, this is not only an invasive procedure with a finite if small risk of pregnancy wastage as well as a somewhat drawn out anxiety provoking process [29–31] for the parents who generally have to wait up to a week for the results and much longer if amnion culture and chromosome analysis is also carried out. For these reasons it is likely to be at least partially replaced by high precision USS now that the apparatus is becoming increasingly sophisticated and versatile and the operators are becoming more skilled [32]. The non-invasive USS is apparently safe and is able to detect also closed NTD as well as an increasing number of other abnormalities.

However, to avoid terminating pregnancies with a normal fetus, or some forms of spina bifida occulta, positive USS findings may well have to be followed by a diagnostic amniocentesis and chemical investigation of the amniotic fluid and occasionally by fetoscopy. Hopefully however, the need for prenatal diagnosis of NTD and selective termination which, after all is only secondary prevention and is not acceptable for some, will become increasingly unnecessary. Primary prevention of NTD using both improvement in the maternal nutrition [33, 34] and preconceptional supplementation with folic acid [35, 36] or multivitamin preparations containing folic acid [37] offered eventually to women not only those at increased risk for NTD, but to all women planning a pregnancy whether at increased risk or not, will hopefully reduce substantially the number of fetuses that develop NTD and reduce the need for prenatal diagnosis and pregnancy screening for NTD [38].

References

[1] Laurence, K. M.: Preparation of neural tube defects by genetic counselling prenatal diagnostic surveillance and pregnancy screening. J. Genetic Hum. 24 (1979) 289 – 299.
[2] Roberts, C. J., B. M. Hibbard, G. H. Elder et al.: Efficacy of a serum AFP screening service for neural tube defect: the South Wales experience. Lancet I (1983) 1315 – 1318.
[3] U. K. Collaborative Study: Maternal serum alphafetoprotein measurement in the antenatal screening for anencephaly and spina bifida in early pregnancy. Lancet I (1977) 1323 – 1332.
[4] Barlow, R. D., H. S. Cuckle, N. J. Wald: A simple method for amniotic fluid gelacetyl cholinesterase determination suitable for routine use in antenatal diagnosis of open neural tube defect. Clin. Chem. Acta. 119 (1982) 137 – 142.
[5] Smith, A. D., N. J. Wald, H. S. Cuckle et al.: Amniotic fluid acetylcholinesterase as a possible diagnostic test for neural tube defects in early pregnancy, Lancet I (1979) 665 – 668.
[6] Wyrill, P. C., D. A. Hullin, G. H. Elder et al.: Prospective study of amniotic fluid cholinesterases: comparison of quantitative and qualitative methods for the detection of open neural tube defects. Prenatal diagnosis 4 (1984) 319 – 327.
[7] Kajii, T.: Pseudomosaicism in cultured amniotic cells. Lancet II (1971) 1037.
[8] Laurence, K. M., A. S. Bligh, K. T. Evans et al.: Vertebral abnormalities in parents and sibs of cases of spina bifida cystica and anencephaly. Proceedings of the 13th Congress of Paediatrics, vol. V (1971) 415 – 421.
[9] Laurence, K. M., J. O. Dew, C. Dyer et al.: Amniocentesis carried out for neural tube indications in South Wales 1973 – 1981: outcome of pregnancies and findings in the malformed abortuses. Prenatal Diagnosis 3 (1983) 187 – 201.
[10] Laurence, K. M., P. J. Gregory: Prenatal diagnosis of chromosome abnormality. In: Pathology Annual, vol. 8 (H. J. Ioachim, ed.), pp. 155 – 188. Raven Press, New York 1978.

[11] Laurence, K. M., P. A. David, M. O. Carter: The major central nervous system malformations in South Wales. I. Incidence local variations and geographical factors, Brit. J. Prev. Soc. Med. **22** (1968) 146–160.

[12] U. K. Collaborative Study: Second report of the U. K. collaborative Study on alphafetoprotein in relation to neural tube defects: Alphafetoprotein measurements in the diagnosis of anencephaly and open spina bifida in early pregnancy, Lancet **II** (1979) 651–662.

[13] Medical Research Council Working Party on Amniocentesis. An assessment of the hazards of amniocentesis, Brit. J. Obstet. Gynaec., 85, Suppl., 2. Wales 1964–66. Brit. J. Prev. Soc. Med. **52** (1978) 59–64.

[14] Wald, N. J., H. S. Cuckle: Alphafetoprotein in the antenatal diagnosis of open neural tube defects, Brit. J. Hosp. Med. **24** (1980) 473–489.

[15] Bell, J. E.: The pathology of central nervous system defects in human fetuses of different gestational ages. In: Advances in the Study of Birth Defects (T. V. N. Persand, ed.), vol. 7, pp. 1–17. MTP Press, Lancaster 1983.

[16] Bell, J. E., A. Gordon, A. F. J. Maloney: Association of hydrocephalus and Arnold Chiari malformation in the spina bifida fetus, Neuropath. Appl. Neurobiol. **6** (1980) 29.

[17] Laurence, K. M.: The natural history of spina bifida: detailed analysis of 407 cases, Arch. Dis. Childh. **39** (1964) 41–57.

[18] Laurence, K. M., B. J. Tew: The natural history of Spina Bifida Cystica and Cranium Bifidum Cysticum: the central nervous system malformations in South Wales Part IV, Arch. Dis. Childh. **46** (1971) 127–138.

[19] Laurence, K. M., J. Morris: The effect of introduction of prenatal diagnosis on the reproductive history of women at risk from neural tube defects, Prenatal Diagnosis **1** (1981) 51–60.

[20] Carter, J., K. M. Laurence: Genetic counselling for neural tube defect high risk couples during pregnancy: is this the optimum time to attend. Biology and Society (in press).

[21] Fearn, J., B. M. Hibbard, K. M. Laurence et al.: Screening for neural tube defects and maternal anxiety. Brit. J. Obstet, Gynaec. **89** (1982) 218–221.

[22] Laurence, K. M.: Towards prevention of neural tube defects: discussion paper, J. Roy. Soc. Med. **75** (1982) 723–728.

[23] Laurence, K. M., N. James, M. Miller et al.: The increased risk of recurrence of neural tube defects to mothers on poor diets and the possible benefit of dietary counselling, Brit. Med. J. **4** (1980) 1592–1593.

[24] Laurence, K. M., H. Campbell, N. James: The role of improvement in the maternal diet and preconceptional folic acid supplementation in the preventation of neural tube defects. In: Prevention of Spina Bifida and Other Neural Tube Defects (J. Dobbing, ed.), pp. 85–106. Academic Press, London 1983.

[25] Laurence, K. M., N. James, M. H. Miller et al.: Double blind randomized controlled trial of preconceptional folate therapy to prevent recurrence of neural tube defects, Brit. Med. J. **2** (1981) 1509–1511.

[26] Smithells, R. W., S. Sheppard, C. J. Shorah et al.: Possible prevention of neural tube defects by preconceptional vitamin supplementation, Lancet **I** (1980) 339–340.

Termination of pregnancy for fetal malformation*

K. M. Laurence, J. Lloyd

Introduction

Much work has been done on the psychological consequences of termination of pregnancy for medico-social reasons carried out generally in the first trimester of pregnancy. Such terminations usually are of pregnancies which are unplanned and unwanted. Handy [1], in a review of the literature, concluded that although some women may experience adverse psychological sequelae, the great majority do not. The importance of counselling and follow-up in preventing such sequelae in those women who may be vulnerable has been stressed by Pare and Raven [2], Lask [3], and more recently by Schmidt and Priest [4]. Few terminations for medico-social reasons are carried out after 20 weeks gestation and there is little information on these. However, Brewer [5] in his series found that the emotional consequences were less marked than might have been expected when late terminations, took place after fetal movements had been felt. With the advent of prenatal diagnostic tests, terminations of a wanted pregnancy usually at or about 20 weeks gestation, with a fetus shown to be abnormal, according to Laurence [6], now accounts for about 1% of total terminations. With the exception of a small study from Manchester [7] which noted the difficulties experienced by patients in coming to terms with the ending of a wanted and planned pregnancy, such terminations do not seem to have been extensively studied.

A retrospective case comparison study was carried out to investigate the psycho-social consequences of such termination. It was designed to demonstrate the attitudes and emotions experienced immediately post-termination and those symptoms still present 6 months later. The hypothesis, which was developed during a pilot study being that women undergoing a late termination for fetal malformation experience an acute grief reaction similar to that following stillbirth or neonatal death.

Methods

The subjects for the study were the 73 women resident in the County of Mid-Glamorgan (in South Wales) who had a termination of pregnancy between 1977

---

* This paper is based on one published in the British Medical Journal (in press).

and 1981 following positive tests either during the alphafetoprotein screening programme for neural tube defect, or because they were known to be at increased risk for the latter or chromosome abnormality. Each had attended one of the antenatal clinics of the four district general hospitals in the Mid Glamorgan Health Authority district and thence being referred by one of twelve consultant obstetricians to the University of Wales for pre-natal diagnostic tests. The terminations were performed at the referring hospital.

The agreement of the relevant obstetrician and general practitioner was sought before a written approach was made to each patient for permission to interview in her own home. Thirteen of the cases could not be contacted either because they had moved out of the area and were inaccessible or had changed their name and could not be traced. Seven of the remaining 60 declined to help in the study and in a further five cases the general practitioners advised against an approach either because of current pregnancy (4 patients) or illness (1 patient). The remaining 48 women were therefore approached and interviewed by the same observer (J. L.) using a semistructured interview schedule, developed following the pilot study in another Health District. This was designed to record:

1. Emotions and attitudes immediately after the termination.

2. Symptoms within 6 weeks, post-termination, and until routine hospital "post-natal" or gynaecological out-patient appointment.

3. Symptoms persisting to such an extent that treatment by general practitioner or a referral to a psychiatrist was indicated.

4. The nature of any follow-up support available within the first 6 weeks post-termination and the timing of any referral for formal genetic counselling.

Data on other personal and social variables which may affect the reaction and its resolution were also collected during the interview. Following the formal part of the interview, ample time was allowed for free discussion. The content of this was noted by the observer in private immediately after the conclusion of the home visit.

Projected comparison groups of women who had previously had a termination for medico-social reasons at a similar late gestational age and those who had experienced a stillbirth without malformation proved impractical. However, comparison groups from within the study group were constructed by categorising from previous obstetric history. Twelve had previously had one or more spontaneous abortions, six had a previous stillbirth or neonatal death and four had a previous termination early in pregnancy for medico-social reasons. Responses following these episodes were recorded in the same manner as for the index termination. All interviews were carried out between August 1982 and February 1983.

Results

The number of acute grief reactions noted after the termination for fetal malformation and after previous stillbirth or neonatal death was high (77% and 84% respectively) (tab. 1) and in sharp contrast to the reactions following spontaneous abortion or termination for medico-social reasons. These results are highly significant (p < 0.001 using Yates correction). The severity of the reaction ranged from mild tearfulness with sadness, to lethargy and insomnia to incapacitating grief with somatic symptoms, and finally to complete withdrawal. Two subjects demonstrated a delayed bereavement reaction but in the main resolution proceeded but at six months 22 women recalled that they still had symptoms of depression with some anxiety. The symptoms leading to treatment were depressive – often with considerable repressed anger.

Fifteen women were seen by one of us (K. M. L.) for genetic counselling at the University Hospital of Wales at the time of referral for the high precision ultrasound scan and amniocentesis. This was frequently seen as part of the distressing diagnostic routine and was not perceived as helpful for the future.

Table 1   Maternal reaction following ending of pregnancy

	Termination for fetal malformation	Stillbirth or neonatal death	Spontaneous abortion	Termination for medico-social reasons
Total number	48	6	12	4
Acute grief	37	5	1	0
Symptoms at six months	22	0	0	0
Treatment needed	10	0	0	0

Table 2   The perception of genetic counselling

	Genetic Counselling at amniocentesis	Genetic Counselling 6 – 16 weeks post-termination
Helpful	5	12
Not helpful	9	3
Equivocal	1	1
Total seen	15	16

Eight of the above together with a further eight, not counselled previously, were referred (by the general practitioner or consultant obstetrician) for genetic counselling at a later date when the emotional crisis was over (tab. 2). This was generally perceived as helpful.

Support immediately post-termination was remarkably sparse. Although all women had a routine hospital out-patient or general practitioner appointment at about six weeks post-termination, only eight of the 48 had any kind of home visit in the first few days after hospital discharge post-termination and in three of these it was a friend or relative in the nursing profession who called. In contrast women who had experienced a stillbirth all had a home visit and all four women who had earlier had a termination for medico-social reasons were also supported by post-termination counselling. However, 29 subjects did visit their general practitioner at some stage in the first six weeks after termination (tab. 3).

Table 3   Reasons for general practitioner attendance post termination

Reason for visit	Number of subjects
Certificate only	7
Routine "postnatal"	2
Mastitis or lactation	7
Haemorrhage	1
Urinary infection	4
Depression	8
Total	29

Discussion

These results suggest that the response to the late termination of a wanted pregnancy challenged as a consequence of advances in prenatal diagnostic techniques often is an acute grief reaction, similar to that following still birth which is akin to that following any death – a bereavement reaction. This is not a psychiatric disorder but is a normal process which may require formal psychiatric intervention or other professional help if resolution does not occur and depression supervenes. Our patients did not have the normal aids to the resolution of grief generally available under other circumstances. Twelve of the 48 women in the study group had not embarked on a further pregnancy by the time of interview and eleven of these demonstrated marked grief reactions which in eight subjects had not resolved at six months and in five this was severe enough to require psychiatric help and three women became severely emotionally disturbed. The severity of the reaction in our study may have been because in general mourning was difficult — there was no grave, no baby, no photograph and only occasionally was the fetus seen. The "death" was passed over, denied, regarded as a failure of pregnancy and the mother was met by a conspiracy of silence. However, 35 of the patients recounted some form of a mourning process. Eleven women volunteered that they had named the fetus, usually secretly and this seemed to help the process. One woman visited the local cemetery regularly and several would have liked some form of burial of formal recognition of the death. The paucity of follow-up at home did not allow conclusions to be drawn regarding the impact of support in this study. However, experience following stillbirth suggests that this is important in the resolution of grief and it is reasonable to assume our group would respond to support [8].

Supportive evidence for the identification of this response as different from that following the more usual termination for medico-social reasons comes from Brewer's study [5]. In his series 25% noted mild symptoms at three months post-termination and not one required any psychiatric help. These patients had pre- and post-termination counselling which may account for the milder reactions and, in any case, the characteristics of their reactions were not suggestive of bereavement.

The lack of coordinated home visiting post-termination was surprising. Most of the terminations for fetal malformation took place on gynaecological wards and liaison between these and midwives in the community, antenatal clinics and general practitioners was not as effective as between the same professionals and the obstetric services. Staff on the gynaecological wards often assumed that these terminations were no different from the termination for medico-social reasons. In view of the rarity of the procedure in each one of the hospitals over several years, the severity of the reaction was unsuspected and the assumption probably made that the elaborate pre- and post-termination counselling arrangements made for terminations for medico-social reasons automatically applied to this different category. Ten of our series had either had previous stillbirth, were of advanced maternal age or had a strong family history of congenital malformation and thus could have been described as embarking on the pregnancy with some insight and might therefore have been, to some degree, prepared. However, eight of these demonstrated an acute grief reaction no different from the others.

It was not possible to measure the impact of genetic counselling at the time of tests on the severity of the reaction to termination as the number of patients seen was too small. Many women stated that they needed more information and advice. Although the routine hospital follow up at 6 weeks was uniformly efficient as a post-operative or postnatal check, there was generally no opportunity for the involved and highly personal attention many needed. For those referred, genetic counselling post-termination was therefore understandably appreciated. A lack of information was also recorded pre-termination. As the pre-natal diagnostic tests took place before the routine ante-natal clinic health education programme could explain parturition and the post-partum routines to the primigravidae, the normal sequelae of childbirth were therefore unexpected. Whether or not this was the first pregnancy, lactation and mastitis were distressing. However, in view of these and the other problems, surprisingly few presented to the general practitioner.

Conclusions

In spite of the flaws in experimental design, the response to termination for fetal malformation under the study conditions was identified as similar to that following perinatal death. From our study, it was apparent that with the advances in pre-natal diagnostic techniques, provision of support after termination had not proceeded at the same rate and services had not developed to meet an unperceived need. There are several implications which follow from this.

1. Better liaison between ante-natal clinics, obstetric departments, gynaecology wards, general practitioners and community services would ensure that patients did not return home without information or support. In some centres, minimal reorganization or services might be required.

2. We would suggest that support should be organised as following perinatal death and that supportive counselling commencing early in the first six weeks post-termination be undertaken by a skilled health care professional (e.g. genetic clinic field workers, health visitor, community midwife or general practitioner). For those patients where resolution fails to ensue, later referral to a bereavement counsellor or psychiatrist might be indicated. Support should be clearly coordinated.

3. For terminations for fetal malformation, genetic counselling is indicated and we suggest that all women, whether or not they had been counselled during pregnancy, should be seen by a skilled genetic counsellor not earlier than six weeks after the termination and preferably at about three months.

4. Following from above, hospital-based and community staff should have appropriate training to understand the nature of the termination under these conditions to enable the patient's needs to be identified and met.

References

[1] Handy, Jocelyn A.: Psychological and social aspects of induced abortion. Brit. J. Clin. Psychol. **21** (1982) 29 – 49.

[2] Pare, C. M. B., H. Raven: Follow-up of patients referred for termination of pregnancy. Lancet **I** (1970) 653 – 658.

[3] Lask, B.: Short-term psychiatric sequelae to therapeutic termination of pregnancy. Brit. J. Psychiat. **126** (1975) 173 – 177.

[4] Schmidt, R., R. G. Priest: The effects of termination of pregnancy. A follow-up study of psychiatric referrals. Brit. J. Med. Psychol. **54** (1981) 267 – 276.

[5] Brewer: Induced abortion after feeling fetal movements: its causes and emotional consequences. J. Biosoc. Sci. **10** (1978) 203 – 208.

[6] Laurence, K. M.: Prenatal diagnosis, selective abortion and the abortion (amendment) bill. Lancet **I** (1980) 249 – 250.

[7] Donnai, P., N. Charles, R. Harris: Attitudes of patients after "genetic" termination of pregnancy. Brit. Med. J. **282** (1981) 621 – 622.

[8] Forrest, G. C., E. Standish, J. D. Baum: Support after perinatal death: a study of support and counselling after perinatal bereavement. Brit. Med. J. **285** (1982) 1475 – 1479.

Importance of computer-assisted cisternography and myelography for surgical treatment of cranial and spinal dysraphic malformations

A. Zieger, G. Düsterbehn, J. Pozo

Introduction

The neurosurgical treatment of cranial and spinal dysraphic malformations tends to prevent infectious complications, to preserve neurological functions and to favour the further development of the nervous system [1, 3, 9, 10]. Successful treatment depends on early detections and exact demonstration of the abnormalities. By computer-assisted cisternography and myelography the high computertomographic spatial resolution is combined with the positive-contrast visualization of the subarachnoidal spaces [4, 7]. These techniques permit a detailed presentation of occult abnormalities of the subarachnoidal spaces and the surrounding structures [2, 12–14]. We have examined the importance of computer-assisted cisternography and myelography for the surgical treatment of cranial and spinal dysraphic malformations.

Material

Since the introduction of computerized tomography (CT) in our hospital in 1978, 92 patients with cranial and spinal dysraphic malformations have been diagnosed and treated (tab. 1). These investigations were performed with a TOMOSCAN 210 and 310. 13 patients have been examined by computer-assisted cisternography and 28 patients by computer-assisted myelography (tab. 2).

Table 1   Cranial and spinal dysraphic malformations

1978 – 6/1984	n = 92
Myelo- and meningoceles	54
Cephaloceles	11
Dermal sinus tracts	12
Combinations	15
(tethering cord, malascensus, diastematomyelia, congenital tumours, syringomyelic cavitations, Dandy-Walker and Arnold-Chiari malformations, occult dysraphic state)	

Table 2   CT-cisternographic and CT-myelographic findings

CT-cisternography	n = 13
Arnold-Chiari malformation	2
Dandy-Walker malformation	1
Syringomyelia, Arnold-Chiari	3
Cephalocele	1
Exclusion	6

CT-myelography	n = 28
Myelo- and meningocele	7
Dermal sinus tract, malascensus, congenital tumour	5
Diastematomyelia, tethering cord, malascensus	6
Congenital tumour, diastematomyelia	4
Tethering cord	1
Exclusion	5

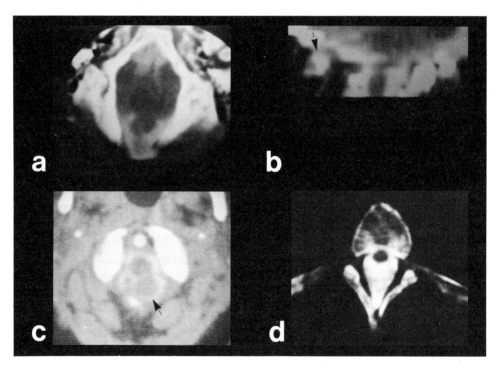

Fig. 1 a – d   CT-cisternogram (a – c), CT-myelogram (d). Suboccipital meningocele associated with a lipofibroma and herniation of cerebellar tonsils (a). Sagittal reconstruction of the same case with extracranial demonstration of contrast medium (arrow) (b). Arnold-Chiari malformation with ectopia of cerebellar tonsils (c). Occult spina bifida with a thoracal meningocele (d).

2 – 10 ml metrizamide of 170 – 270 mg/ml iodine concentration were intrathecally injected. The investigations were carried out in infancy and childhood mostly and in only eight adults. The examinations were performed, only if no reliable clues about the localization and the extent of the nervous tissue partizipation could be obtained by roentgenograms and unenhanced CT scans.

Results

By *CT-cisternography*, obliteration and compression of the subarachnoid spaces, non-communicating cysts, cavitations of the cervical spine and the level of cerebellar tonsil herniation (fig. 1c) could be precisely visualized. Also the exact size of cephalocele with associated congenital tumour could be clearly demon- strated (fig. 1a, b).

By *CT-myelography* cavitations of the spinal cord, myelomeningoceles (fig. 2f), dermal sinuses and fistulous tracts (fig. 2e), tetherings cord with malascensus, diastematomyelias with bony spurs (fig. 2c, d) and the exact intradural extent of congenital tumour could be revealed (fig. 2a, b).

The presence of nervous system abnormalities in cases of *occult* dysraphic malformations could be demonstrated or excluded by both methods. The use of sagittal reconstructions (fig. 1b, 2b) could be helpful to demonstrate the total extent of congenital tumours.

Discussion

Since the introduction of CT-cisternography by Greitz and Hindmarsh [7] and CT-myelography by Dichiro and Schellinger [4] numerous reports in the literature have emphasized the importance of these methods for the diagnosis of cranial and spinal dysraphic malformations [2, 5, 8, 11 – 14]. CT-cisternography and CT-myelography are safe and effective techniques which provide dynamic as well as morphologic information not readily available by routine CT-scanning alone [6, 8]. These techniques will be used if no exact information can be obtained by conventional radiological methods of the nervous tissue participation or the subarachnoidal space obliteration in developmental disorders [5, 6, 8, 13].

Our series shows that in cases of tethering cords, dermal sinuses and fistulous tracts, malascensus, splitted cords, congenital tumours, syringomyelic cavitations and myelomeningoceles the size and localization of nervous tissue abnormalities will be precisely demonstrated by CT-myelography. In cases of cranial dysraphic malformations, subarachnoid space obliteration, non-communicating cysts and

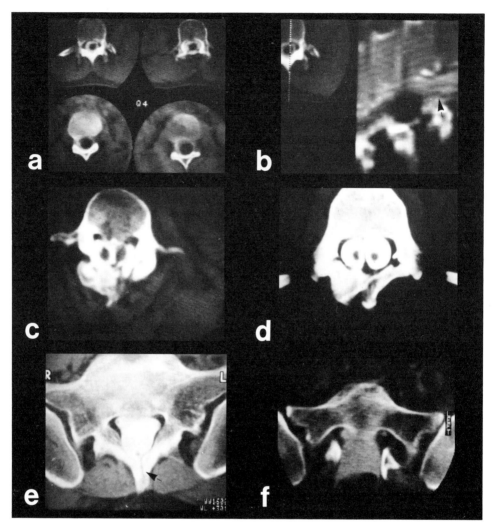

Fig. 2 a – f   CT-myelogram (a – f). Intramedullar lipoma of the conus (a). Sagittal reconstruction of the same case with lipoma and a tethering cord (b). Diastematomyelia (c, d) with malascensus and a bony spur (c). Intradural dermal sinus tract with an occult osseous channel at S₁ (e). Lipomeningocele without demonstration of nervous tissue structures within the contrast enhanced cele (f).

the level of the ectopia of the cerebellar tonsils and occult cephaloceles, will be exactly visualized by CT-cisternography.

It has been pointed out in the literature that early detection and surgical treatment improve the prognosis of dysraphic malformations of the neuro-axial compartments [1, 3, 9, 10]. Both CT-cisternography and CT-myelography make it possible to detect potentially treatable cranial and spinal dysraphic malformations and permit prophylactic surgical treatment.

In our series occult dysraphic malformations were detected in only eight adults. The complex cranial and spinal dysraphic state was effectively revealed by CT-cisternography and CT-myelography mostly in infancy and childhood. Surgical treatment could be performed directly and carefully using microsurgical techniques and gentle reconstructive methods. Therefore a further development of the nervous system and the neurological function could be preserved or improved.

Because of their increased risk, CT-cisternography and CT-myelography should be performed very selectively [15, 16]. Both methods can visualize low concentrations of contrast medium not seen in conventional cisternography and myelography.

Conclusion

CT-cisternography and CT-myelography are of considerable help in clarifying the extent and type of spinal and cranial dysraphic malformations in infancy, childhood and adulthood. The relationship of the subarachnoidal spaces and the nervous tissue can be accurately demonstrated. Both methods permit the early detection of developmental malformations not seen in conventional cisternography and myelography or unenhanced CT-scanning, especially in occult dysraphism. Therefore surgical treatment can be performed early, more directly and carefully, using microsurgical techniques and gentle reconstructive methods.

References

[1] Campbell, J. B.: Congenital anomalies of the neural axis. Surgical management based on embryologic considerations. Am. J. Surg. 75 (1948) 231 – 255.
[2] Claussen, C. D., F. W. Lohkamp, U. Banniza v. Bazan: The Diagnosis of Congenital Spinal Disorders in Computed Tomography (CT). Neuropädiatrie 4 (1977) 405 – 417.
[3] Cohn, G. A., W. B. Hamby: The surgery of cranium bifidum and spina bifida. A follow-up report of sixty-four cases. J. Neurosurg. 10 (1953) 297 – 300.
[4] DiChiro, G., D. Schellinger: Computed tomography of the spinal cord after lumbar intrathecal introduction of metrizamide (computer-assisted myelography). Radiol. 120 (1976) 101 – 104.
[5] Diebler, C., O. Dulac: Cephaloceles: Clinical and neuroradiological appearance. Associated cerebral malformation. Neuroradiology 25 (1983) 199 – 216.
[6] Di Lorenzo, N., L. Bozzazo, D. Antonelli et al.: Arnold-Chiari Malformation Detected by Unenhanced Multiplanar CT Scan. Surg. Neurol. 16 (1981) 340 – 345.
[7] Greitz, T., T. Hindmarsh: Computer assisted tomography of intracranial CSF circulation using water-soluble contrast medium. Acta radiol. (Diagn.) 12 (1974) 497 – 507.

[8] Goldstein, S. J., J. W. Walsh: Positive-contrast Computed Cranial Tomographic Encephalography in Children. Surg. Neurol. **19** (1983) 174 – 180.

[9] Heimberger, R. F.: Early repair of myelomeningoceles (spina bifida cystica) J. Neurosurg. **37** (1972) 594 – 600.

[10] Ingraham, F. D., D. D. Matson: Neurosurgery in Infancy and Childhood. C. Thomas Pub.; Springfield 1954.

[11] Inone, Y., A. Hakuba, K. Fujitani et al.: Occult cranium bifidum. Radiological and surgical findings. Neuroradiology **25** (1983) 217 – 223.

[12] Kendall, B. E., D. Kingsley: The value of computerized axial tomography (CAT) in craniocerebral malformations. Brit. J. Radiol. **51** (1978) 171 – 190.

[13] Prömper, K. H., G. Friedmann: Spinale Fehlbildungen. In: Computertomographie der Wirbelsäule und des Spinalkanals (P. Thurn, G. Friedberg, eds.), pp. 39 – 47. Enke Verlag, Stuttgart 1983.

[14] Sator, K., R. Richert: Konventionell-radiographische und computerassistierte Zisternographie der hinteren Schädelgrube mit Metrizamid. Fortschr. Röntgenstr. **130** (1979) 472 – 478.

[15] Skalpe, I. O.: Adverse effects of water-soluble contrast media in myelography, cisternography and ventriculography. A review with special reference to metrizamide. Acta radiol. (Suppl.) **355** (1977) 359 – 370.

[16] Yu, Y. L., G. H. du Boulay: Is there an increased risk of early side effects in post-myelogram computed tomography? Neuroradiology **26** (1984) 399 – 403.

III   Surgical treatment of spinal dysraphias — technique and results

Methods and results of the neurosurgical treatment of spinal dysraphias

M. Schwarz, D. Voth, J. Brito, G. Kessel, E. G. Mahlmann, M. Henn

Introduction

Treatment of an open myelomeningocele (MMC) demands urgent surgical intervention in the neonatal period. The treatment may be indicated for ethical, general medical, surgical-technical, but also social reasons. A clear-cut decision on medical grounds alone is possible if severe malformations of other organs are present at the same time. However, the malformation of the CNS may be so extensive that it is *a priori* incompatible with life. Similarly an operation on a small sacral myelocele may only be indicated if it is possible to hope for a near complete *restitutio ad integrum*, or if additional neurological complications can be avoided. Admittedly, the majority of cases of myelomeningoceles display more or less severe neurological deficiencies at birth, and further complications must be expected in the follow-up period, a decision to operate lies between these two extremes [2, 4, 9, 10, 12].

Material and methods

Between 1974 and 1984, 78 children with spinal dysraphias were operated on in our clinic. For the present summary we have selected those children whose histories we were able to document as far as their immediate postoperative course is concerned or the further course by regular follow-up examinations. In this way 46 male infants, or 59%, and 32 female infants, or 41% were observed.

Table 1   Height localisation and extent of the MMC related to the vertebral column sections. The extent of the lesion was determined preoperatively by X-ray pictures of the vertebral column in postero-anterior and lateral view

Thoracolumbosacral	2
Thoracolumbar	19
Lumbosacral*	48
Lumbar	9

* of these 3 lipomyelomeningoceles, 2 meningoceles, 1 lipoma.

In 6 patients (the thoraco-lumbar manifestation group), there were 3 cases of lipomyeloschisis, 2 meningoceles and 1 lipoma. As these 6 patients were found as having closed dysraphias they were operated on later (tab. 1).

As the term myelocele always implies the prolapse of parts of the spinal cord and cauda equina, an open myelomeningocele must be regarded as an open lesion in the central nervous system. For this reason appropriate surgical measures must be implemented as soon as possible.

The aim of the operation is

1. removal of the cyst in the case of cystic forms,
2. a careful covering of the cord and nerve roots, while retaining functioning neural tissue, and
3. leakage free sutures.

Indication for an early operation

Earliest possible surgical treatment is necessary within the first 24 hours, or not later than within 48 hours at the most; a mild bacterial invasion is evident on the newborn infant's skin [1, 5, 11]. Both the size of the defect and the profuse leakage of C.S.F. favour bacterial invasion and the spread of bacteria, particularly if the infant still requires incubator care. One factor which should not be disregarded in connection with the prevention of infection is the premature rupture of the amnion. In such cases, pre- and perioperative antibiotic treatment should begin as soon as possible. A further reason for an early operation is the already visible reaction of the rudimentary spinal tissue and the adjoining structures. As a result of the incipient epithelialisation in the border zones, a development of granulation filaments and trabeculae can be seen leading to a fixation of the *area medullo-vasculosa*. If the operation is carried out later, it will hardly be possible to prepare the epithelial layer of the cicatricial scute without traumatising the latter, thus causing additional lesions.

In view of these complications we performed early treatment within the 48 hour limit in 60 cases, or 83%. 12 infants were not treated until later, either because there were contraindications or because the necessary consent for the operation had been refused. The operation was carried out within 12 hours after birth on 29 infants, within the first 24 hours on a further 25 infants, and the remaining 6 children were operated on between 24 and 48 hours after birth.

Contraindications to an early operation [7, 8, 9]

1. Myelomeningoceles which cannot be covered plastically,
2. additional severe malformations of other organ systems and of the CNS, and
3. the newborn infant's inoperable state.

The 48 hour limit may be exceeded without hesitation [14] if there is adequate covering and if the danger of a rupture of the cele in the case of *hydrocephalus internus* can be reduced by an early shunt implantation. In the case of noted myelomemingoceles having a large extent [6] this must be specially noted.

Operational technique — anaesthesia — positioning

As every myelocele varies in size and internal extent, the operating technique used by us is based on a case of a lumbosacral MMC.

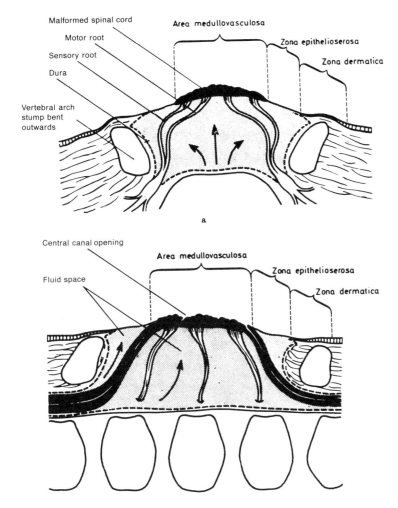

Fig. 1   Diagram of an MMC seen in longitudinal and cross section showing the important anatomic structures and the course of the nerve roots (taken from [3]).

The infant is positioned on the operating table under insufflation anaesthesia in a ventricumbent posture. Body heat losses are compensated by an electric blanket. The extremities are protected against heat losses, as far as possible, by cotton wool bandages. The base of the cele is then peritomised (fig. 1) in the area of the normal cutis and subcutis. The cele sac is then opened up laterally and the contents are first inspected. The *zona epithelioserosa*, the *area medullovasculosa* and the nerve roots are exposed [3].

Particular care should be taken when separating the *zona epithelioserosa* (fig. 2) in the vicinity of the cranial end of the *area medullovasculosa* as the rise of the

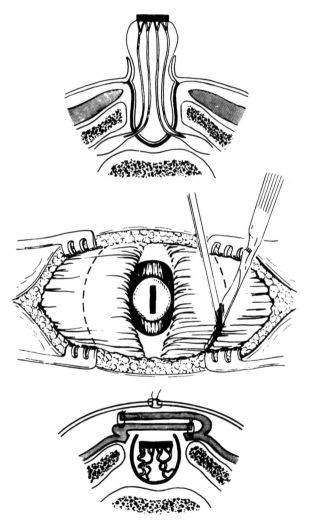

Fig. 2   Reconstruction of the dural tube with the fascia of the *musculus erector trunci* (taken from [13]).

spinal cord and the nerve roots is steeper at the level of the beginning of the defect than caudally. This part of the operation should be carried out microsurgically. Each individual root appearing in the *area medullovasculosa* should be traced in its peripheral course; if it is found that it has a blind ending (by electric stimulation or dissection), it may be cut through. After the dissection has been completed, the rudimentary cord is then repositioned into the spinal canal and the dura, mobilised from both sides, is sutured.

Frequently insufficient native dura is present for suturing. In such cases, the thoracolumbar fascia is exposed on either side of the spinal canal by a wide flap incision, and is then folded over the defect, either doubly or singly (fig. 1). In addition, a strip of lyophilised dura can be sown over the whole opening as a second covering and sealed with fibrinous adhesive [13].

The suture or reconstruction of the dural tube becomes difficult if an extensive myelomeningocele is present in the thoracolumbar area having a wide spinal canal and a slender preformed *musculus erector trunci* (fig. 3). In this case, a

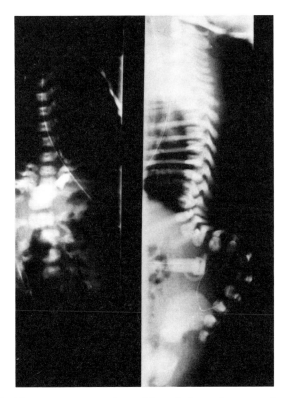

Fig. 3   X-rays: postero-anterior and lateral views of an extensive MMC in the thoracolumbosacral region — wide spinal canal without kyphoscoliosis.

sufficiently large muscle-fascia flap should be prepared. The entire skin should be exposed without cutting, including the subcutaneous tissue down to the caudal scapula tips, and medially to the osseous edge of the fissuration. A medial suture has to made with the muscle fascia flaps on the other side. In the case of kyphotic malformations, the rudimentary and in part high-angled arch parts are exposed and removed using the bone-cutting forceps (fig. 4). This is necessary as a precaution against necrosis in a skin suture. Suturing of skin still presents a problem in cases of larger celes. Lateral relieving incisions in the skin or transverse relieving incisions in the vicinity of the interscapular region have not been carried out in our clinic for some time. Covering of skin defects caused by these relieving incisions with amnion or with cele sac cuts leave ugly scars. Transverse or arch shaped relieving incisions, including the cele to form a Z- or S-shaped displacement give better results.

By means of adequate mobilisation, i.e. so-called subcutaneous scalping of the healthy skin at the periphery, including the subcutaneous adipose tissue in a

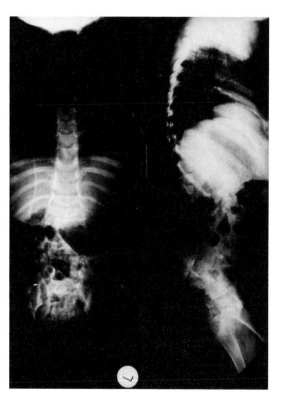

Fig. 4   X-rays: A MMC in the thoracolumbar region, postero-anterior and lateral views, showing severe kyphoscoliosis.

cranial direction to the scapula tips, and laterally to the mid-axillary line, always allows a craniocaudal oblique or transverse primary skin suture. The suture should be made on two levels: subcuticular sutures should be avoided in the defective area, i.e. externally recognisable by the teleangietatic areas. The skin suture is made using monophile suture material, so that the sutures can be left for 10 – 11 days. As a rule, the insertion of a subcutaneous drainage is dispensed with. A Redon drainage with a slight suction is fitted for 24 hours if extensive subcutaneous scalping is present.

Postoperative complications

Two surgical complications can cause problems in the postoperative phase:

1. Impairment of wound healing due to necrosis,

2. C.S.F. fistula with consecutive infection.

The congenital *hydrocephalus internus* contributes an important complication in the formation of a C.S.F. fistula (tabs. 2 and 3). The diagnosis of the infants was generally carried out prior to the operative treatment of the cele by means of ultrasonic examination or, in some cases, in order to exclude any other severe CNS malformation, by cranial computer tomography.

In 4 cases a shunt was implanted after treatment of the cele under the same anaesthesia. In the other case with progressive *hydrocephalus,* a shunt operation was carried out within 6 – 8 days of the MMC.

Table 2   MMC and *hydrocephalus internus* – localisation and number of myelomeningoceles (MMC)

Localisation and number of celes		Hydrocephalus
Thoracolumbosacral	2	2
Thoracolumbar	19	19
Lumbosacral	42	36
Lumbar	9	6

Table 3   Myelomeningoceles and Arnold-Chiari II malformation – localisation and frequency

Localisation and frequency		Arnold-Chiari
Lumbosacral	42	10
Thoracolumbar	19	7
Lumbar	9	2

MMC and vertebral column deformation

Severe vertebral column deformations in the sense of kyphoscoliosis, kyphoses or skolioses were found on 20 infants, especially with thoraco-lumbo-sacral localisation in two cases, with a thoracolumbar cele site in 18 cases. 11 infants displayed slight deformation with lumbosacral myelomeningocele.

Summary

From 1974 to 1984, 78 newborn infants with spinal dysraphias were treated surgically in the Neurosurgical Clinic in Mainz. The operation was indicated on ethical, general medical, surgical-technical and also social grounds. 83% of the myeloceles were closed within the first 48 hours. It was possible to reduce complications, such as ascending infections and granulation tissue formation by performing an early operation. A shunt operation was carried out in 63 cases to relieve an existing *hydrocephalus internus*. In 19 cases an Arnold-Chiari II deformation was present.

References

[1] Eckstein, H. B.: Problems of Primary Closure of Myelomeningoceles. Proc. Roy. Soc. Med. **64** (1971) 1145 – 54.

[2] Edward, J., G. McCarthy, P. McCarthy: Implications of a selectice policy in the management of spina bifida. J. of Pediatr. Surg. **16**, No. 2 (April) (1981) 136 – 138.

[3] Gerlach, J., H. P. Jensen: Mißbildungen des Rückenmarks. Handbuch der Neurochirurgie, vol. VII/1, pp. 308 – 351. Springer, Berlin – Heidelberg – New York 1969.

[4] Hemmer, R.: Klinik und Therapie der dysraphischen Fehlbildungen und des Hydrocephalus. In: Klin. Neurochirurgie (H. Dietz, W. Umbach, R. Wüllenweber, eds.), vol. 2, pp. 12 – 31. Georg Thieme Verlag, Stuttgart – New York .

[5] Katoua, F., E. Paraicz (Neurosurgical Institute Budapest): Pre- and postoperative problems in myelodysplasia. Prog. Pediatr. Surg. **8** (1975) 119 – 134.

[6] Lorber, J.: Ventriculocardiac shunts in the first week of life. Results of a controlled trial in the treatment of hydrocephalus in infants born with spina bifida cystica or cranium bifidum. Developmental Medicine and Child Neurology Suppl. **20** (1969) 13 – 20.

[7] Lorber, J.: Results of treatment of myelomeningocele. An analysis of 524 unselected cases, with special reference to possible selection for treatment. Dev. Med. Child Neurol. **13** (1971) 279 – 303.

[8] Lorber, J.: Spina bifida cystica. Results of 270 consecutive cases with criteria for selection for the future. Arch. Dis. Child **47** (1972) 854 – 873.

[9] Lorber, J.: Early results of selective treatment of spina bifida cystica. Br. Med. J. **4** (1973) 201 – 204.

[10] Maier, W. A.: Operativer Verschluß großer Myelomeningocelen. Zeitschrift für Kinderchirurgie, Suppl. **29** (1982) 42 – 45.

[11] McLone, D. G., A. J. Raimondi, M. W. Commers: The results of early treatment of 100 consecutive newborns with myelomeningocele. Z. Kinderchirurgie **34**/2 (1981) 115 – 117.

[12] Milhorat, T.: Pediatric Neurosurgery. Philadelphia 78, 137 – 151.

[13] Schürmann, K., D. Voth: Neurochirurgie. In: Spezielle Chirurgie für die Praxis (F. Baumgartl, K. Kremer, H. W. Schreiber, eds.), vol. I, part 2, pp. 831 – 1019. Georg Thieme Verlag, Stuttgart 1975.

[14] Sharrard, W. J., R. B. Zachary, J. Lorber et al.: A controlled trial of immediate and delayed closure of spina bifida cystica. Arch. Dis. Child 38 (1963) 18.

[15] Zachary, R. B.: Recent advances in the management of myelomeningoceles. Prog. Pediatr. Surg., vol. 2 (1971) 155 – 169.

Selective treatment in spina bifida cystica

H. Collmann, F. Hanefeld, A. Mielfried, D. Rating, B. Rühe, W. Stoeckel

The problem whether every child suffering from spina bifida cystica should be subjected to vigorous treatment has been discussed and led to considerable controversy [2, 3, 7 – 10, 13, 19, 22]. Various aspects are involved including ethical [2, 7, 8, 9, 17, 22] and legal considerations [18], selection criteria [3, 14, 20, 21], the fate of the nontreated children [6, 11, 14, 15, 20] and the implications to their families [5].

These cases have only reluctantly been discussed in Germany up to the present time [1, 4, 11]. Encouraged by the work of John Lorber and his team [13 – 16] we started to practise selective treatment in 1974. We were particularly interested in the problem of the unoperated survivors, since any decision against full treatment implies that an unoperated child will not survive for any length of time.

The five departments cooperating in this study could not reach a consensus as to the strict adoption of Lorber's criteria for selection [14 – 16], as there were objections against the proposed motor level of L3 in addition to the risk of making general decisions in cases of special individual malformations. We therefore took the following adverse criteria as guidelines: paralysis below D12, gross hydrocephalus with frontal brain mantle below 10 mm, untreatable associated malformations and severe perinatal asphyxia. In borderline situations we some-times accepted a high lumbar level L1 to L3 and in these cases we even took social circumstances into account. Severe kyphoscoliosis and a thoracolumbar localisation of the lesion are not shown in this list as we were never confronted with these features on their own.

The basis for selecting a particular child was a meticulous clinical examination carried out by a senior pediatrician and an experienced neurosurgeon separately. It included x-rays and ultrasound or computer tomography of the skull.

This was followed by a detailed and frank interview with – as a rule – both parents. It was started by a senior member of the spina bifida team with objective briefings about the infant's handicaps and their consequences to psychomotor development and social independence. Possibilities and limits of surgical and conservative treatment were then discussed. Finally a cautious prognosis of survival was given should the parents decide against surgical treatment. At the end of the interview an advice of an explicitly personal character was offered, whether surgical closure of the defect should be performed. The parents were given up two days to consider the information before they reached a decision. In case of deciding against active treatment the parents were advised to keep the infant in hospital care [5, 9, 16].

During the last 10 years 68 newborns with myelomeningocele were treated following these guidelines. In 28 an examination as well as an interview resulted in a decision for treatment. 35 had one or more adverse criteria and were not considered for surgical closure of the lesion. The remaining 5 infants had been operated on previously at other centers in spite of adverse criteria. Two of the 28 operated children died during early childhood because of shunt-related cerebral hemorrhage, and bacterial meningitis unrelated to the shunt. The other children were to some extent outpatients and only few had disabling brain dysfunction, although most of them had shunt-treated hydrocephalus (tab. 1). No parents definitely refused total care when it was suggested. In contrast to these observations we examined 13 children who were operated on in spite of adverse criteria, most of them before the period of selection in our own department (tab. 1). All

Table 1   Prognosis of vigorously treated meningomyeloceles. Capabilities of 28 children of the present series who were selected for treatment, compared with 13 other children operated on in spite of adverse criteria. Most of the latter were treated before introduction of selection at our department. (Parentheses: Number of patients evaluable.)

| | adverse criteria | |
	absent n = 28	present n = 13
died	2	5
at least partially able to walk	25 (27)	0 (11)
gross cerebral palsy	3 (27)	9 (11)
gross mental retardation	2 (27)	8 (11)

of them had complete paraplegia, often combined with severe kyphosis. In addition nearly all were handicapped with severe cerebral palsy and mental retardation. Five of them succumbed between the first months of life and up to 10 years due to shunt infection (2 patients), renal failure, pulmonary infection and head injury.

35 newborns in the non-treatment group presented with the following adverse criteria: complete thoracic level in 21 infants, severe hydrocephalus in 8, perinatal

asphyxia in 6 and associated malformations in 4. Social considerations played an additional role in 5 children with a defect at a high lumbar level. The parents opposed any operation despite adverse criteria. Most children of this group were nursed in the hospital and return to their families regularly resulted in severe emotional distress for the whole family. Until now 29 of the 35 unoperated children died, mainly during the first 3 to 6 months of life. The cause of death was asphyxia during the first days of life (4 infants), ascending infection (12 infants) or progressive hydrocephalus (9 infants). In 4 cases the cause of death was not established.

However, so far 6 children, 17% of the untreated survived. Their ages range from 2 months to 4 years. Two are in a serious condition and are not expected to live much longer. A third child presented no ethical problems, because his small thoracic lesion healed rapidly and − due to absence of a Chiari malformation − no hydrocephalus was expected. One boy has been operated on at the age of 13 months in order to avoid extreme head enlargement, as further survival was considered most probable. Up to now his psychomotor development seems to be only slightly retarded. We will suggest the same 'wait and see treatment' in a 6 months old girl who is now in a stable condition. A 13 months old boy survived a severe ascending infection without antibiotic treatment. He is now microcephalic and extremely disabled by cerebral palsy, visual impairment and seizures in addition to a complete paraplegia.

Looking more closely at the individual cases it seems realistic to estimate about 10 per cent survival rate in untreated survivors. These figures approximate those of other centres [9, 10, 12, 19, 21] although extreme figures of no survival [16] and 70 per cent survival [6] have been reported as well.

The following problems confront doctors taking care of the unoperated children:

1. Non-treatment − what does it mean? There is agreement that no antibiotics should be used and no shunt should be inserted only for facilitation of care [3, 9, 16]. But there are doubts about the use of nasogastric feeding tubes and the use of analgesics and sedatives. We use tube feeding and analgesics.

2. Concerning the severe emotional distress to the whole family it seems to us unreasonable to burden the parents with the care for their unoperated child. But if the child is cared for in a hospital the parents should be contacted at intervals and be offered psychological support.

3. Any decision − whether total care or against active treatment − should be realized fully, even in the case of an erroneous primary prognosis. We therefore suggest like others [9, 16] to reconsider the prerequisites of the initial decision if an unoperated child survived for 6 months or more.

Selection for treatment will never be able to solve the complex and excruciating problems of severe meningomyelocele, that the affected children and their families have to face. At present this may be an acceptable way to relieve suffering even at the cost of not preserving life and of increased suffering in some of the non-treated survivors. There is reason to hope that selective treatment of severe spina bifida will before long be superseded by effective means of prophylaxis.

References

[1] Bettex, M.: Indikationen und Kontraindikationen in der Behandlung der Myelomeningozele und des Hydrocephalus. Z. Kinderchir. **27** (1979) 120 – 124.

[2] Black, P. McL.: Selective treatment of infants with myelomeningocele. Neurosurgery 5 (1979) 334 – 338.

[3] Brocklehurst, G.: Spina bifida for the clinician. William Heinemann Medical Books, London 1976.

[4] Bundesärztekammer, Wissenschaftl. Beirat: Empfehlungen zur Versorgung von Kindern mit Spina bifida. Dtsch. Ärztebl. **26** (1977) 1727 – 1735.

[5] Duff, R. S., A. G. M. Campbell: On deciding the care of severely handicapped persons: With particular references to infants. Pediatrics **57** (1976) 487 – 493.

[6] Feetham, S. L., H. Tweed, J. S. Perrin: Practical problems in selection of spina bifida infants for treatment in the USA. Z. Kinderchir. **28** (1979) 301 – 306.

[7] Freeman, J. M.: To treat or not to treat. In: Practical management of meningomyelocele, pp. 13 – 22. University Park Press, Baltimore 1974.

[8] Freeman, J. M.: Early management and decision making for the treatment of myelomeningocele: A critique. Pediatrics **73** (1984) 564 – 566.

[9] Gross, R. H., A. Cox, R. Tatyrek et al.: Early management and decision making for the treatment of myelomeningocele. Pediatrics **72** (1983) 450 – 458.

[10] Guiney, E. J., P. MacCarthy: Implications of a selective policy in the management of spina bifida. J. Pediatr. Surg. **16** (1981) 136 – 139.

[11] Haensel-Friedrich, G., M. Schmidt, E. Engel et al.: Outcome of 97 children with myelomeningocele: Surgical versus conservative treatment. Neuropediatrics **15** (1984) 242.

[12] Hide, D. W., H. P. Williams, H. L. Ellis: The outlook for the child with a myelomeningocele for whom early surgery was considered inadvisable. Dev. Med. Child Neurol. **14** (1972) 304 – 307.

[13] Lorber, J.: Results of treatment of myelomeningocele. An analysis of 524 unselected cases, with special reference to possible selection for treatment. Dev. Med. Child Neurol. **13** (1971) 279 – 303.

[14] Lorber, J.: Spina bifida cystica. Results of treatment of 270 consecutive cases with criteria for selection for the future. Arch. Dis. Child. **47** (1972) 854 – 873.

[15] Lorber, J.: Early results of selective treatment of spina bifida cystica. Br. Med. J. **4** (1973) 201 – 204.

[16] Lorber, J., S. A. W. Salfield: Results of selective treatment of spina bifida cystica. Arch. Dis. Child. **56** (1981) 822 – 830.

[17] Newcastle Regional Hospital Board. Ethics of selective treatment of spina bifida. Report by a working party. Lancet I (1975) 85 – 88.

[18] Robertson, J. A., N. Fost: Passive euthanasia of defective newborn infants: Legal considerations. J. Pediatr. **88** (1976) 883 – 889.

[19] Shurtleff, D. B., P. W. Hayden, J. D. Loeser et al.: Myelodysplasia: decision for death or disability. J. Med. **291** (1974) 1005 – 1011.
[20] Smith, G. K., E. D. Smith: Selection for treatment in spina bifida cystica. Brit. Med. J. **4** (1973) 189 – 197.
[21] Stark, G. D:, M. Drummond: Results of selective early operation in myelomeningocele. Arch. Dis. Child **48** (1973) 676 – 683.
[22] Zachary, R. B.: Life with spina bifida: Br. Med. J. **2** (1977) 1460 – 1462.

Complications in plastic surgical treatment of spinal dysraphias

G. Keßel, D. Voth, M. Schwarz, E. G. Mahlmann, J. Brito

Introduction

Within the framework of operative procedures dealing with dysraphic malformations the plastic wound toilet deserves special attention. Deficient technique in this area causes severe complications, such as p.o. meningitis. This infection can easily occur if a leakage of CSF is present due to failure of imperfect dural sutures. In this instance the prognosis is considerably worsened and in addition to sensory-motor signs including bladder and rectal disturbances further neurological symptoms can develop [1, 2]. For these reasons the operational technique of the wound toilet of the spinal malformation will be discussed including the type of complications and frequencies observed in our surgical unit [3, 4, 5].

Operational procedures

The range of the skin incision has to be considered first to make provisions for the size of the defect allowing tension-free sutures. In case this proves necessary the skin flap made, should allow further extension for a plastic mobile skin flap. The following operational steps, such as the incision of the prolapse, the preparation of the zona epithelio-serosa and medullo-vasculosa including the reposition of spinal portions and nerve roots will be discussed elsewhere in this book. This account will deal only with the closure of the dura. In most cases it will be possible to achieve a watertight closure by using single stitches. However no pressure or tension should be applied to endangered nerve roots. Under these conditions – almost favourable – it is possible, by carrying out a winglike incision of the lumbo-sacral resp. thoraco-lumbar fascia and liberating sufficient fascia for a double covering and closing of the defect.

In order to achieve a liquor-tight closure this approach is most important if sufficient dural material is not available for a primary suture. This type of closure offers good protection for the spinal cord and its roots in case necrotic tissue appears or a secondary wound healing in the skin area is the result. Again it must be emphasized that a tension-free closing is necessary. Those malformations which do not exceed a diameter of half the width of the back have a good chance

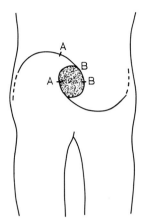

Fig. 1   Preparing a rotation flap for covering large defects.

to be closed by a transverse suture after mobilising the cutis and subcutis. The transverse oder trans-oval incisure is the method we prefer as well.

If a tension-free closure is not possible, the defect has to be closed by a plastic skin operation which we execute as follows: the incisure is extended (fig. 1) and the cutis and subcutis freely mobilised obtaining a flap which can be rotated and sawn in. Larger wound areas are subjected to a Redon-suction-wound drainage for 24 hours.

To return to the problem of the best possible way for closing the dura by forming a muscle flap, we have to mention the use of lyophilised dura. In 78 operations we have used in 57 cases (78%) lyodura, either for closing a dural gap or mainly as an additional layer on top of the musculo-fascial flap.

Resulting complications

Besides the development of a CSF leak and in consequence the possibility of meningitis further complications are septicaemia, a rupture of sutures, skin necrosis, subcutaneous seromas, haematomas, wound infections, abscess formations followed by the rejection of lyodura (tab. 1).

In treating 78 cases we have seen 3 cases of CSF leaks. Two of these children had not received a CSF shunt. In one child the fistula occured when the shunt failed after a ventriculo-atrial junction. In each case the fistula had to be closed by operation.

Two patients had received lyodura but showed no increased risk of complications (tab. 2).

Table 1   Myelomeningoceles. Complications encountered in plastic surgery

1.	CSF fistula
2.	Meningitis, sepsis
3.	Suture failure
4.	Skin necrosis
5.	Seroma, haematoma
6.	Wound-infection, abscess formation
7.	Rejection of lyophilised dura

Table 2   Operative care of MMC. Complications (I)

Total operative interventions	78
CSF fistula	3
(2 with lyodura)	
Meningitis, sepsis	2

Table 3   Operative care of MMC. Complications (II)

Total operative interventions	78
Dehiscence of sutures	11*
slight skin necrosis	
Extensive necrotic lesions	3**
(2 with lyophilised dura)	

*   Uneventful course
**   1 child died after abscess formation and sepsis

Table 4   Operative care of MMC. Complications (III)

Operations	78
Seroma, haematoma	6*
Rejection of lyodura	2
and local fistulas	

* After puncture uneventful course

Two children – both without CSF fistula – developed meningitis and severe sepsis after a shunt was made. The meningitis could not be attributed with certainity to the primary operation (tab. 2). In 11 children suture failure and skin necrosis occured, but the skin lesions were small. Paying stricter attention to steril wound handling all lesions healed quickly.

Extensive necrotic lesions were seen thrice, two in cases where lyodura had been used. One child (no lyodura was used in this instance), became septic and died (tab. 3). In six babies subcutaneous seromas or haematomas were noted, but drainage by puncture secured healing. Two children rejected the lyodura by forming a local fistula and in one existed a CSF fistula before the second event (tab. 4).

Summary

This brief contribution attempts to characterise the complications occuring in the management and operative treatment of spinal dysraphia. These observations cover the whole range from a relatively harmless disturbance in wound healing to severe complications, such as meningitis, abscess formation and sepsis terminating in death. However taking everything into account one can state that the frequency and degree of severity of complication is limited, provided the most careful wound toilet is made.

References

[1] French, B. N.: Midline Fusion defects and defects of formation. In: Neurological surgery (J. R. Youmans, ed.), vol. III, pp. 1236 – 1380. Saunders, Philadelphia 1982.

[2] Gullotta, F.: Fehl- und Mißbildungen. Klinische Neurochirurgie, vol. II, pp. 2 – 12. Thieme Verlag, Stuttgart – New York 1984.

[3] Hemmer, R.: Klinik und Therapie der dysraphischen Fehlbildungen und des Hydrozephalus. Klinische Neurochirurgie, vol. II, pp. 12 – 31. Thieme Verlag, Stuttgart – New York 1984.

[4] Maier, W. A.: Operativer Verschluß großer Myelomeningozelen. Z. Kinderchirur., Suppl. 29 (1982) 42 – 45.

[5] Milhorat, Th.: Paediatric Neurosurgery, pp. 137 – 169. Philadelphia 1978.

Lumbo-sacral lipoma in spina bifida occulta

Clinical and radiological features and operation results

K. E. Richard, P. Sanker, P. van den Bergh

Introduction

A congenital lumbosacral intraspinal lipoma is one possible manifestation of the occult spinal dysraphies. The pathological anatomy is known from the early descriptions by Johnson 1857 [11], Gowers 1875 [8], and von Recklinghausen 1886 [16].

Based on the case of a 25 year old shoemaker Heinrich Kieffer, von Recklinghausen in 1886 presented his classical description of the clinical neurological picture and the complex pathological anatomy of the lumbosacral lipoma in spina bifida occulta (fig. 1). On page 251 we read: "1. Das untere Ende des Rückenmarks, der Conus medullaris, liegt nicht wie normal im zweiten Lenden-, sondern im zweiten Kreuzbeinwirbel. 2. Der Rückgratskanal ist weiter wie normal. 3. Dieser weite Theil wird aber vollständig erfüllt, nicht nur durch das Rückenmark, sondern noch durch eine wie Fettgewebe erscheinende Masse, welche das Rückenmark gegen die vordere Kanalwand drängt, ... und auch im übrigen Sacralkanal die Nerven der Cauda equina größtentheils einbettet, nur den Conus medullaris freiläßt." (See fig. 1.)

And on page 254: "7. Das Verhältnis der frühen embryonalen Periode ist ... dadurch erhalten worden, daß *das untere Rückenmarksende im Sacralkanal* an der Stelle, wo jetzt noch das Myofibrolipom seine *Anheftung* an die Bogentheile der Lenden- und Sacralwirbel vermittelt, *-festgehalten wurde.*"

Hackenbroch [9] an orthopaedic surgeon in Cologne in 1936 mentioned "Fesselung" (tethering) of the cauda equina and of the spinal cord by myo-lipofibroma. It seems inexplicable why Matson [12], a respected American neurosurgeon, considered that the surgical treatment of this abnormality was only occasionally indicated and then for cosmetic reasons. His concept determined the surgical practice for a long time to come [13].

Recent advances in diagnostics and the use of surgical visual aids have furthered new interest in the clinical, neurosurgical and microanatomical issues of this process, widely considered to be a malformation tumor [19]. The development of myelography [7] and computer-tomography [14] have offered additional helps

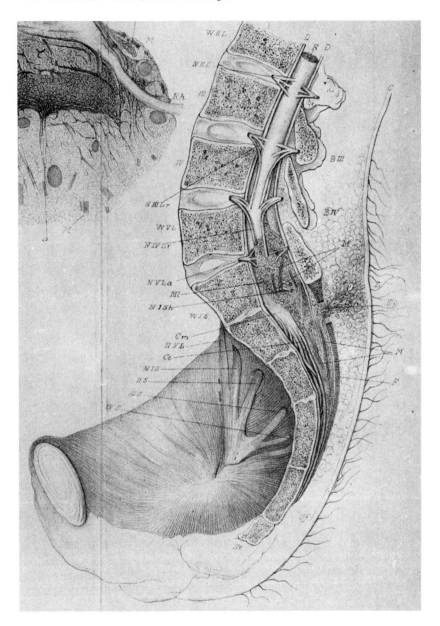

Fig. 1   Detail from plate IX from v. Recklinghausen's publication showing a lipomatous tumor in the conus area as well as the compression of the cauda and the adhesion of the cauda at the dorsal soft-tissue layers.

for a microsurgical approach. The intraoperative use of evoked potentials has improved the careful surgical approach of tumor-related nerve fibers [4].

Based on the analysis of the pre- and post-operative disturbances as well as on the correlation between the patient's age at the time of surgery and the longterm results as compared to the results of other authors (tab. 2). The authors will attempt to demonstrate clues for the optimal timing of surgical treatment. Furthermore, we present the diagnostic methods and the surgical techniques used by us.

Patient material

At the Department of Neurosurgery of the University of Cologne, 14 patients (4 male, 10 female) with a lumbosacral lipoma have been admitted up to the present time. 13 patients were surgically treated. Surgery was abandoned in a 21 year old patient with advanced non-progressive paraplegia and a neurogenic bladder.

At the time of surgery the patients were from 3 months to 57 years of age. Whereas most spinal myelo- and meningoceles were operated on under 3 months, surgery in lumbosacral lipomas was performed after the first year of life except in one case, while 2 patients were operated on in early and 1 patient in late (57 years) adult life.

Results

Preoperative neurological findings (fig. 2)

All patients presented with a more or less pronounced vaulting in the lumbosacral area. This was already observed at birth in all but one. In some cases, relatives or the patient himself had noticed a rapid increase in size of the tumour. Neurological deficits were only absent in 2 children, age 3 months and 2 years. Bladder and bowel emptying disturbances had developed in 8 patients, incontinence being the most frequent feature. Another 6 patients presented with foot and/or leg muscle weakness, three of them with a typical "equinovarus" deformity. 3 patients presented clearcut and 4 others slight gait disturbances. Segmental sensory disturbances of the legs were less frequent. In 2 older children and in 2 adults increasing exercise-related pain in the calf and feet had appeared.

The *duration of the symptoms* was variable and was related to the patient's age at the time of examination.

In a 57 year old surgeon, lower back pain radiating down the left leg was present since the age of 25. But only when paresthesiae occurred during longlasting operations, that an excision of the lipoma was decided upon.

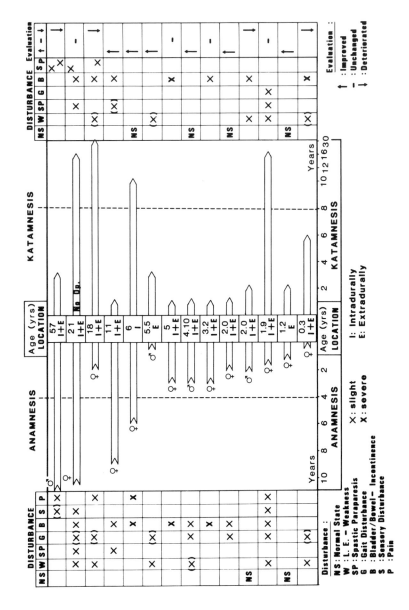

Fig. 2   Anamnesis, pre-operative neurological findings, age at time of surgery, extra-/intraspinal tumor location, katamnesis and treatment results in 14 patients.

Ancillary investigations

Plain X-rays of the lumbar spine usually showed an increased interpedicular distance, a missing vertebral arch or excavation of the dorsal surface of the vertebral bodies, often with an abnormal fusion.

Lumbar myelography showed an enlarged thecal sac with a low conus, a horizontal nerve root course and a communication between the lumbosacral subarachnoid space and the subcutaneous tissue inside the lipoma.

High-resolution metrizamide *computed tomographic myelography* offered the best definition. A stalky connection between the low conus medullaris and the extraspinal tissue, partially showing negative density, characteristic of fat tissue was present.

Operative results (figs. 2, 3)

Excision of the lipomas was successful in 6 patients: in 3 the preoperative deficits (gait and bladder disturbances) were completely resolved; 1 remained free of complaints and deficits and in 2 the spasticity and bladder disturbances or leg weakness improved (fig. 2). The results in 3 other operated patients were satisfactory: so far surgery had stopped further progression of the neurological defects.

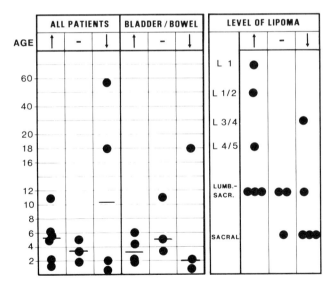

Fig. 3   Relationship between the operative results and age at time of surgery, pre-operative bladder and bowel disturbances, and the location of the lipoma: ↑ good/improved; − unchanged; ↓ bad, deteriorated.

The postoperative neurological state deteriorated in 4 patients. The painful parasthesia in the 57 year old surgeon persisted.

The results obtained were mostly good in children even when bladder disturbances were already present (fig. 3). They were satisfactory for lumbar and lumbosacral lipomas. They were poor in the 2 adult patients and for low sacral lipomas at all ages.

After 1970 all lipomas were removed by microsurgical techniques with good results.

Surgical technique

After transverse incision above the center of the tumor the lipoma is loosened from the surrounding tissues with sharp and blunt dissection. The lipoma stalk is then dissected through the paraspinal fascial defect up to the bony vertebral arch. Subsequently laminectomy of 1 or 2 dorsal arches above the vertebral defect is performed. The dura covering the spinal cord is opened and the lipoma progressively reduced in size till only a small rest remains. The filaments of the cauda are carefully saved. Complete removal cannot be accomplished because of the inseperable connection with the pia mater and the dorsal spinal cord at the conus level.

Usually, the dural defect has to be closed by a graft allowing the ascent of the conus together with the small lipoma stump. Preferably, we use fascia lata from the thigh, because closure with lyophilized dura is never waterproof even with the addition of fibrin glue.

To minimize the accumulation of spinal fluid, the patient is treated with compressive dressings and is kept in prone position for 5–7 days.

Spinal fluid accumulations in the dead space of the tumor bed should be treated with punctures. In one case, however a lumbo-peritoneal shunt system had to be implanted.

After wound healing and mobilization the patient gets up at the 7th–10th day. 3–4 weeks after surgery, a CT control study provides a control of the results, especially whether the fixation in the conus-cauda area has been dealt with successfully.

Discussion

Von Recklinghausen's observation that the normal ascent of the conus medullaris is prevented by its close connection with the tumor tissue, has been frequently confirmed [1–6, 9, 10, 13, 15, 17, 18]. In the Anglo-Saxon literature the concept "tethered conus" [6] is used today. The goal of surgical therapy is the early "untethering" ("Entfesslung") of the conus by an extensive resection of the lipoma. Bassett [2] and Bruce [3] advocate surgery as early as in first weeks after birth.

According to Chapman [4], surgery should be carried out very soon after the patient has first presented at the neurosurgical clinic, irrespective of whether neurological deficits exist or not.

Most patients were operated on in their infancy. The majority of our patients though was slightly older at the time of surgery (tab. 1).

The aim of early surgery is to prevent the development of neurological defects, which is to be expected during growth. The impact of tumor resection upon bladder and bowel disturbances, present in 50% of the cases according to the literature, was less favourable than upon weakness. Although improvement of

Table 1   Patients' age at the time of surgery reported in the literature and in the author's patient material

	N	0 – 1.9	2 – 5.9	6 – 10.9	11 – 20	21 – 40	>40 Yrs
Bassett	9	5	1	–	3	–	–
Swanson	9	3	2	2	2	–	–
Dubowitz	12	1	9	1	1	–	–
Bruce	42	27	3	8	4	–	–
N	72	36 (50%)	15 (21%)	11 (15%)	10 (14%)	–	–
Cologne	13	3 (23%)	6 (46%)	1 (8%)	2 (15%)	–	1 (8%)

Table 2   Operative results reported in the literature and in the author's patient material

Author	Year	N	Asymptom. improved (good)	Stabili- sation (satisfact.)	Deterio- ration (bad)	Repeat operation	Postop- compli- cations
Bassett	1950	9	5	1	0	2	1
Swanson	1962	9	2	3	2	2	–
Dubowitz	1965	12	5	1	6	–	–
Rogers	1971	18	9	8	1	3	–
Bruce	1979	40	25	13	2	–	4
James	1981	60	7	46	7	–	–
Pierre-Kahn	1983	32	10	19	3	–	–
McLone	1983	42	28	10	4	6	6
Chapman	1983	17	3	11	3	–	1
N		239	94 (39%)	112 (47%)	28 (12%)	13 (5%)	12 (5%)
Cologne	1984	13	6 (46%)	3 (23%)	4 (31%)	0	3 (23%)

pain can generally be obtained, regression of the frequently occurring wasting and of foot deformities is not likely to occur [1].

In recent years (tab. 2) the results obtained in increasing numbers of patients are encouraging. According to Bruce [3] the probability of functional deterioration without surgery is 80%, whereas after surgery some 40% were either free of complaints or had improved neurological function. In 47% stabilization of the functional defect could be obtained, i.e. further deterioration was prevented but progression could not be stopped in 12%. McLone pointed out the risk of relapse because of scar formation [13].

In summary, conditions for satisfactory results are:

- surgery early in infancy, ideally before the development of neurological disturbances [3, 4, 10, 13];

- careful radiological clarification of the spatial relationship between lipoma and conus-cauda area [4, 14];

- careful microsurgical technique, eventually completed by intraoperative recording of somato-sensory evoked potentials [4].

Conclusion

The basic pathophysiology of the lumbosacral lipomas in spina bifida occulta has been understood since the early studies of von Recklinghausen: the lower spinal cord is held tight in the sacral canal by tumor tissue invading the conus medullaris.

Characteristic consequences are foot deformities appearing during growth, gait disturbances, bladder and bowel difficulties and pain.

Experience gained in recents years only have shown that surgical resection of the lipoma and release of the conus in early infancy in some cases could prevent the development of severe neurological defects, whereas in most cases improvement or at least an arrest of further progression of these was obtained.

References

[1] Anderson, F. M.: Occult spinal dysraphism: A series of 73 cases. Pediatrics 55 (1975) 826 – 835.
[2] Bassett, R. C.: The neurologic deficit associated with lipomas of the cauda equina. Ann. Surg. 131 (1950) 109 – 116.
[3] Bruce, D. A., L. Schut: Spinal lipomas in infancy and childhood. Child's Brain 5 (1979) 192 – 203.
[4] Chapman, P. H.: Congenital intraspinal lipomas. Anatomic considerations and surgical treatment. Child's Brain 9 (1982) 37 – 47.

[5] Dubowitz, V., J. Lorber, R. B. Zachary: Lipoma of the Cauda equina. Arch. Dis. Childh. **40** (1965) 207–212.

[6] Fitz, Ch. R., D. C. Harwood-Nash: The tethered conus. AJR **125** (1975) 515–523.

[7] Gold, L. H. A., St. A. Kieffer, H. O. Peterson: Lipomatous inversion of the spinal cord associated with spinal dysraphism: myelographic evaluation. Am. J. Roent. Rad. Ther. Nucl. Med. **107** (1969) 479–485.

[8] Gowers, W. R.: Myo-lipoma of spinal cord. Trans. path. Soc. Lond. **27** (1876) 19–22.

[9] Hackenbroch, M.: Beitrag zur Kenntnis der Geschwulstbildungen im Lumbosakralkanal bei Spina bifida occulta. Med. Klin. **35** (1936) 1179–1181.

[10] James, C. C. M., L. P. Lassman: Spina bifida occulta. Orthopaedic, radiological and neuro-surgical Aspects. Academic Press, Grune and Stratton, Orlando, FL-London 1981.

[11] Johnson, A.: Fatty tumor from the sacrum of a child, connected with the spinal membranes. Trans. path. Soc. Lond. **8** (1857) 16.

[12] Matson, D. D.: Neurosurgery of infancy and childhood. Charles C. Thomas, Springfield, 1969.

[13] McLone, D. G., S. Mutluer, Th. P. Naidich: Lipomeningoceles of the conus medullaris. In: Concepts in Pediatric Neurosurgery **3** (1983) 170–177.

[14] Naidich, Th. P., D. G. McLone, S. Mutluer: A new understanding of dorsal dysraphism with lipoma (Lipomyeloschisis)-Radiologic evaluation and surg. correction. AJR **140** (1983) 1065–1078.

[15] Pierre-Kahn, A., D. Renier, C. Sainte-Rose et al.: Les lipomes lombo-sacrés avec spina bifida. Corrélations anatomo-cliniques. Resultats thérapeutiques. Neurochirurgie **29** (1981) 359–363.

[16] Recklinghausen, F. von: Untersuchungen über die Spina bifida. Virchows Arch. Path. Anat. Physiol. **105** (1886) 243–330 and 373–455.

[17] Rogers, H. M., D. M. Long, S. N. Chou et al.: Lipomas of the spinal cord and cauda equina. J. Neurosurg. **34** (1971) 349–354.

[18] Swanson, H. S., J. C. Barnett: Intradural lipomas in children. Pediatrics **29** (1962) 911–926.

[19] Walsh, J. W., W. R. Markesbery: Histological features of cogenital lipomas of the lower spinal canal. J. Neurosurg. **52** (1980) 654–569.

Encephaloceles — their location, morphology and surgical treatment

M. Henn, D. Voth, M. Schwarz, G. Keßel, E.-G. Mahlmann

Introduction

In contrast to the occurrence of dysraphias in the region of the vertebral column, cephalo-celes are rare and reported to be present in 1:2500 and 1:25000 among normal births [7]. A preference for one sex has not been reported. During 1974 – 1984, 14 patients suffering from cephalo-celes were operated on, 2/3 of these cases were admitted after being born.

In these malformations bony defects are present in the middle of skull, frequently between the chondro- and desmo-cranium. The contents of the herniation allow a classification according to pathological-anatomical principles. These enclosures can consist of meningo-celes, meningo-encephalo-celes and encephalo-meningo-cysto-celes in case portions of the ventricles are present [2, 4].

The various aspects of encephalo-celes, including the classifications and subdivisions seen in our patients. The first principle of the classification is the localisation. Cele-formations of the convexity have to be separated from fronto-basal-celes. Without any doubt in the Western hemisphere occipital-celes are more frequently found [1, 7]. These herniations can be divided further in supratentorial-celes including cerebellar portions. A combination can occur in the

Table 1 Meningoencephaloceles (localisation) 1974 – 1984 – n = 14

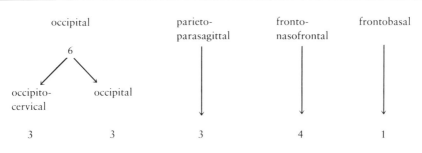

Further cerebral malformations e.g. lipoma of corpus callosum and facial skeleton cleft palate in 4 patients

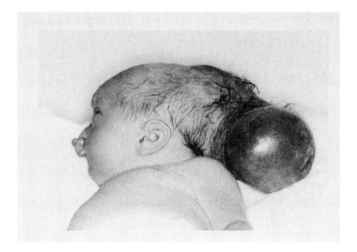

Fig. 1   Large occipital encephalocele.

upper cervical regions between a split cranium and spina bifida [6, 7]. Table 1 summarises the locations found in our patients and shows the preference for occipital malformations in spite of our limited number of cases (fig. 1). After the occipital malformations we encounter the fronto-ethmoidal-celes; the fronto-basal-celes can be subdivided further, but our patients showed spheno-ethmoidal encephalo-celes (fig. 1).

Further malformations

In the region of the brain (A) and facial skeleton (B) [1, 7] we see other malformations, these are:

(A) 1. A deformed ventricular system
    2. Lipoma of the Corpus callosum
    3. Agenesia of the Corpus callosum
    4. Teratoma

(B) 1. Cleft lip and palate
    2. Dysplasia of the auricle
    3. Atresia of the outer meatus acusticus.

Diagnostic considerations

The clinical inspection of the herniation gives no clue concerning its content. Difficulties in swallowing or breathlessness may be pointers for the presence of

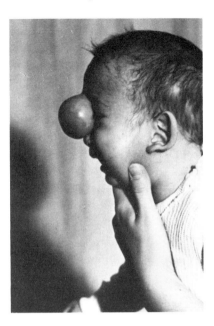

Fig. 2   Naso-frontal encephalocele.

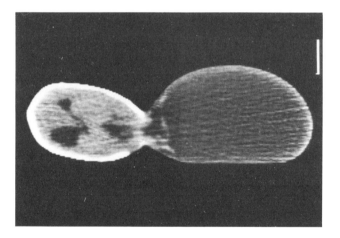

Fig. 3   CT of a giant occipito-encephalocele. Hermiated brain tissue is present within the encephalocele and the deformed ventricular system is visible.

a fronto-basal cele, as this was the case in one child. It is important to use *X-rays*
or tomography for exploring the fronto-basal region in order to detect bone
defects. *CT examination* has to follow to limit the content of the prolapse and
the extent of the ventricular system (figs. 1 and 2). An *EEG* will tell whether the
prolaps contains functionally active cerebral portions. *VEP* (visually evoked

potentials) similarly are able to verify functional visual cortex. *Angiography* [7] is capable to verify whether the posterior cerebral artery is inside the prolapse in cases of large occipital encephaloceles (fig. 3).

Pre-operative neurological findings

Besides the above enumerated malformations of brain and facial skull the pre-operative neurological signs vary considerably. Occipito-cervical celes with cerebellar and brainstem involvement have an unfavourable outlook and are accompanied by increased muscle tone, disturbance of swallowing and of temperature regulation [7].

12 children were sent to our clinic for a plastic surgical treatment. Apart from their state of consciousness the behaviour of the children appeared unremarkable crying vigourously, bilateral movements were present and their general condition was good. However some patients had increased tone, or atrophic musculature, forced head posture, while others were somnolent. 2 children with large occipito-encephaloceles became inpatients only after 7 months resp. 7 years. In the first case of a supra-tentorial encephalocele, containing cerebral cortex, a microcephalus and a beginning suture closure with optic atrophy was present. The 7 year old child had an occipito-cervical-encephalocele and showed at operation a cerebellar dysraphia, probably responsible for gait ataxia.

Indication for operation and operational procedure

In the cases of 5 patients with open celes and CSF leakage an operation was performed under the protection of antibiotica. Severe malformations of additional organs however excludes an operation in all cases.

The general condition of the children was good enough to permit plastic operative care. The others — closed encephaloceles — were to be operated on, as soon as possible and were classified as postponed but urgent operative cases. In these cases the priority was the procurement of reasonable starting conditions for operating, such as being well fed, no infections or bed sores and the exclusion of additional severe malformations.

The operative procedures follow the rules of plastic surgery and the prevention of CSF leaks. The prolapse is circumcised leaving enough healthy skin for defect covering. The dura is traced to the bony defect. This is followed by opening the top of the prolapse with a vertical incision and an exploration of the content. Frequently glio-vascular tissue is encountered, which must be removed. Whenever possible an inspection of the intra-cranial space should follow to look for malformation in the occipito-cervical region. Finally a suture of the available

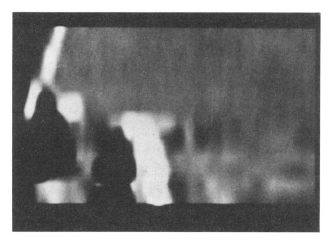

Fig. 4   CT of fronto-basal encephalocele, showing a distinct bone defect in the anterior fronto-basal
area.

dura is carried out or a reconstruction with a galea-periost flap a covering with lyodura and a tension-free skin suture, using a mobilised scalp flap if necessary.

A case of a fronto-basal encephalocele was cared for by bifrontal craniotomy and intra-dural repair. The fronto-basal defect present in the region of the sphenoid and reaching to the anterior clinoid process was closed by using a "Kieler Knochenspan" (fig. 4).

Macroscopical and microscopical findings

The tissues removed in 13 cases of meningo-encephaloceles mainly consisted of glial cells, frequently connected with the intact cerebrum by cellular bridges. In general the tissue showed abnormally structured brain parenchyma, resembling cerebral cortex or cerebellum, glia cell islands with ependyma or choroid plexus inclusions [3].

Complications

a) **Meningitis**: In two cases a post-operative meningitis occured, which healed without further complication.
b) **Hydrocephalus**: The most important after-effect was hydrocephalus, needing to be drained [7].

Table 2 shows that 8 patients out of 14 had a shunt operation. The hydrocephalus could develop quickly with clear signs of intra-cranial pressure during the post-

Table 2   Meningoencephaloceles 1974–1984

Complications:	*hydrocephalus* needed drainage in 8 cases p.o.
	the interval OP → shunt was up to 10 months

operative stay in hospital. In some cases the CT-controls taken in the follow up period showed a gradual increase in ventricular size. Even after 3 years one case needing drainage was found, but epidural control of ventricular pressure helps in the decision for making a shunt.

Summary

From 1974–1984 we had to attend to 14 cases of cephaloceles of different locations, 13 of which showed in the histological examination an encephalocele. In agreement with the literature a preponderance of the occipital location was seen by us. The aim of the operative treatment is a plastic – CSF leak preventing-removal of the prolapse. In case of an open cephalocele with an existing CSF leak, the need for operating is paramount, while in closed-celes the operation is also necessary but can be postponed. The most important p.o. complication is the occurrence of a hydrocephalus.

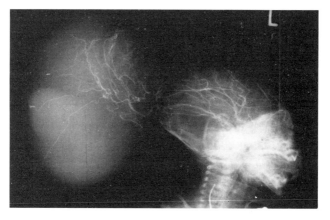

Fig. 5   Large occipital encephalocele. Angiographic illustration of vessels from the territory of the posterior cerebral artery within the occipital cele (pictures from the University Clinic, Giessen).

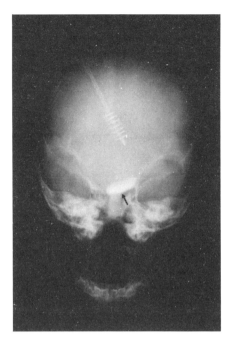

Fig. 6   Plain X-ray picture: Fronto-basal encephalocele, having been closed by "Kieler Knochenspan" (arrow).

References

[1] Bushe, K. A., P. Glees: Chirurgie des Gehirns und Rückenmarkes im Kindes- und Jugendalter. Hippokrates-Verlag, Stuttgart 1968.
[2] Doerr, W.: Organpathologie, Bd. III. Georg-Thieme-Verlag, Stuttgart 1974.
[3] Friede, R. L.: Developmental Neuropathology. Springer-Verlag, Berlin – Heidelberg – New York 1975.
[4] Gerlach, J., H.-P. Jensen, W. Koos: Pädiatrische Neurochirurgie. Georg-Thieme-Verlag, Stuttgart 1967.
[5] Milhorat, Th.: Pediatric Neurosurgery. Philadelphia 1978.
[6] Suwanela, C., N. Suwanela: A morphological classification of sincipital encephalomeningoceles. J. Neurosurg. **36** (1972) 201 – 211.
[7] Youmans, J. R.: Neurological Surgery. Saunders Company, Philadelphia 1982.

Diagnosis and treatment of the tethered spinal cord syndrome

N. Sörensen, M. Ratzka, M. Büsse

Introduction

Early in fetal life, the spinal cord and spinal canal are of the same length. The differential growth of the spine and the spinal cord causes progressive ascent of the conus medullaris. Embryological studies disclosed [1] that between 9 and 16 weeks, there is a rapid ascent of the conus, combined with atrophy of the terminal

a   b

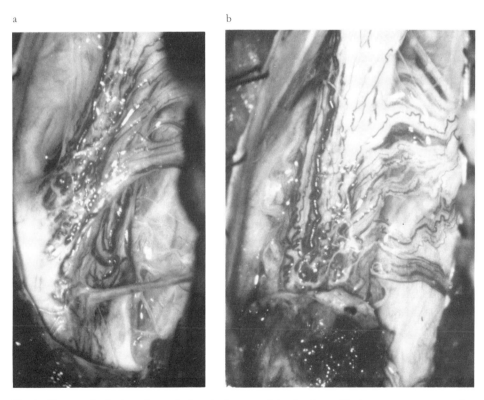

Fig. 1   Elongated spinal cord, attached to the bottom of the dural sac. The lower roots are ascending (a); after freeing in the broad based attachment to the dura the cord migrates cephalically and the roots run in a transverse direction (b).

portion of the cord forming the filum. At 40 weeks after gestation, the conus is situated at the L3 level, and by 2 months of postnatal age, it reaches the adult L1 – 2 level.

Diagnosis and Treatment

A thickened filum terminale may tether the conus below the L1 – 2 level and prevent further ascent of the cord. As the child continues to grow, traction on the cord increases and serious neurologic symptoms result (motor or sensory loss in the lower limbs; bowel and bladder incontinence; low back pain of sciatic distribution; spinal and leg or foot deformities).

About 50% with tethered cords have a cutaneous evidence of spina bifida (hairy patch, dimple, subcutaneous lipoma).

Myelography with positive contrast water-soluble dye and postmyelographic CT scanning will show the intraspinal, intra and extradural malformation [3]. At operation [2] the spinal cord and the nerve roots are untethered by freeing the attachments to the dural sac (fig. 1), to fibro-lipomatous tissue in lipomyelome-

a   b

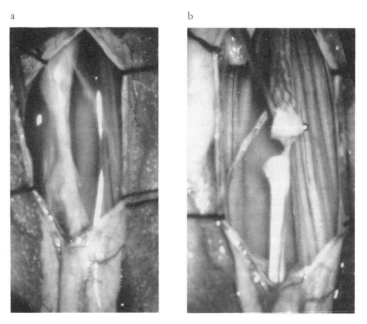

Fig. 2   Exposed thickened filum terminale with a small lipoma (a); filum terminale during coagulation and transection. Dissection of small sacral roots surrounding the filum terminale must be avoided (b).

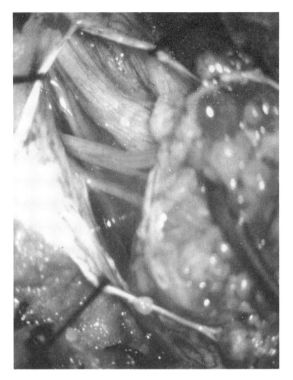

Fig. 3   Lipomyelomeningocele, freeing the attachment to the surrounding dura before duraplasty.

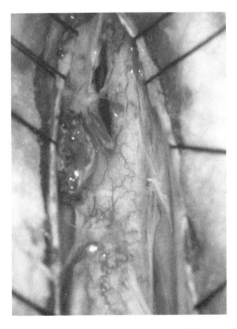

Fig. 4   Diastematomyelia after resection of a fibrocartilagenous spur.

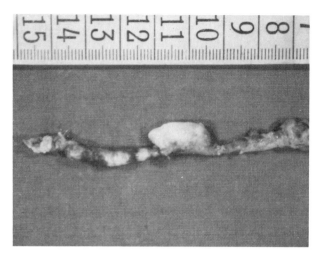

Fig. 5   Resected dermal sinus tract, which had been attached to the conus medullaris.

ningocele (fig. 3), by dividing a thickened filum terminale (fig. 2), by extirpation of a dermal sinus tract (fig. 5) or by resection of a cartilaginous or bony spur in diastematomyelia (fig. 4).

To prevent serious neurological disturbances in the growing child with tethered cord syndrome the operation should be performed as soon as the diagnosis is made. Some recovery of lost neurological function is possible.

References

[1] Barson, A. J.: The vertebral level of termination of the spinal cord during normal and abnormal development. J. Anat. **106** (1970) 489–497.
[2] James, C. C. M., L. P. Lassmann: Spina bifida occulta. Academic Press, London – Toronto – Sydney 1981.
[3] Pettersson, H., D. C. F. Harwood-Nash: CT and myelography of the spine and cord. Springer Verlag, Berlin – Heidelberg – New York 1982.

The operative treatment of spinal deformities in cases of meningomyelocele

J. Harms, R. Grey, K. Zielke

Spinal column deformities in myelomeningocele are of great significance, because they impair the ability to sit, to stand and to walk. Their treatment places considerable demand on operative techniques. Apart from diastematomyelia and spondylolisthesis, which often occur with the meningomyelocele, it is particularly the kyphosis, the scoliosis and the lordosis with which the spinal surgeon is confronted.

Apart from the pure paralytic from of meningomyelocele one often finds defects of segmentation as well as combined defects, which can severely complicate the condition and make treatment very difficult.

Kyphosis

There are pure paralytic and pure congenital forms, as well as a mixed form. Shurtleff estimates that the chances of developing kyphosis in cases with a thoracic lesion are between 1:7 and 1:10, whereas with lumbar lesion it is less then 1:20 [5].

In contrast, with lumbar lesions, only in 1% is kyphosis found at birth. In about 2 to 5% of these a kyphosis of more than 30 degrees is to be expected after 10 years.

Indication for operation

The following aspects must be taken into consideration when deciding to correct the kyphosis by surgical means:

- Increased progression of the kyphosis,
- chronic skin ulceration,
- maintaining the ability to sit,
- improving functions of micturition and of defecation.

Paralytic form

The paralytic form poses no great therapeutic difficulty as long as it is approached early enough and there are no existing structural changes.

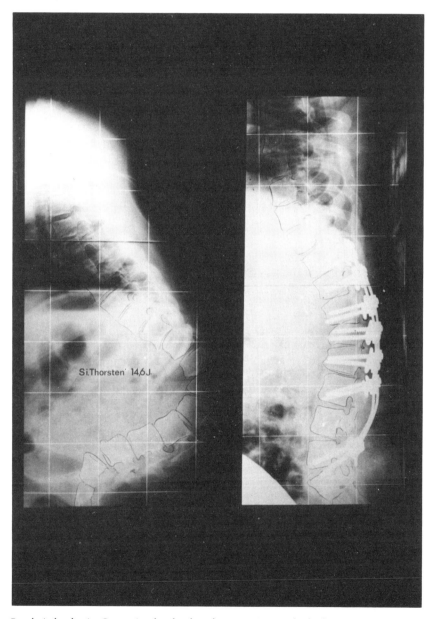

Fig. 1   Paralytic kyphosis. Correction by the dorsal compresion method of Zielke.

Here we employ the dorsal and ventral erection method: as a rule both methods are used in combination as in the treatment of other forms of kyphosis not associated with meningomyelocele. To be precise, ventrally many segments must be supported by a graft and dorsally compression instrumentation is used. Here the dorsal compression method of Zielke with the aid of transpedicle screws proved itself to be efficient (fig. 1).

Congenital kyphosis or mixed form

In these forms the operative technique is determined by the age of the patient at the time of the operation.

The following methods of treatment can be tabulated in the correction of kyphosis:

0 – 3 years: ventral fusion at the apex of the kyphosis (anterior strut grafting)
5 – 10 years: Hall's method, for details, see below.

older than

10 years: dorso-ventral instrumentation and fusion, the Zielke/Rodegerdts-instrumentation is used dorsally and ventrally the Zielke distraction rod or the Slot distraction device.

If the kyphosis is diagnosed and treated early, that is to say up to 3 years of age, a correction is not accomplished in most cases, but a progression can be prevented. If this occurs then later the area of fusion must be extended.

Between the ages of 5 and 10 the kyphosis accompanying meningomyelocele can be treated by the method of Hall [3, 4]. The operation consists of many phases, all done at once. First there is the excision of the dilated dural sack over the apex of the kyphos in a caudal direction. Cranially, where the spinal cord begins to appear normal, the dural sack is closed and the dilated part of the sack is excised. Here the possibility of bleeding from the epidural venous plexus is great. This plexus is in direct contact with bone and it may be difficult to stop the bleeding.

The next step is to proceed from dorso-lateral to the ventral side and then dissect the anterior longitudinal ligament at the apex of the kyphos and excise the bony apex. The end vertebrae which are now parallel to each other must be stabilised (fig. 3) either by the Harrington compression system or better still, by the Zielke compression system.

Then follows an intervertebral and dorsal fusion. It is of extreme importance to carry out the fusion accurately, otherwise relapse will follow (fig. 2).

In patients over 15 years of age the combined ventro-dorsal method is used. Figure 2 shows the correction of the kyphosis, by the case of ventral distraction

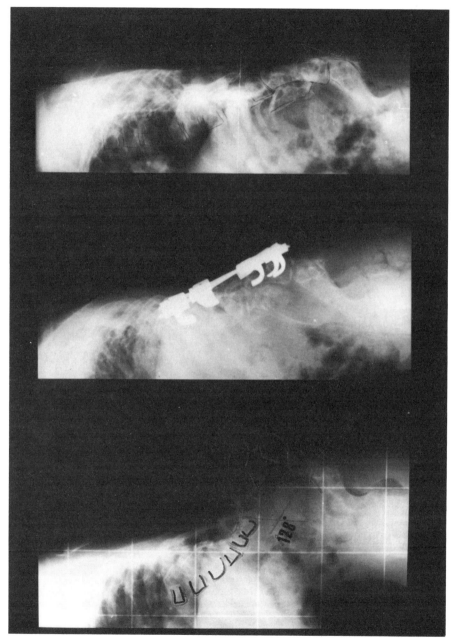

Fig. 2   Combined paralytic and congenital kyphotic deformity. Corrected by the method of Hall.

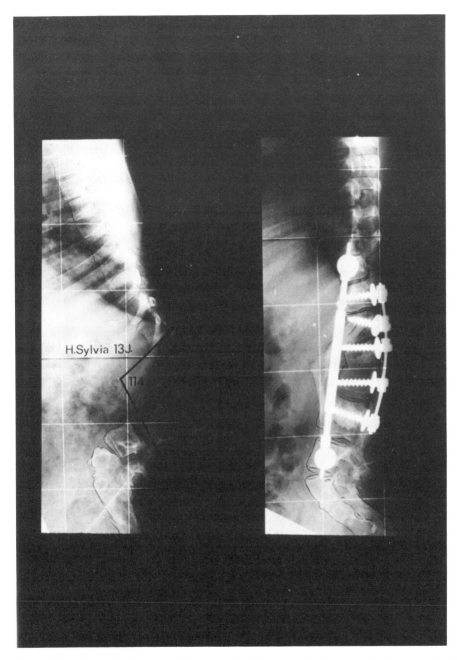

Fig. 3   Paralytic kyphosis, corrected by a combined anteroposterior approach. Anterior the Zielke-
distractor, dorsal compression rod.

with a fibular graft, ventral derotation spondylodesis and followed by compression with the Zielke method combined with transpedicular screws [6].

Without any doubt we are dealing here with big operations whose success demand wide knowledge of the surgical techniques. Such operations should be carried out by surgeons well versed in vertebro-spinal surgery.

Scoliosis

Scoliosis in subjects with meningomyelocele is seen mostly in the patients with paralysis. A pelvic obliquity is usually present. A further characteristic is the progression with age and an increase of neurological deficit.

As with kyphosis, Shurtleff has demonstrated that scoliosis requiring surgical treatment is determined by the extent of the neurological lesion accompanying the myelomeningocele.

When the lesion is thoracic then within a few years 80% develop a scoliosis which requires therapy while in contrast with a lumbar lesion the scoliosis requires therapy in less than 9%.

Table 1   Scoliosis (30°) depending on the neurological lesion (Shurtleff)

	Thoracic	high lumbar	low lumbar	sacral
4 years	17%	14%	3%	3%
10 years	22%	22%	18%	3%
15 years	81%	44%	23%	3%
20 years	88%	81%	23%	9%

Indications for operative treatment

Scoliosis greater than 35 degrees —
increasing pain —
decreased pulmonary function —
increase of neurological symptoms.

The aim of the therapy is to establish a spinal column as stable and as straight as possible both in the sitting and in the standing position, and to avoid pelvic obliquity. A further goal is the maintenance of good pulmonary function which is part of good scoliosis therapy.

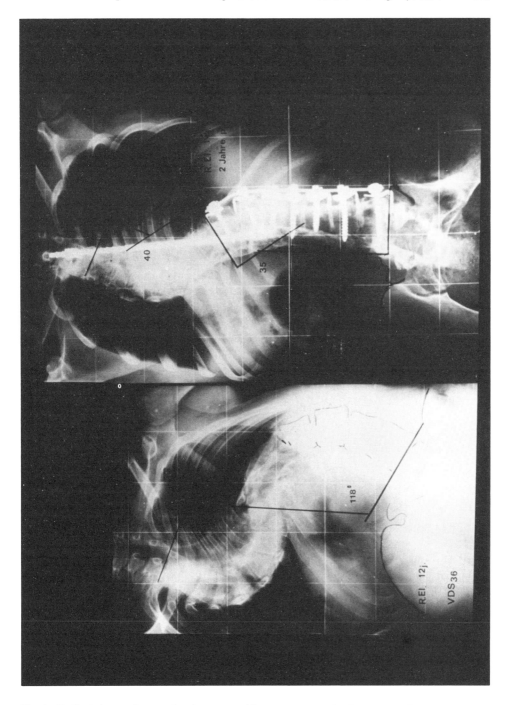

Fig. 4   Scoliosis by meningomyelocele, corrected by antero-posterior instrumentation.
         Anterior VDS-Zielke-system, posterior Harrington-distraction rod.

Operative techniques

The usual therapeutic procedures used in the treatment of "normal" scoliosis can be employed only to a limited extent in the scoliosis in patients with meningomyelocele.

Therefore the earlier results were disappointing. The big breakthrough in the scoliosis therapy by meningomyelocele came about in 1969 when Allen Dwyer introduced the technique of anterior spine fusion.

The Dwyer method [1, 2] was improved in 1974 when Zielke introduced the ventral derotations spondylodesis (VDS). Also in 1974 O'Brien recommended a dorso-ventral instrumentation of the spinal column whereby the Dwyer method or the VDS could be used for the ventral part. For the dorsal segment a modified Harrington method is used. The advantage of the combined instrumentation is the better stabilisation of the correction. In most cases a levelling of the pelvis can be achieved.

A further advantage is that the patients need be kept in plaster cast and corset for a shorter time. Plaster cast is essential when a double curve is present.

The results of a dorso-ventral surgical treatment of a case of extreme scoliosis is illustrated in figure 4. It shows that the pelvic obliquity is corrected, as well as a very impressive correction of the lumbar and thoracic scoliosis was achieved through the VDS of the lumbar region and the Harrington method in the thoracic region.

Using the combination of these methods of treatment even the most severe deformities can be satisfactorily corrected.

Lordosis

Apart from the kyphosis a rare but very pathological lordosis of the lumbar spine is sometimes found.

The aetiology cannot always be explained. It is frequently associated with contraction of the hips producing flexion as compensatory lordosis.

Very occasionally it results from an overcorrection of a lumbar kyphosis. Surprisingly, many develop after lumbo-peritoneal shunt operations. The pathogenesis is not known in such patients.

Correction of the lumbar lordosis is very difficult because correction by means of Harrington rods results in a complete blocking of the lumbo-sacral junction so that a tilting of the pelvis becomes impossible. In such cases the modified

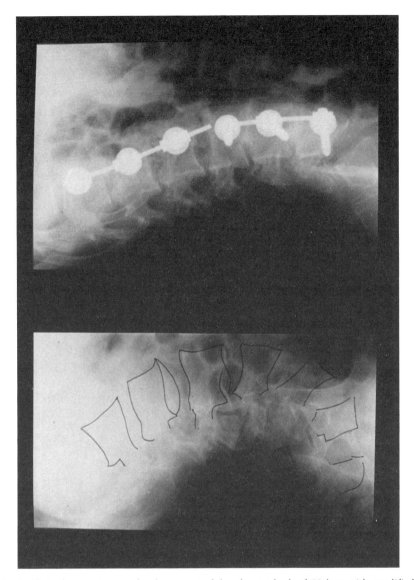

Fig. 5   Lordosis by meningomyelocele, corrected by the method of Hakey with modified VDS-
        system.

VDS technique put forward by Hakey in 1981 has proven itself. Here the ventral derotation spondylodesis by Zielke is used in a lordosing direction.

The use of this method requires detailed knowledge of the VDS system. The result of one such correction is shown in figure 5.

Conclusion

Kyphosis, scoliosis and lordosis are frequent in meningomyelocele. Their therapy requires excellent knowledge of spinal surgery. By the use of the instrumentation which is at our disposal today, good and stable correction can be achieved.

References

[1] Dwyer, A. F.: An anterior approach to scoliosis – a preliminary report. Clin. Orthop. 62 (1969) 192.

[2] Dwyer, A. F.: Experience of anterior correction of scoliosis. Clin. Orthop. 93 (1973) 191.

[3] Hall, J. E., W. P. Bobechko: Advances in the management of spinal deformities in myelodysplasia. Clin. Neurosurg, 20 (1973) 164–173.

[4] Hall, J. E., R. Martin: The natural history of spine deformity in myelomeningocele. A study of 130 patients. Paper Presented to Canadian Orthopaedic Association, Bermuda, June 1970.

[5] Shurtleff, D. B., R. Goiney, L. H. Gordon et al.: Myelodysplasia: The natural history of kyphosis and scoliosis. A preliminary report. Dev. Med. Child Neurol. 18 (suppl. 37) (1976) 126–133.

[6] Zielke, K.: Personal communication.

IV Interdisciplinary problems of spinal dysraphias

Incidence of spina bifida occulta and its importance in orthopaedic diseases

A. Härle

Introduction

Since Virchow described spina bifida occulta (SBO) for the first time in 1875, embryologists and clinicians became interested in this radiologically demonstrable anomaly. Whereas from 1890 to 1930 many publications on defect vertebral arches were appearing and a possible correlation with many diseases was discussed, no special interest was shown in spina bifida occulta during the period after 1950, particularly noticeable in the field of orthopaedics. However a laudable exeption is the monograph by James and Lassman [6].

The data about the incidence of SBO differ greatly in the German from those in the English literature, reaching from 2%, see Eisenstein [3] to 54% in Karlin [2] (tab. 1). Their analyses are based on very divergent series and examination techniques; explaining the reason for the substantially different results. Whereas Karlin evaluated X-rays from a clinical sample, Eisenstein's investigations are based on anatomical specimens from South Africa. In case that there were racial

Table 1   The reported incidence of spina bifida occulta differs widely in the literature

Sutow	(1956)	28.0%
Kohler	(1928)	10.0%
Roederer	(1926)	33.0%
James	(1972)	5.0%
Kammel	(1960)	21.9%
Hintze	(1922)	10.0%
Graessner	(1916)	16.0%
Lorber	(1967)	5.0%
Wynne-Davis	(1979)	6.7%
Meyerding	(1931)	25.0%
Perret	(1963)	20.0%
Wheeler	(1920)	15.4%
Sutherland	(1922)	5.2%
Gillespie	(1949)	4.8%
Karlin	(1935)	54.0%
Eisenstein	(1978)	1.9%

Table 2   There is a decrease of the radiological spina bifida occulta parallel with ageing up to 20
years

	Hintze n = 700	Kammel n = 3,209	Meyer n = 1,400
Up to 5 years	81.0%	73.0%	72.0%
Up to 10 years	66.0%	50.0%	42.0%
Up to 15 years	44.0%	40.0%	–
Over 20 years	10.0%	21.9%	24.0%

differences in the incidence of SBO, a correlation and comparison of the results from different continents is hardly feasible.

Another reason for the diverging data are the variation in ossification times of the vertebral arches during growth which were often falsely interpreted as partial radiological clefts of vertebral arches. Hinze [5], Kammel [8], and Meyer [10] worked out the correlation between age and incidence of radiologic SBO (tab. 2). In all of these three studies, the incidence of SBO is decreasing with increasing age; accordingly, apparent clefts of the vertebral arches were found to be present in 70 – 80% of the children up to 5 years, in 40 – 60% up to 10 years, and in 10 – 24% above 20 years of age.

These studies demonstrate the importance of the ossification times of the vertebral arches. However, the investigators must have made some mistakes concerning the interpretation of the radiographs, particularly in the younger age groups; for the radiological SBO incidence up to the age of 10 years might have to be 100%, as the ossification of the vertebral arches is still incomplete.

A too high occurence will also be found if the sample of patients is not representative for the general population and it is striking that Kammel [8] and Meyer [10] found a percentage being nearly twice as high as Hinze's [5] results who based his study mainly on skeletons in the anatomy department.

A further reason for the different data on incidence is the difficulty to verify cleft formations, if only AP radiographs are available. In most of the works, a description of the decisive criteria is missing, making a subsequent clarification impossible where the border between 'normal' and 'pathologic' was fixed.

Material and methods

With this background, a correlation of SBO and orthopaedic diseases is hardly possible. For this reason, we have again started an extensive study. To obtain results representative for the general population, we did not evaluate records of orthopaedic patients. For more exact control we chose at random two series each of which should show a characteristic caused by random events. Trauma was selected as the first series, and spontaneous occurrence of a bacterial or viral inflammation as the second series. Accordingly, the records of only such patients were analysed, whose attendance at our hospital had a direct relationship to one of these events. It is presumed that accidents and spontaneous viral or bacterial inflammations affect an individual at random, creating statistically reliable control series.

The results were separately analysed for females and males. The age limit was fixed 16 years for females and 18 years for males.

The patients were classified into one of the 3 following categories: 1. normal, 2. evident clefts of the vertebral arches and 3. asymmetric arches without real spinous processes (fig. 1). In the last group, oblique clefts of the vertebral arches are for the most part present, and was seen in oblique radiographs (fig. 2). To obtain objective measurements, the distances between the pedicles of the vertebral arches L4 to S3 were determined. A standard film/focus distance of 1 m was fixed. If the film/focus distance diverged, it was multiplied with an average factor being seperately calculated for males and females from comparative radiographs.

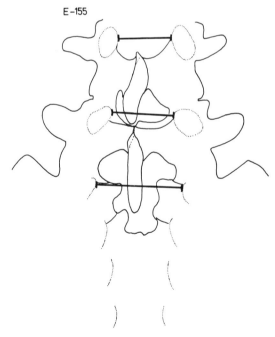

E-155

Fig. 1   Spina bifida occulta at the S1 level; the interpeduncular distance is measured as the shortest connection line.

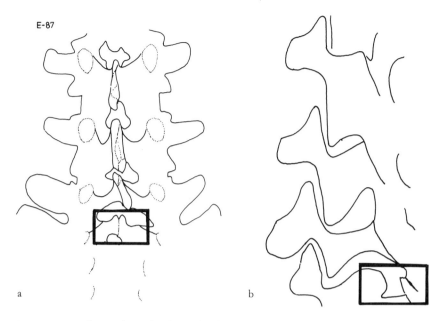

E-87

a   b

Fig. 2   Asymmetric arches at the S1 level (a); the oblique view shows that there is a cleft present at the spinal process (b).

From more than 5.000 clinical records, 470 X-rays of female and 469 of male patients were evaluated, about half of those belonged to the inflammation or the trauma series. Regarding the easily recognizable clefts of vertebral arches of above 1 mm, the evaluation showed comparable results (tab. 3). The incidence was 16% in the trauma group and 18% in the inflammation patients. This represents a mean incidence of 17% in men. Comparable results were found for women, or were identical in both of the collectives with real clefts of vertebral arches, amounting to 9% in the inflammation and to 9% in the trauma group with a mean of 9%.

These sexual differences already apparent in the preliminary analyses in approximally the same ratio, allows the conclusion that SBO has a sex-linked preference.

Table 3   -The incidence of spina bifida occulta in the two groups (inflammation and trauma) is quite equal

| | Men | | Women | |
	with cleft	asymmetric	with cleft	asymmetric
Inflammation group	18,2%	9.9%	9.4%	7.1%
Trauma group	16.2%	7.0%	9.2%	6.9%
Both group	17.2%	8.5%	9.3%	7.0%

Results

An asymmetric formation of vertebral arches was found in 9.9% of the male patients in the inflammation group and in 7% in the trauma group (average 8.5%). In the females being 7.1% in the inflammation group and 6.9% in the trauma group (average 7%).

Most of the radiological features were found at the first sacral vertebra (tab. 4); 96.9% of all real clefts of vertebral arches were here located, whereas they were observed at L5 in 2.3% and at L4 in 0.8%. Asymmetric arches showed a slightly differing incidence pattern of distribution; L5 was involved in 14.8% and S1 in 85.2%. The segments S2 and S3 were not analysed, because this region is often scarcely visualized.

In males the mean distances between the pedicales of the vertebral arches showed comparable results (tab. 5).

The mean distance of the pedicles of the vertebral arch S1 was 38 mm in the inflammation group and of 37 mm in the trauma group. In the groups of 'cleft formation' and 'asymmetric vertebral arches' the figures were almost the same. Statistical analysis indicated later that there were some differences between the mean distances of the pedicles in the three categories ('normal', 'clefts of the vertebral arches', and 'asymmetric vertebral arches') in both groups. However, in comparison with the normal group, evidently higher mean values were found

Table 4   Lumbosacral spina bifida occulta is mostly found at the S1 level

	Clefts		Asymmetric arches		Both	
L4	1	0.7%	—	—	1	0.4%
L5	3	2.3%	12	14.8%	15	7.1%
S1	126	96.9%	69	85.2%	195	92.4%

Table 5   Spina bifida occulta is combined with a significant increase of the interpeduncular distance at the S1 level of compared with normal findings in men (p > 0.01)

	Normal	Clefts	Asymmetric arches
Inflammation group	38.0	41.4	40.7
	± 2.1	± 2.8	± 2.7
Trauma group	37.6	41.0	41.6
	± 2.9	± 3.4	± 3.3
Both group	37.8	41.1	40.9
	± 2.6	± 3.2	± 3.0

in the category with clefts of vertebral arches, being 41.2 mm, in contrast to those with asymmetric vertebral arches, being 41 mm.

The same observations applied to females (tab. 6). In the 'normal' category the mean distance of the pedicles was 36.1 mm in the inflammation group and 36.3 mm for the trauma series. Higher mean distances were seen in the 'cleft' (40.3 mm) and in the 'asymmetric vertebral arch' group (39.4 mm) than in the 'normals'.

A comparison of the results from females and males showed constantly higher values in men for all samples or groups; the differences range from 2 – 5%. This may be caused by the different skeletal development in both of the sexes, concerning size and weight. The generally supposed co-existence of spina bifida and pes cavus, of 75%, Beck [1], appears to be confirmed by these findings, and a pathogenetical relation may be assumed. Although spina bifida cystica and occulta are generally considered to be distinct entities, Lorber [9] showed an interesting relationship; namely the incidence of the occulta type is obviously higher in parents of cystica children than in his normal controls, and in males, the factor is about five and a half times higher. An increased incidence of spina bifida occulta combined with spondylolisthesis is evident (tab. 7). In our 293 cases of spondylolisthesis SBO was present in 52% of the males and 49% in the female patients. These results agree very well with the 49% found by Wynne-Davies [11]. The ratios of the male dominance are 1.8:1 in the spina bifida in

Table 6   Spina bifida occulta is combined with a significant increase of the interpeduncular distance at the S1 level of compared with normal findings in women ($p > 0.01$)

	Normal	Clefts	Asymmetric arches
Inflammation group	36.1	40.1	39.2
	± 2.1	± 2.3	± 2.0
Trauma group	36.2	40.5	39.4
	± 2.7	± 2.8	± 3.1
Both group	36.2	40.3	39.3
	± 2.4	± 2.6	± 2.7

Table 7   Spina bifida occulta is increased in patients with spondylolisthesis, especially in female patients

	Men (n = 202)			Women (n = 104)		
	Total	SBO	%	Total	SBO	%
L4/L5	50	15	30.0	30	7	23.3
L5/S1	130	76	58.5	66	42	63.6
Both segments	180	91	50.6	96	49	51.0

Table 8   Spina bifida occulta represents an unfavourable prognistic sign in female patients with spondylolisthesis at the L5/S1 segment

| | Men | | Women | |
| | with | without | with | without |
	spina bifida		spina bifida	
L4/L5	20.3°	18.7°	21.0°	22.6°
L5/S1	25.4°	18.7°	45.2°	24.6°

agreement with each other. The highest concordance spondylolisthesis was at segment L5/S1 (63.6% in women and 58.5% in men), whereas the mean values of olisthesis at segment L4/L5 was 23% and 30% respectively.

However, the close relation between spina bifida occulta and spondylolisthesis is not limited to an associated picture, but are also related to the degree of the spondylolisthesis, too [4]. Different mean values of spondylolisthesis were found at segment L5/S1 in female patients, if series with and without SBO were made. The mean value of spondylolisthesis amounted to 21° in the group without spina bifida: it was more than twice as high with SBO, being 45.2°. Higher degrees of spondylolisthesis were also found in the male spina bifida group. However, the mean value of 24° in the spina bifida group was not significantly different from that of the group without spina bifida, being 18°. In olisthesis at segment L4/L5, no significant difference was detectable in the groups with and without spina bifida for either of the sex (tab. 8).

Discussion

The pathogenetic role of SBO in spondylolisthesis may be shown, firstly, through impaired vertebral arches, which provide a diminished insertion area for the intersegmental muscles and, secondly, through disturbed muscle coordination due to neurological disorders. This results in mechanical stresses for the lumbar spine if they are not moderated and kept in tolerable limits. The coincident presence of spina bifida and spondylolisthesis at segment L5/S1 in a girl must be considered to be an unfavourable combination, and higher degrees of spondylolisthesis are to be expected. For this reason, particularly careful serial observation of further development should be made.

Cowell [2] when dealing with the connexions between spina bifida and scoliosis found an incidence of SBO of 34% in 100 patients with scoliosis. Objections must be raised to his control collective, however, as all relatives with a scoliotic angle outside 10° were used. This is not representative for the general population, and furthermore no exact age limits were fixed. If parents with scoliosis were classified according to the characteristic of SBO, a coincidence of 16% was found in mothers, whereas SBO without scoliosis was observed in only 5%. In fathers, no significant differences of SBO incidence with scoliosis was shown. Other investigators, however, refuse to accept pathogenetic relations between SBO and scoliosis and this problem is still unresolved.

Possible relations of SBO with other orthopaedic diseases, such as Scheuermann's disease, disk hernation, and low back pain generally, can only be proved by means of extensive investigations. We have started such an analysis for patients with disk herniation, but no definite conclusions can as yet be drawn.

Conclusions

Reviewing our present findings and their relevant literature, we can assume that a definite relation of SBO exists with some orthopaedic diseases, for the incidence of SBO is higher in orthopaedic patients than in the general population.

References

[1] Beck, O.: Spina bifida occulta und ihre ätiologische Beziehung zu Deformitäten der unteren Extremität. Ergeb. Chir. Orthop. 15 (1922) 491–568.
[2] Cowell, M. J., H. R. Cowell: The incidence of spina bifida occulta in idiopathic scoliosis. Clin. Orthop. 118 (1976) 16–18.
[3] Eisenstein, S.: Spondylolysis – A skeletal investigation of two population groups. J. Bone Jt. Surg. 60-B (1978) 489–494.
[4] Härle, A., G. Hitzler: Die Häufigkeit der Spina bifida occulta und ihre ätiologische Bedeutung bei der Spondylolisthesis. Z. Orthop. 118 (1980) 466.
[5] Hintze, A.: Die Fontanella lumbo-sacralis und ihr Verhältnis zur Spina bifida occulta. Archiv klin. Chir. 119 (1922) 409–454.
[6] James, C. C. M., L. P. Lassman: Spina bifida occulta. Orthopaedic, radiological and neurological aspects, pp. 4–6. Academic Press, London 1981.
[7] Karlin, I. W.: Incidence of spina bifida occulta in children with and without enuresis. Am. J. Dis. Child. 49 (1935) 125–129.
[8] Kammel, W.: Häufigkeit und klinische Bedeutung der Spina bifida occulta. Z. Orthop. 92 (1960) 449–452.
[9] Lorber, J., K. Levick: Spina bifida cystica. Incidence of spina bifida occulta in parents and in controls. Arch. Dis. Child. 42 (1967) 171–175.
[10] Meyer, H.: Die Bedeutung der Spaltbildung im knöchernen Wirbelkanal in der Ätiologie orthopädischer Leiden. Verh. Deutsch. Orthop. Ges. 19. Kongr. (1924) 107–117.
[11] Wynne-Davies, R., J. H. S. Scott: Inheritance and spondylolisthesis. A radiographic family survey. J. Bone Jt. Surg. 61-B (1979) 301–305.

The indication for operative improvement of lower limb function in children with myelomeningocele

J. Correll, H. M. Sommer

In practise operative treatment for the functional improvement in the lower extremities of children with myelomeningocele differs widely. The aim of the treatment is a return of function. The operation itself must encompass the relationship of patient cooperation and the planned improvement of function. Besides the pathological-anatomical considerations, the time and the degree of operative procedures must be considered in view of the child's anticipated outcome [2, 3, 6]. Nearly all patients with a myelomenigocele have a wide range of pedal deformities. The degree of palsy is responsible for the reduction of function. Mainly those disabilities brought to the attention of the surgeon have a partial or a complete spastic palsy. Completely paralysed feet being without any innervation usually give no problems. A foot having weak palsy develops a rather normal outer shape and the necessary orthopaedic devices do not pose insoluble problems. In contrast, a partial innervation of the muscles of the foot will cause a deformity of varying degrees, as a balanced influence is not present [13, 15].

The decision for orthopaedic intervention should be based on the surgical indication for operative measures regarding instability, deformities of the foot, patient's age, and the expected improvement of function achieved by the operation. The aim must be to achieve the best possible result concerning foot function in relation to the present state of the child, preferable in early childhood. It must be pointed out that surgical treatment performed too late can lead to further and extreme operative measures which are a bad basis for more operations later on. The initial operation in early childhood should be undertaken to correct present foot deformities. At this young age soft tissues operation, e.g., tendons, muscles, ligaments, and capsules can be performed with the aim of maximal deformity correction. Transfer of muscles and tendons must be planned with great care and forethought. The ensuing function gained from such a transfer can be calculated seldom exactly [5, 7].

The aim of an early operative treatment should be, as much as possible, to achieve a positive influence on foot form development during adolescence. Further measurements should be carried out correcting the inward or outward deformity of the lower leg. However, a foot deformity correcting operation should precede in any case. The time to correct the rotational deformity is when the child starts to stand up. Until the foot has completed its growth pattern, no operation on the bony parts should be done [14].

Intensive conservative therapy should precede operative intervention, in particular physiotherapy on a neuro-physiological basis is very important, followed by passive remodelling treatment. The conservative treatment modalities can be completed by orthopaedic devices such as correcting splints.

In the older child the time for operative measures must be decided upon in relation to the degree of the foot deformity to be corrected. The tendency for improvement or at least a steady state under conservative treatment must be considered. Until pre-puberty an indication for an operation must be oriented by functional considerations. It must be considered if the foot function can be improved by deformity correcting measures (e.g. by correction of a rotational deformity of the lower leg) or if the deformity is so extensive that even with an orthopaedic foot wear, a sufficient stabilization of the foot cannot be achieved. However, this will be seldom the case. In this early stage pressure sores can force an operative intervention especially in those cases when the pressure sores are not amenable to conservative measures, and the patient has to be immobilized for long periods, or suffering from osteomyelitis.

During and after puberty a final correcting operation can be attempted to achieve a lasting result. This type of operation in the form of wedge osteotomies of the tarsus and hind foot or a T-arthrodesis is indicated in the adult foot in order to enable wearing optimal orthopaedic shoes for satisfactory function. The aim of these procedures must be to achieve marginal stability of the foot with a good fitting shoe. Pressure sores must be avoided in any case [1].

In ambulatory pediatric patients using orthopaedic devices, the operative measures are mainly directed avoiding pressure sore problems. Non-ambulatory patients are seldom operated on but rather fitted with a good shoe which protects the foot from exterior forces.

In contrast to foot interactions operations involving the knee joint are rare. An operation for a fixed flexion deformity of the knee caused by muscular imbalance should be done only with the intention that a gait improvement can be gained. The knee in flexion contracture can provoke a hip flexion contracture. The operated knee flexion contracture has a beneficial influence on the hip joint. A child needing orthopaedic devices should be operated on only when the knee-flexion-contracture prevents special fittings, and further immobilisation is anticipated.

In operating, hamstring lengthening combined with a posterior dissection of the knee joint capsule is performed. A supracondylar correction osteotomy is seldom indicated, but this enables the fitting with an orthopaedic apparatus without causing further problems [8].

The correction of the extension contraction and even in the extreme form of the genu recurvatum is a rare operation. The strong quadriceps muscle enables the knee joint to stabilize and allows for vertical mobility. In cases of a very strong knee recurvation or patients confined to a wheel chair, quadriceps tendon lengthening gives the possibility of an improved function. Axial deviations such as varus or valgus knees are seldom operated on. However, a strong deformity in a patient who walks without technical aids demands a correction.

The unilateral overload of the joint with its increasing instability must be equalized with a correction osteotomy. A child fitted with an orthopaedic apparatus must be operated on when a further fitting for support is not possible or when problems such as pressure sores, develop.

Operational procedures on soft tissue and bone of the hip joint have now to be discussed. A soft tissue operation is indicated when a limited range of motion of the hip joint hinders function. Total release of the anterior hip muscles should be performed when a flexion deformity and eventually an abduction deformity prevents the wearing of calipers. The same must be considered if a thoracic palsy with reflex activity has caused the deformity.

A palsy at lumbar level leads to the lengthening of hip flexors if active hip flexion power should be preserved. Symmetrical flexion deformity of the hips may influence the vertebral spine by developing a hyperlordosis. The asymmetrical deformity can be responsible for a scoliosis. The anterior 'hip release' can enhance stretching of the spine.

Sometimes an abduction deformity which prevents wearing of aids must be operated on. A Z-shaped lengthening or a dissection of the tensor fasciae latae and the tractus ilio-tibialis must be performed. The indication to dissect the adductors must be discussed, when an adduction deformity impairs aids wearing or gait. In combination with a muscular imbalance, a subluxation or even a luxation can develop. The tenotomy of the adductors gives the possibility to easier exercise but bears the risk of recurrence [6].

Bony operative measures should be performed on the hip joint only during adolescence if gait and standing without orthopaedic devices is possible. Sometimes the wearing of a caliper must be achieved with the help of an operation. After growth stops, osteotomies of the coxal end of the femur may be necessary to enable caliper fitting. We have to recognize that a mere correction of bones at the hip joint by derotation and varus osteotomy or osteotomy of the pelvis cannot improve muscular balance. The latter has to be corrected. Thus in correcting a subluxation or luxation of the hip, a soft tissue operation must be performed additionally. The most important is the posterolateral transfer of the iliopsoas muscle after Sharrard [12]. The results of the iliopsoas transfer are generally favorable; but it is extremely important to consider some parameters.

Table 1   Authors results of 84 transfers of the iliopsoas muscle due to subluxated or luxated hip joints in 50 patients with MMC. The follow-up is on the average 10.5 years. No muscle transfer was performed without open reduction or coxal osteotomy of the femur

	Stable	Sub- or reluxated
Operated hips: follow-up of 10.5 years	49	35
Iliopsoas-transfer without osteotomy of the pelvis	34	32
Iliopsoas-transfer with osteotomy of the pelvis	15	3

These are: The patient's age, the level of palsy, and the necessary additioned operations. Our own experience in 50 patients with 84 operated hips showed that without a bone operation at the hip joint a subluxation or luxation of the hip could not demonstrate long term improvement from a posterolateral transfer of the iliopsoas muscle alone. The aim of a stable hip joint can be achieved, when bony deformities of the upper femur and hip joint are corrected in the same procedure with the muscle transfer. Our own results show a good follow-up in 15 out of 18 hips after 10.5 years [9, 12], (tab. 1), (fig. 1a – e).

a
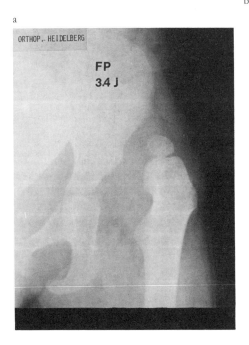

b
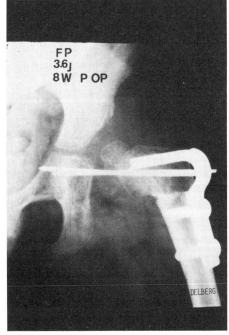

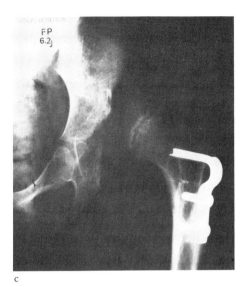

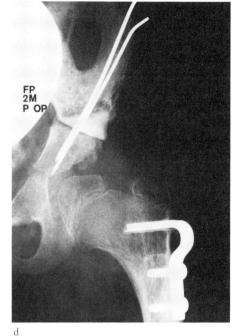

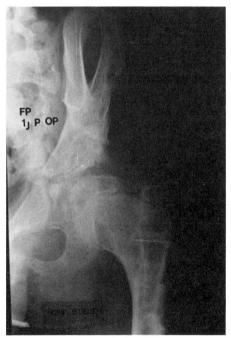

Fig. 1   Follow-up of 4.5 years of a community walker:
a) dislocation of the left hip joint pre-op, age: 3.4 yrs.;
b) 8 weeks after open reduction and derotation-varus-osteotomy;
c) after mobilisation reluxation, patient 6 years old pre-op.;
d) 2 month after Salter-osteotomy of the pelvis and postero-lateral transfer of the iliopsoas muscle;
e) 1 Year post-op, full weight-bearing, gait without devices, no reluxation.

The paralytic luxation of the hip during the postnatal and early childhood period is not an indication for operating. Treatment should be conservative without any immobilizing devices. Frequently we see an outwards abduction-flexion deformity of the hip after a hip joint immobilizing treatment. The child should be encouraged by motivation to stand erect and walk. This is best accomplished during the second or third year of life.

The indication for an operative treatment in children with myelomeningocele forces us to consider procedures which are quite unusual compared to problems in children without myelomeningocele. The functional results must be the most important consideration. An eventual less than perfect X-ray result must be considered of lesser importance. The success of an operation depends, in addition to the correct technique, on intensive, and long-term pre- and post-op. physiotherapy. The main condition for success is the full cooperation of the medical team caring for the patient [10, 11].

References

[1] Duckworth, T., R. P. Betts: The valgus foot in spinal dysraphism. Z. Kinderchir. **31** (1980) 402 – 409.
[2] Feiwell, F.: Surgery of the hip in myelomeningocele as related to adult goals. Clin. Orthop. Rel. Res. **148** (1980) 87 – 93.
[3] Feiwell, E.: Selection of appropriate treatment for patients with myelomeningocele. Orthop. Clin. North Amerika **12** (1981) 101 – 106.
[4] Frank, J. D., J. A. Fixsen: Spina bifida, Brit. J. Hosp. Med. **24** (1980) 422 – 435.
[5] Goldner, J. L., W. A. Somers, R. J. Ruderman: Management of true congenital talipes equinovarus in myelodysplasia. Z. Kinderchir. **31** (1980) 413 – 420.
[6] Katzen, N.: The total care of spina bifida dystica. Surg. Annual, New York **13** (1981) 325 – 331.
[7] Menelaus, M. B.: The orthopedic management of spina bifida cystica. Livingstone, Edinburgh – London – New York 1980.
[8] Menelaus, M. B.: Orthopedic management of children with myolomeningocele: a plea for realistic goals. Dev. Med. Child Neurol. (Suppl.) **37** (1976) 6.
[9] Parsch, K., K. P. Schulitz: Die orthopädische Frühbehandlung des Kindes mit Spina bifida cystica. Z. Orthop. **109** (1971) 458 – 467.
[10] Parsch, K.: Was hat die Psoastransposition für die Rehabilitation des Spina bifida-Kindes gebracht? Z. Orthop. **120** (1982) 405.
[11] Sharrard, W. J. W.: Paralytic deformity in the lower limb. J. B. J. S. **49B** (1967) 731 – 747.
[12] Sharrard, W. J. W.: Posterior iliopsoas transplantation in the treatment of paralytic dislocation of the hip. J. B. J. S. **46B** (1964) 426 – 444.
[13] Sharrard, W. J. W., I. Grosfield: The management of deformity and paralysis of the foot in myelomeningocele. J. B. J. S. **50B** (1968) 457 – 465.
[14] Silk, F. F., D. Wainwright: The recognition and treatment of congenital flat foot in infancy. J. B. J. S. **49B** (1967) 628 – 633.
[15] Smith, T. W. D., T. Duckworth: The management of deformities of the foot in children with spina bifida. Dev. Med. Child Neurol. (Suppl.) **37** (1976) 105.

New methods of treating lumbar kyphosis, hip instability and dislocation in spina bifida patients

A. Härle, H. H. Matthiaß

Lumbar kyphosis presents a severe deformity in about 10% of patients with myelomeningocele, caused by neurological disorders extending from the lower thoracic to the sacral region. At birth, the curvature may measure up to 70°, and has usually a progressive tendency, especially under the action of gravity. Patients with this deformity offer additional skin problems at the apex of the curvature and are mostly unable to stay and wear braces. Even when sitting these children have problems as the center of gravity is displaced forward, which affects their capability to keep a balance. Ulcer formation over the prominent kyphosis is frequent and causes severe problems for treatment including the risk of meningitis or spondylitis. The extensive kyphosis also interferes with respiratory function and causes an "abdominal narrow" syndrome which may affect the urine drainage.

The aims of the treatment in congenital lumbar kyphosis are:

1. Straightening and stabilization of the vertebral column in order to achieve a balance in sitting and to bring the center of gravity backwards;
2. settlement or at least an essential reduction of the bony prominence at the kyphotic apex to prevent further ulceration;
3. increase of trunk height to improve the respiratory and urological functions.

Sharrard [10] first suggested the resection of vertebral bodies from the apex of the kyphotic spine. This surgical technique was generally accepted with slight alterations concerning the number of resected segments and the osteo-synthesis material used for stabilization. In the seventies, this procedure was used worldwide including in our institution. As reported in the literature, we also had to encounter cases with severe recurrence of lumbar kyphosis after resection of vertebral bodies causing extensive skin problems at the kyphotic apex. McKay [6] used an entirely different technique in the middle of the seventies; he pulled the spine to the plate by U-bolts after removal of the anterior longitudinal ligament and disk. The aim of this treatment is the complete return to normal spinal statics, and the elimination of kyphotic acting forces due to the displaced center of gravity. Moreover, a considerable elevation of the thoracic area and an increase of the abdominal cavity leading to a functional improvement of gut and bladder.

With this considerations in mind, we developed a spinal plate being adequate to our operative techniques, which is anteriorly applied and forces the lumbar region in a lordotic posture. After transthoracic exposition in the Riseborough technique [8], removal of the 10th rib, and ligation of the segmental arteries in the kyphotic region was performed. This area is also exposed posteriorly by a second incision. The spaces of the discs are incised anteriorly and an osteotomy of the bony substance which is posteriorly in the area of the dorsolateral vertebral elements, is made. This procedure is carried out at the apex of the kyphotic curvature at two or three segments. Only in case of kyphotic angles above 120° we remove one or two vertebrae at the apex of the kyphotic curve. U-bolts are then introduced from anterior and hooked in a plate placed between the U-bolts and the vertebral body; the U-bolts are screwed up with a lordotic formed plate while the lumbar spine is pulled in a lordotic posture. The clefts gaping at the osteotomy are so closed and the contact areas used as prerequisite for the later consolidation, are enlarged. If a complete return to a normal position is successful (by fixation of a lumbar lordosis), the soft tissue problem is usually solved, and the dorsal nuts are not prominent below the skin (fig. 1).

A case illustration demonstrates the problems and failures of the treatment for lumbar kyphosis. At the age of nearly 2 years, removal of the vertebral body L3 and dorsal stapling after the Blount technique, was performed in this boy because of a 90-degree kyphosis. As the stapling became loose and displaced during the following weeks, anterior spinal fusion was additionally performed with application of a plate, leaving a significant residual kyphosis of about 60°. In the

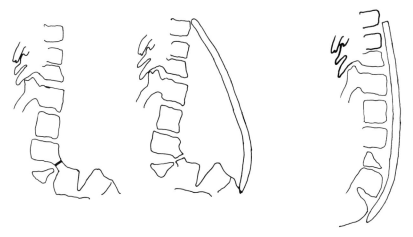

Fig. 1   The lumbar kyphosis is osteomized ventrally at the apex, then after mobilization pulled to the lordotic shaped plate.

following years, the lumbar kyphosis progressed slowly, but continuously. In addition a detachment of the screws occured due to a double fracture of the plate. A kyphotic angle of 110° had again developed in March 1981. The Riseborough technique was performed by anterior exposition with a removal of the plate and an anterior osteotomy of the bony bar stretching over one vertebral body. After cautious mobilization, a partial straightening of the spine could be achieved, and a lordotic positioning of the lumbar region achieved by means of this clasping technique. The posteriorly removed osseous parts were anteriorly packed into the gaping osteotomy area. Postoperatively, the boy was first bedded in a prone position for 14 days. After unproblematic healing of the dorsal wound he got a Risser cast in a lying position for 3 months, and subsequently a sitting Risser cast for further 9 months. After having finished the plaster cast treatment the spine which showed also a scoliotic deformation was stabilized by means of a trunk brace. No relapse of the kyphosis occurred during the 4½-year follow-up period, and a stable fusion of the lumbar region is present. Furthermore, the boy obtained a good sitting ability (fig. 2).

A 12-year old girl was affected with a severe lumbar kyphosis of 150°, bringing the thorax nearly in contact with the pelvis anteriorly. For several years, a

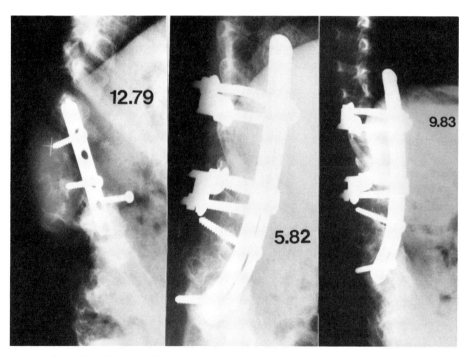

Fig. 2   The 110° kyphosis could be straightened to a lordotic curve, which is maintained unchanged over a period of 4 years.

dorsal exulceration was present with temporary excretion of spinal fluid and a permanent threat of meningitis. In her case, a wedge-shaped excision of two vertebral bodies was carried out. Nevertheless, it was difficult to obtain a normal position of the lumbar region in view of the extreme deformation and tightness of the abdominal wall. However, by means of the U-bolt technique we succeeded in pulling the lumbar spine to the lordotic plate, fixing it in this posture with residual kyphosis of about 10 degrees. This treatment was followed by a 9-month plaster cast fixation, and after 1 year, a solid ossification had been achieved in the area of the osteotomy of the vertebral bodies. After bilateral release of extension contractures of the hip, the girl's sitting ability is now very satisfactory. The elevation and enlargement of the abdominal cavity obtained by means of this procedure is illustrated by AP radiographs. The loop-like course of the ventricular drainage is after the operation for the most part straightened and associated with a gain of height of the abdominal cavity of 10 cm.

Our results of treatment are in contrast with the control findings after vertebral body excision and dorsal pinning as reported by Lowe [4] and Linseth [3]. In both of the series the mean kyphotic angle amounted to about 60° post-operatively and deteriorated during the following year to a mean value of about 75° (tab. 1).

Hip dislocation resp. instability is mostly found in patients with neurologic disturbances at the segments L2 − S1. Dependent on the degree, a weakness of the hip abductors develops besides the failure of the hip extensors; from the predominant activity of the hip flexors and adductors a muscular imbalance results causing hip dislocation already in the first years of life or during the school-age. As treatment of this muscular imbalance the transposition of the iliopsoas muscle from the minor trochanter to the greater trochanter has been

Table 1   The 3 groups concern different methods of vertebral excision; an essential recurrence of kyphosis is encountered in each group after surgery (nach [3])

	Angle preop.	Angle postop.	Angle 1 year
Group 1 n = 5	113°	74°	100°
Group 2 n = 8	119°	50°	81°
Group 3 n = 12	113°	46°	67°
All	115°	53°	78°

Table 2   The stability of the hip joint could be established in about a third of the treatment group after iliopsoas transfer (after [2])

	Success	Failure
Dislocated hips (n = 6)	2 (33%)	4 (67%)
Subluxated hips (n = 19)	5 (26%)	14 (74%)
All (n = 25)	7 (28%)	18 (72%)

recommended. This transposition could be performed to the anterior side of the greater trochanter by the technique after Mustard [7], or as a posterolateral transposition after Sharrard [9] through a fenestration in the ala of the ilium. By the latter method, a better abduction and a reduction of the flexion action of the psoas muscle is achieved (tab. 2).

Some considerations about the situation of the hip can be demonstrated by means of a bio-mechanic model. The spheroid hip joint being primarily unstable is stabilized by four functional groups of muscles: adductors, flexors, abductors, and extensors. This joint could be simply compared to a four-legged table. In case of a myelomeningocele with a paralysis in the lumbar region, two of these functional groups, the extensors and abductors, would fail. This would lead to a complete instability of the table model, for the table could hardly be balanced in normal position on two legs. After the Sharrard technique, the iliopsoas muscle which is mainly a flexor, is postero-laterally transferred and acts then as abductor. Parts of the iliac muscle and the spina muscles remain as residual flexors. However, the flexion ability is considerably limited. In our bio-mechanic model, this result would be adequate for a three-legged table being primarily designed as four-legged table by the architect. Consequently, the table is unstable and may easily tip over by overloading. For that reason McKay [5] dealt with a new method of hip stabilization, using an operative procedure being already applied in the treatment of poliomyelitis after Thomas [11], namely the transposition of the obliquus abdominis muscle on to the greater trochanter. The aim of this method is to achieve a hip stabilization being based on three groups of muscles. In this procedure, a new muscle, the obliquus abdominis externus muscle, is used, and also the adductors are as far as possible dorsally transferred. In myelomenigocele patients with paralysis in the lumbar region, the use of a normally – that is from the lower thoracic area – innervated abdominal muscle seems to be advantageous for support of the weak hip abductors. Additionally, the flexors may be left in their original location, although they must be lengthened or detached in order to avoid their possible predominance.

For bio-mechanical reasons, we consider the operative technique after McKay in myelomeningocele patients at least worthy of discussion. First of all, some annotations shall be given about the operative procedure which includes the transfer of the obliquus abdominis externus muscle to the greater trochanter and the retroposition of the adductors to the tuber ossis ischii; mostly by open reduction and reconstruction of the acetabular roof, or possibly by de-rotational varus osteotomy of the coxal end of the femur, carried out in combination.

The skin incision is started in the anterior axial line at the level of the eighth rib, continued to the anterior iliac spine and then turned to the anteromedial side of the thigh. After removal of the skin from the abdominal fascia, a 1.5 cm wide strip of the obliquus abdominis externus muscle, which becomes broader in craniolateral direction, is detached at the symphysis closely medially to the inguinal ring. If possible, four muscle insertions at the ribs should be comprehended. The second step of the operation is the open reduction resp. the additional reconstruction of the acetabular roof (fig. 3).

A further skin incision follows over the greater trochanter with exposition of the trochanter and canalization under the glutaeus medius. This tunnel is widened to let pass two fingers, then the aponeurosis of the obliquus abdominis externus muscle is drawn through the hole to the trochanter and fixed in a bore hole

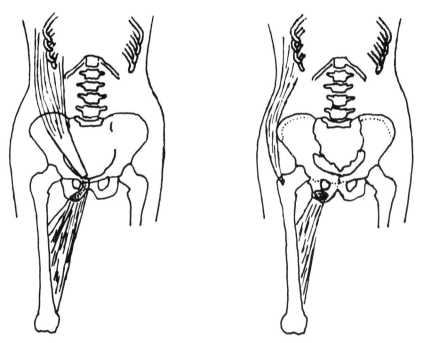

Fig. 3   The obliquus abdominis externus is transferred to the greater trochanter and the adductors displaced backwards around the tuber ossis ischii.

Table 3   After hip dislocation in myelomeningocele children a stable hip joint could be established in 11 out of 12 cases

		Hip stable	Hip instable
Spina bifida	n = 12	11	1
Tumors	n = 2	2	0
Polio	n = 2	2	0
	n = 16	15	1

under slight tension. A possibly necessary derotational and varus osteotomy must be planned in such a way that the blade does not cut the thread aponeurosis of the tendon. The last step is the removal of the adductors from the anterior pubic ramus and the fixation of the dorsal and caudal side of the tuber ossis ischii. Postoperatively, the children get a hip spica cast for four weeks. Then physiotherapeutic exercises are started to activate the obliquus abdominis externus muscle by means of acoustic feedback. After 10 days of training, the children are mostly able to contract the muscle actively, and ambulant continuation of the physiotherapy is then possible. The action of the transferred obliquus abdominis externus muscle can be recognized by a striking traction at the waist, if the child is able to carry out the required motion for hip abduction. If the retroposition of the adductors was sufficient, comparatively satisfying extension may be also achieved and even the ability to extend the legs against the gravity.

Our experience with this operative technique is based on 12 dislocated hips in patients with lumbar myelomeningocele, 2 tumour patients and two female polio patients. In 11 of the 12 myelomeningocele patients stability of the hip could be achieved within a mean follow-up of two years. In one case, dislocation occurred again after the transposition and reconstruction of the acetabular roof, although there was a sufficient formation of the acetabular roof present, at that time (tab. 3).

A final valuation is not yet possible because of the low number of cases and the short follow-up period.

Jackson [2] indicated a successful rate of posterolateral iliopsoas transfers for dislocated or unstable hips of 30% in a follow-up study, and he stated that only very few patients were able to perform active abduction. Freehafer [1] reports similar results, and in his opinion, no better hip stability is obtained after iliopsoas transfer than after tenodesis. Based on our experience until now, we intend to apply the above described operative procedure also in future, because the method of iliopsoas transfer as formerly used by us, was not fully satisfactory.

References

[1] Freehafer, A. A., J. C. Vesseley, R. P. Mack: Iliopsoas muscle transfer in the treatment of myelomeningocele patients with paralytic hip deformities. J. Bone Jt. Surg. **54** (1972) 1715–1729.
[2] Jackson, R. D., T. S. Padgett, M. M. Donovan: Posterior iliopsoas transfer in myelodysplasia. J. Bone Jt. Surg. **61**A (1979) 40–45.
[3] Linseth, R. E., L. Stelzer: Vertebral excision for kyphosis in children with myelomeningocele. J. Bone Jt. Surg. **61**A (1979) 699–704.
[4] Lowe, G. P., M. B. Menelaus: The surgical management of kyphosis in older children with myelomeningocele. J. Bone Jt. Surg. **60**B (1978) 40–45.
[5] McKay, D. W., K. V. Jackman, S. S. Nason et al.: McKay hip stabilization in myelomeningocele. Dev. Med. Child Neurol. **18** (Suppl. 37) (1976) 168–169.
[6] McKay, D. W.: The McKay plate for kyphosis of the spine. Dev. Med. Child Neurol. **18** (Suppl. 37) (1976) 169.
[7] Mustard, W. T.: Iliopsoas transfer for weakness of the hip abductors. J. Bone Jt. Surg. **34**A (1952) 647–650.
[8] Riseborough, E. J.: The anterior approach to the spine for correction of deformities of the axial skeleton. Clin. Orthop. **93** (1973) 207–214.
[9] Sharrard, W. J. W.: Posterior iliopsoas transposition in the treatment of paralytic dislocation of the hip. J. Bone Jt. Surg. **46**B (1964) 426–444.
[10] Sharrard, W. J. W.: Spinal osteotomy for congenital kyphosis in myelomingocele. J. Bone Jt. Surg. **50**B (1968) 466–471.
[11] Thomas, L. I., T. C. Thompson, L. R. Straub: Transplantation of the oblique muscle for the abductor paralysis. J. Bone Jt. Surg. **32**A (1950) 207–216.

Neuro-urological findings in dysgenesis of the sacrum

J. Weißmüller, K. M. Schrott, A. Sigel

In neural tube defects urological complications are often decisive for the prognosis. The problems of bladder emptying, incontinence, urinary tract infection, and protection of renal function demand continuous urological care.

Anomalies of the urinary tract coexist in about 43% of cases having spina bifida cystica. Dysgenesis of the sacrum is present in about 20%, while in spina bifida about 20% of the cases suffer of a dysgenesis of the sacrum [13] (tabs. 1 and 2).

Dysgenesis of the sacrum is an aspect of the caudal regression syndrome [3, 4, 7], which can be subdivided in

a) complete sacral agenesis,
b) incomplete sacral agenesis,
c) hemisacrum (total – partial),
d) dysplasia of the sacrum.

The osseous sacral anomaly belongs to the decompensated numerical anomalies (tab. 3) of the vertebral column with agenesis or hemiagenesis of a variable number of vertebrae [7] (fig. 1). Structural anomalies in the deformity of the sacrum occur in different degrees and are referred to as dysplasia of the sacrum [6, 13].

Generally speaking the extent of the osseous anomaly correlates with a corresponding anomaly of the neural structures of the bladder, the rectum, the floor

Table 1 Correlation anomalies in spina bifida. Some coexisting anomalies in 101 children (E. D. Smith, Melbourne 1965)

Vertebral column	Sacral agenesis	18
	Vertebral anomalies	18
Urogenital tract	Megaureter, hydronephrosis	26
	(22 × reflux)	
	Vesicoureteric reflux	8
	Double kidney	3
	Hypospadia, urethral malformations	4
	Ectopia of bladder	2

Table 2   Correlation anomalies in dysgenesis of the sacrum. Coexisting anomalies in 125 cases of
the literature

Skeleton		
	Clubfoot	49
	Vertebral anomalies	46
	Atrophy of lower extremities	26
	Spina bifida	20
	Luxation of hip joint	19
	Curvature of the spine	13
	Meningomyelocele	13
Urogenital tract		
	Vesicoureteric reflux	19
	Hydronephrosis	11
	Diverticula of the bladder	5
	Solitary kidney	5
	Urethral malformations	5
	Ectopic kidney	2
	Stricture of ureter	2
	Double kidney	2
Gastrointestinal tract		
	Atresia of anus	17
	with fistulas	6
	Inguinal hernia	6
	Rectourethral fistulas	3
	Umbilical hernia	2
	Omphalocele	2
	Deformation of the bowel	10
	Hydrocephalus	4

Table 3   Classification of vertebral anomalies [7]

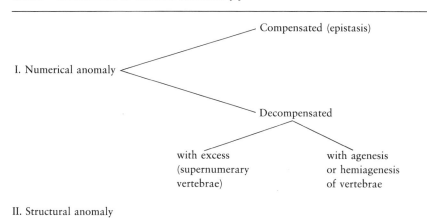

I. Numerical anomaly — Compensated (epistasis)

Decompensated

with excess (supernumerary vertebrae)   with agenesis or hemiagenesis of vertebrae

II. Structural anomaly

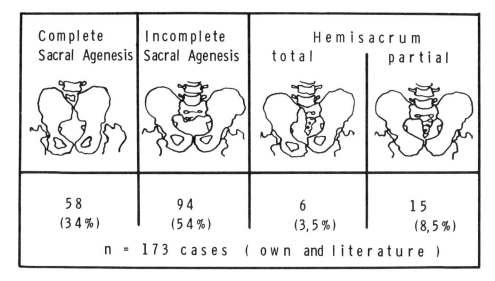

Complete Sacral Agenesis	Incomplete Sacral Agenesis	Hemisacrum	
		total	partial
58 (34%)	94 (54%)	6 (3,5%)	15 (8,5%)
n = 173 cases (own and literature)			

Fig. 1   Classification and frequency of the decompensated numerical sacral anomalies [13].

of the pelvis, and of the lower extremities. If only one or more vertebrae are absent, several neuro-urological disturbances are found in more than 50% [1, 8, 9].

In sacral dysgenesis defects of the peripheral sacral roots are maintly found and rarely a dysplasia of the sacral spinal cord [5, 10]. Due to the fact, that the motor roots are more frequently affected, the sensory defect is less marked than in meningomyelocele. The type of neurogenic bladder disturbance is characterised by complete or incomplete, lower nuclear or infranuclear, parasympathetic and somatic neuron lesions, but the sympathetic nerves can be intact.

The urological consequences of a *complete lesion* are the so-called autonomic bladder, laxity of the urethral sphincter, and therefore dribbling or stress type of incontinence. The partial resistance of the bladder neck by intact sympathetic nerves allows continence to a certain degree and sympathicomimetic drugs can reinforce this condition [11]. Voiding can be accomplished by abdominal muscle contraction or Credé manoeuver and is mostly without residual urine. The unfortunately more frequent *incomplete lesion* with its disturbed neural interactions often causes detrusor-sphincter-dyssynergia. These cases present the greater problem in therapy.

If sacral dysgenesis coexists with lumbar dysraphia, *mixed upper and lower neuron lesions* occur. Only in the complete upper neuron lesion is automatic reflex bladder with complete bladder emptying the rule. Reflex-incontinence, residual urine, dilatation of the upper urinary tract, urinary tract infection, development of the Christmas tree appearance of the trabeculated bladder, and a secondary stenosis of the terminal ureters or a vesico-ureteric reflux frequently occurs.

This fatal disease progress explains the patient's early consultation of a urologist during his first year of life in more than 50% [1, 2]. Visible anomalies of the bowel, a sacral dimple or voiding disorders and urinary tract infection necessitate the several X-ray examinations − including a.p. and lateral X-ray pictures of the sacrum − which enables the detection of the sacral dysgenesis. This diagnosis always demands further examinations [12] to detect correlating neurological and urological defects or other malformations present in a high percentage of patients. Urological therapy has to conform to the same rules as those generally applied to neuro-urological disorders:

1. Protection of renal function;
2. conservative pharmacological or surgical therapy in order to improve the social hardships resulting from incontinence.

References

[1] Auvinet, F., J. P. Chabrolle, J. Valayer et al.: Les malformations sacro-coccygiennes. Sem. Hop. Paris 55 (1979) 159 − 164.

[2] Blumel, J., M. C. Butler, E. B. Evans et al.: Congenital Anomaly of the Sacrococcygeal Spine. Arch. Surg. 85 (1962) 132 − 143.

[3] Bors, E., A. E. Comarr: Neurological Urology, pp. 207 − 209. Karger Verlag, Basel 1971.

[4] Duhamel, B.: Malformations ano-rectales et anomalies vertébrales. Arch. Fr. Pediatr. 16 (1959) 534 − 540.

[5] Durham Smith, E.: Congenital sacral defects. In: Congenital malformations of the rectum, anus and genito-urinary-tract (F. D. Stephens, ed.), pp. 82 − 96. Livingstone, Edinburgh − London 1963.

[6] Foix, C., P. Hillemand: Dystrophie cruro-vésico-fessière par agénésie sacro-coccygienne. Rev. Neurol. 40 (1924) 450 − 468.

[7] Köllermann, M. W.: Urologische Probleme bei anorektalen Fehlbildungen. In: Lehrbuch der Kinderchirurgie (A. Sigel, ed.), p. 307. Thieme Verlag, Stuttgart 1971.

[8] Mariani, A. J., J. Stern, A. U. Khan et al.: Sacral Agenesis: An Analysis of 11 Cases and Review of the Literature. J. Urol. 122 (1979) 684 − 686.

[9] Parkkulainen, K. V.: Sacrococcygeal and urological anomalies in connection with congenital malformations of anus and rectum. Ann. Pediat. Fenn. 3 (1957) 51 − 57.

[10] Price, D. L., E. C. Dooling, E. P. Richardson: Caudal Dysplasia (Caudal Regression Syndrome). Arch. Neurol. 23 (1970) 212 − 220.

[11] Schrott, K. M., A. Sigel: Neue Aspekte der Pharmakotherapie der neurogenen Blase. Verh. Ber. Dtsch. Ges. Urol. 27 (1976) 142.

[12] Schrott, K. M., A. Sigel: Diagnostik neurogener Blasenentleerungsstörungen unter simultaner Zystourethrographie, Zystosphinkteromanometrie und Pharmakotestung. Verh. Ber. Dtsch. Ges. Urol. 28 (1977) 315 − 320.

[13] Weißmüller, J., K. M. Schrott, A. Herrlinger: Sakrale Dysgenesie und ihr neuro-urologisches Fehlkorrelat. Urologe A 21 (1982) 327 − 334.

The artificial sphincters, their role in the treatment of urinary incontinence caused by meningomyelocele (MMC)

F. Schreiter, F. Noll

Introduction

The treatment of urinary incontinence is difficult in children with meningomyelocele. Continence cannot always be achieved by intermittent self-catheterisation and supporting medical therapy.

The psychic disintegration becomes more relevant in adolescence when the children get conscious of the social and psychological significance of their incontinence.

The supra-vesical urinary diversion is often the only possible way to achieve continence. However, this procedure is a severe interference with the self-image of the growing child.

The treatment of incontinence in MMC-patients with the artificial sphincter has to be seen with reference to this background.

Material and method

In 1975 – 1984 18 patients (7 female, 11 male) with MMC and urinary incontinence were treated with the artificial sphincter. The youngest patient was 7 years old and the eldest 26 years at the time of implantation. 15 patients had an a-reflexive and 3 a hyper-reflexive detrusor muscle. In 3 patients a vesico-renal and a vesico-ureteric reflux was seen. 5 patients had an infra-vesical obstruction (4 sphincter-detrusor-dyssynergie, 1 bladderneck-sclerosis). In 6 patients 10 preliminary operations were necessary (see below):

4 × Sphincterotomy
1 × Y – V-plastic
3 × Reflux operations
1 × Ileal augmentation of the bladder to increase its capacity
1 × Undiversion of a sigmaconduit.
12 patients did not need any preparatory operations.

Selection of the patients

A meticulous selection of the patients plays a prominent part in the postoperative success. All patients undergo a thorough urological, urodynamic, neurological and psychological examination.

Selection principles:

1. No urinary tract infection. A urinary tract infection has to be cured before sphincter implantation. Patients with chronic UTI, which can not be eliminated with antibiotics, have to be rejected. Otherwise infection of the synthetic material is almost certain.
2. Failure of intermittent self catheterisation.
3. The bladder capacity has to exceed 200 ml.
4. The urodynamic study has to prove a normo- or hypoactive detrusor reaction. In patients with hyperactive detrusors, which cannot be controlled pharmacologically, continence can not achieved. Furthermore the risk of an outflow obstruction from the upper urinary tract is obviously raised.
5. Any infra-vesical obstruction has to be eliminated before sphincter implantation (sphincterotomy or bladderneck resection).
6. The vesico-ureteric reflux is no absolute contra-indication. Regarding certain conditions reflux operations are also possible in neuropathic bladders.
7. Patients with outflow obstruction from the upper urinary tract are primarily not candidates for sphincter implantation.
8. The patients should have normal intelligence, as we expect sufficient dexterity. Otherwise they will not be able to handle the prothesis adequately.

Results

All patients after sphincter implantation which are:

1. totally continent,
2. could drain their bladder without residual urine left and
3. have no chronic UTI

were rated as a good success.

16 of 18 patients (88.8%) fulfilled these conditions and will have good long term results. In 2 cases (11.2%) failure was caused by infection of the prothesis. Both declined a re-implantation.

We had postoperative complications in 7 out of 18 patients (tab. 1). They required 11 re-operations. 5 mechanical defects of the prothesis causing leakage and 6 infections or operative-technical faults made these necessary.

The number of defects due to the prothesis itself will be definitely lower in future, since using the new modell AS 800 we have not seen any material defects.

Table 1   Artificial sphincter in MMC patients complications in 7 of 18 patients

Reoperations (n = 11)	
1. Mechanical defects	
leakage at	
cuff	2
pump	2
ballon	1
connecting tubes	1
	5
2. Infections and operative-technical faults	
change of cuffsize	1
infections	3
re-implantations	1
kinking of the tubes	1
	6

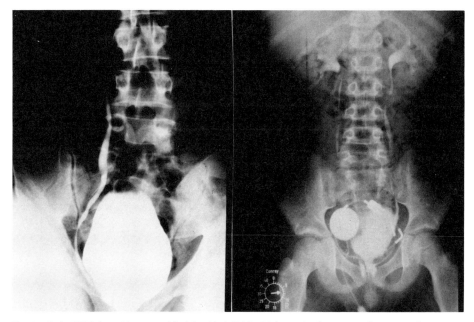

Fig. 1   Left: VRR in a 22 years old girl with MMC. Right: UG after antireflux procedure (Cohen) and implantation of artificial sphincter AS 792.

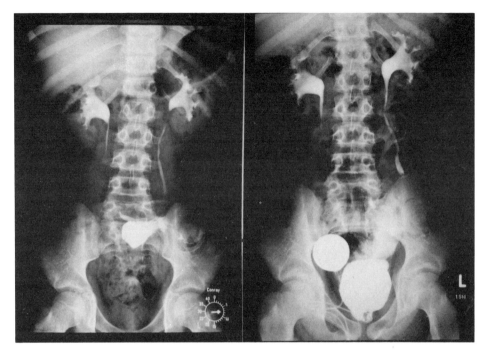

Fig. 2   UF of a 23 years old boy after subtotal cystectomy (left), ileal extension of the bladder and implantation of an artificial sphincter AS 800 (right). Self-catheterisation (little residual urine once a day).

Particularity of the indication and future aspects

The vesico-ureteric-renal reflux is in itself no contraindication for the implantation of an artificial sphincter. We have carried out an anti-reflux operation in 3 cases with a high degree of success (2 times both sides, 1 time only one side, 2 times following Cohen's technique, 1 time Politano – Leadbetter's technique (fig. 1)).

The hyperactive low compliance-bladder is an absolute contra-indication for the implantation of a Scott-sphincter. Continence cannot be achieved and an outflow obstruction of the upper urinary tract with dilatation of calices, pelvis and the ureter is often the result.

A 12 year old boy with hyperactive detrusor muscle was treated by the following procedure: Subtotal resection of the hyperactive detrusor, ileal extension of the bladder to increase capacity and to reduce intra-vesical pressure, implantation of a Scott-sphincter (AS 800). The result is shown in figure 2.

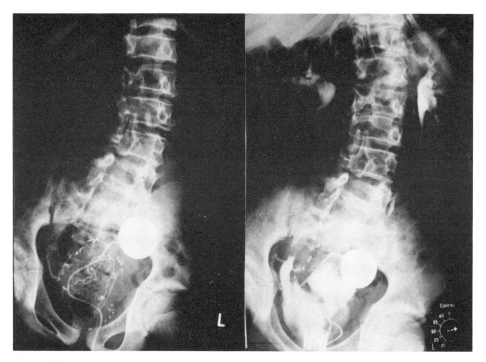

Fig. 3   Left: Sigma-conduit in a 13 years old boy with MCC. Right: UG after re-routeing and implantation of artificial sphincter AS 800.

The patient is continent with a slender upper urinary tract. He empties the bladder almost completely. Only small amounts of residual urine have been measured.

If the bladder is still in situ (After supravesical urinary diversion) and infravesical obstruction is absent a reconstruction of the urinary system is possible. This was carried out on a 13 year-old boy, whose urine was diverted in a sigma-conduit using anti-reflux techniques. We have attached the bladder to the conduit and implanted an artificial sphincter to attain continence. The boy is dry in daytime with tolerable nightly incontinence. He empties his bladder every 3 – 4 hours without residual urine. A reflux is not visible (fig. 3).

First clinical experience [6] and experiments carried out on animals [7] have shown, that the application of the artificial sphincter to intestinal loops is possible. It may be possible in future that continence is attainable by a total replacement of the bladder using intestinal loops and an artificial sphincter. A clinical evaluation is as yet not possible and requires more experience.

Discussion

The well known long term results with the artificial sphincter ranging from 80 to 95% success [1, 2, 3, 4] agrees with our experience in treating patients with MMC and urinary incontinence (88.8% good results). The discussion of these results has to refer to our experiences with the alternative methods of treatment of MMC patients.

The intermittent catheterisation leads only in 66% to "social continence". Furthermore if the intervalls were not correctly choosen the patients will not achieve continence, suffer from recurrent UTI's, show a greater amount of wear and soiling of their clothes and also injuries to the urethra specially in male patients due to a wrong catheterisation technique are often seen [1].

The supra-vesical urinary diversion poses a lot of problems (tab. 2). The outlook is no better for colonic conduits. The late complications have been studied by Elder 1979 who examined the cases operated by Moch.

Table 2   Late problems in ileal conduits

Author	No. of cases	Desease of parenchyma	Stenosis ureter	Stenosis stoma	Stones
Schwarz and Jeffs	95	49	11	32	13
Shapiro et al.	90	30	22	38	9
Pitts and Mucke	242	35	31	31	14

(acc. to [1])

The uretero-sigmoidostomy with reflux prevention is not possible for the treatment of urinary incontinence in patients with neuropathic rectal incontinence including in patients with MMC. A similar caution attitude should be applied to bladder neck operations or sling procedures often used for the treatment of stress incontinence in the female.

The use of intestinal loops for enlarging a contracted bladder together with a partial detrusor resection for treating a drug refractory detrusor hyper-reflexia extends the applicability of artificial sphincters.

But patients with spinal cord injuries are often unable to tolerate severe surgical procedure. The reconstruction of the lower urinary tract with re-attachment of the supra-vesically diverted urinary tract to the still existing bladder or urethra is another interesting application of the artificial sphincter [5].

Conclusion

The treatment of neuropathic urinary incontinence in patients suffering from MMC with an artificial sphincter is superior to a conservative treatment. We obtained good results in 88.8% of our MMC patients and are successfull in 88.2% in patients suffering from neurogenic bladder disturbancies or other in spinal cords injuries.

Our experience with the ileal bladder augmentation or the replacement of the bladder by intestinal loops justifies an optimistic outlook that neuropathic urinary incontinence can be treated in many cases in the near future. This will contribute decisively to the social re-integration of the disabled patients.

References

[1] Light, J. K., M. Hawila, F. B. Scott: Treatment of urinary incontinence in children: The artificial sphincter versus other methods. J. Urol. **130** (1983) 518 – 521.
[2] Gonzales, R., C. A. Sheldon: Artificial Sphincters in children with neurogenic bladders: Long-term results. J. Urol. **128** (1982) 1270 – 1272.
[3] Schreiter, F., M. Bressel: Operative treatment in incontinence secondary to myelodysplasia by an artificial sphincter. Z. Kinderchir. Band 22, Heft 4 (1977) 560 – 565.
[4] Barrett, D. M., W. L. Furlow: The management of severe urinary incontinence in patients with myelodysplasia by implantation of the AS 791/792 urinary sphincter device. J. Urol. **128** (1982) 484 – 486.
[5] Light, J. K., F. N. Flores, F. B. Scott: Use of the AS 792 artificial sphincter following urinary undiversion. J. Urol. **129** (1983) 548 – 551.
[6] Light, J. K., F. B. Scott: Total reconstruction of the lower urinary tract using bowel and the artificial urinary sphincter. J. Urol. **131** (1984) 953 – 956.
[7] Engelmann, H. U., T. P. Feldermann, F. B. Scott: Evaluation of the artificial sphincter AS 800 for continent urinary diversion. Proceeding of I.C.S. 1984.

Assessment of intelligence of school-aged children with spina bifida under hospital supervision

N. Rückert, G. Hänsel-Friedrich, G. Wolff

Introduction

Empirically based information on the intellectual and psycho-social development of children with spina bifida is necessary for the following reasons:

1. the widespread misconception that children with spina bifida are usually mentally retarded;
2. the discussion of interrupting pregnancy or selective treatment, based on estimation of the childrens' intellectual capacity;
3. the anxiety of the parents concerning the mental, physical and social development of their children with spina bifida;
4. the urgent demand of the hospital staff for data needed in order to give the parents a valid prognosis at the beginning of the treatment;
5. the need for giving the children the best possible help in kindergarten, school and in preparation for a profession;
6. in particular the assessment of cognitive dysfunctions of children with spina bifida and the relative quality of their motor, cognitive and speech competence.

Due to the multiplicity and variety of these reasons for assessing the child's intellectual ability, it is mandatory that an appropriate test should be available to be part of a comprehensive psychological evaluation. It must be stressed that emotional factors have an influence upon cognitive performance and that the attitude of the child and its parents to the test affects the test results.

In evaluating cognitive performance in children with spina bifida by using the newly revised German version of the Wechsler-Intelligence-Scale for Children (HAWIK-R), we concentrated on the first and the last of the above mentioned aspects:

1. The patient's general level of intellectual performance in this revised test form. There is ample evidence that using the old version of the HAWIK resulted in wrongly upgraded measurements [12, 22].
2. The problem of whether the revised intelligence test will yield statistically and clinically relevant information on the profile of a child's relative strengths and weaknesses of its cognitive ability.

A number of empirical findings is available on the general intellectual ability and specific cognitive functioning of children with spina bifida:

According to Anglo-American publications the full scale IQ of patients from unselected samples range predominantly at a low normal level around an IQ score of 85 to 90 [2, 5, 15, 16, 18]. Regarding the differences between verbal-IQ and performance-IQ these studies showed a higher verbal competence when compared to visual-cognitive and visual-motor performance in the children with spina bifida [8, 15]. A corresponding discrepancy between the verbal and performance IQ was also found in a German study [6], however with a higher mean full scale IQ of 97. In another German study [10] a mean IQ also above 90 is reported.

In most samples there is a higher proportion of patients with full scale IQs below − 1 standard deviation as compared to healthy control samples. Correspondingly more research has been oriented towards looking for specific factors causing impairment in cognitive functioning. Various factors have been named: for example, the presence of hydrocephalus [5, 7], the type of hydrocephalus (communicating or occlusive) [21], the number of shunt infections and/or revisions [2, 5, 18], the level of lesion [10], or the social status [15].

Recently there has been more research on specific neuropsychological aspects. Regarding manual skill, memory and attention, children with spina bifida are said to show only relatively slight differences when compared to healthy children. For example, a higher proportion is reported to be bimanual, an attribute, which decreases however after the age of 6 years [14]. A disability in the movement of the left hand on finger tapping [8] and slight defects regarding attention span and short term memory have been reported in combination with increased impulsiveness [18]. However performance in long term retainment of pictures and stories was as good as in normal controls [3].

The present paper reports on the first findings regarding general and differential intellectual abilities based on the application of the HAWIK-R [19] in patients with spina bifida who are in care at our hospital.

Patients and methods

The HAWIK-R was given to 16 children (9 girls, 7 boys) with spina bifida aged 7 to 12 years (Mean age: 9.7 years). These children had already been tested in 1979, eight of them with the German version of the Wechsler pre-school and Primary Scale of Intelligence (HAWIVA) and the old WISC (HAWIK), respectively. The results were compared with the results of the present study by means

Table 1   Pairs of subtest combinations for individual profile analysis

1. PC + In + DS + Vo + BD + Ar	vs.	Cp + OA + PA + Si + Cd
2. In + Cp + Ar + Si + Vo + DS + PC + PA	vs.	Cd + BD + OA
3. In + Cp + Ar + Si + Vo + DS	vs.	PC + PA + BD + OA + Cd

Abbreviations: In = Information; Cp = Comprehension; Ar = Arithmetic; Si = Similarities; Vo = Vocabulary; DS = Digit Span; Cd = Coding; PC = Picture Completion; PA = Picture Arrangement; BD = Block Design; OA = Object Assembly.

of transforming the IQs into C-scores (M = 5) corresponding to the four subtests of the HAWIVA.

The present psychological evaluation was carried out on all of the children by the same investigator and including behaviour observations of the children and interviews with the children and their parents. The purpose of the evaluation was to collect a differentiated performance profile. This was used for supportive counseling readily accepted by the parents and the children, which were mainly cooperative. We believe, that the test results can be accepted as being representative of their present level of intelligence.

For individual profile analysis three different pairs of subtest combinations (tab. 1) were calculated and checked for their statistical and clinical significance [4, 20]:

1. Comparison of the first and second part of the test as an indication of the child's ability to sustain continuous cognitive strain.
2. Comparison of the test-performance in those subtests, which require visuo-motor coordination, and the test performance in the remaining subtests.
3. Comparison of verbal and performance (non-verbal) scales.

Three single case analyses are briefly presented discussing the clinical usefulness of a total IQ score as compared to an analysis of the test profile.

We finally included a number of relevant medical parameters for the assessment of the degree of representativity of the present sample.

Results

Clinical data

Fifteen of the children had a myelocele and one had a meningocele. The respective level of lesion is shown in figure 1. Thirteen children developed hydrocephalus which required a shunt-operation. The shuntsystem was inserted within two months after birth (tab. 2). Of the thirteen children five had had one, four two

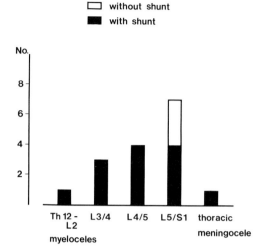

Fig. 1   Level of lesion, N = 16.

Table 2   Age at the moment of first shunt operation and frequency of following revisions

Days	Patients	Revisions
1 – 14	6	9
15 – 28	4	2
29 – 42	2	3
43 – 56	1	2

Table 3   Mobility

Locomotion	N
Walks unaided or with orthopedic shoes	7
Walks with appliance	6
Wheelchair	3

and one child three shunt revisions. Two children had epileptic seizures requiring anticonvulsive treatment.

The patients' present modes of locomotion are as follows (tab. 3).

In regard to the laterality thirteen children are right-handed, two are left-handed, and one child, aged 7, showed no definite dominance.

Psychological data

School entry was delayed by one year in three children. Twelve children presently receive regular schooling, three visit a school for the physically handicapped (one of these in a class for slow learners). One child, presently in a regular school, repeated one class. One child (aged 7.2) still visits a pre-school-class.

The results of the intelligence test are shown in table 4. Mean subtest scores are presented in figure 2.

Table 4   IQ-scores on the HAWIK-R (N = 16)

	Median	Mean	S.D.
Verbal scale	96	95.81	15.65
Performance scale	83	81.13	16.52
Full scale	86	86.69	19.55

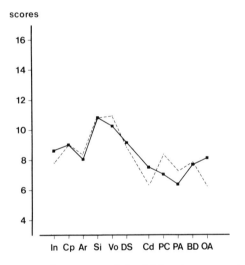

Fig. 2   Mean subtest scores of the children in our sample (———) and in the group of Lonton & Sklayne (– – –).

A comparison between our 1984 results and the test results of the same children tested in 1979, each transformed into C-scores, is shown in figure 3.

Apart from assessing at the general level of intellectual ability the test results were also analysed regarding subtest variability in each child. The first parameter was the maximum difference between any two subtests (tab. 5). A range of ≤

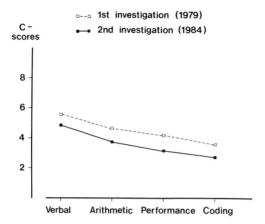

Fig. 3   Comparison of intellectual performance of the same children (N = 8) in the Hawiva/Hawik vs. Hawik-R.

Table 5   Intertestvariability on the Hawik-R

Range	Frequency (%)
5 – 6	3 (19%)
7 – 8	5 (31%)
9 – 10	8 (50%)

9 points is indicative of increased performance fluctuation and can be taken as an expression of partial cerebral dysfunction [11, 12].

Individual profile analysis of the subtest combinations brought about the following results (fig. 4).

With respect to perseverance a clinically significant reduction of achievement towards the end of the test procedure was observed only in one child suffering from seizures. Compared to the other intellectual abilities the visuomotor coordination of most of the children was not reduced. Comparison between the verbal and the performance scales, however, showed statistically lower results in the non-verbal abilities of twelve children. This was clinically significant in seven of them. Of the four children without a significant difference two, living without a shunt, had high scores on the performance scale. The remaining two children who have a shunted hydrocephalus performed poorly also on the verbal scale. It was reported that they had difficulties in verbal participation in school classes. Eight of twelve children with a significant difference between verbal and performance IQs were said to have corresponding difficulties in drawing, solving puzzles and in arithmetic.

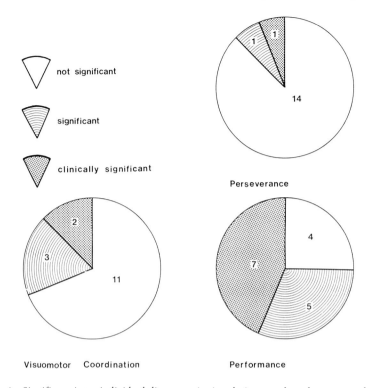

Fig. 4 Significant intra-individual discrepancies in relation to selected neuro-psychological functions (N = 16).

Table 6 Scores of three children on the Hawik-R

Patients Sex/Age	Subtest scores											Verbal Perf. Full Scale IQ		
	In	Cp	Ar	Si	Vo	DS	Cd	PC	PA	BD	OA			
M / 9.3	7	6	9	7	5	9	5	8	4	8	13	83	83	81
F /10.1	10	6	9	9	8	10	5	6	4	10	7	91	75	81
M /10.5	7	8	6	13	12	11	6	9	6	4	6	97	73	84

(Abbreviations: see table 1)

Similar full scale IQs can obviously result from quite different subtest profiles (tab. 6): The first boy, presenting school problems, showed relatively low performance in the verbal and the non-verbal subtests as well. The girl not only showed a significant reduction in performance towards the end of the test procedure but also a significantly low performance in the non-verbal subtests. A similarly high discrepancy between the verbal and performance IQs can be seen in the second boy. In his case this discrepancy is mainly due to deficiencies in spatial visualization.

Discussion

Compared to larger samples [10, 15] the present group of patients seems rather typical when judged by their medical and psychological characteristics. Regarding the general level of intellectual performance the results correspond to those Anglo-American studies quoted above. It must be assumed that earlier studies using the old version of the HAWIK resulted in measurements being wrongly upgraded [12, 20]. This is also shown in the comparison between our 1979 and 1984 investigation (fig. 3). Concerning specific intellectual functions, Figure 2 not only shows a similar subtest profile compared to that found by London [15], but also illustrates the different levels of achievement in the verbal and performance scale. The difference is mainly due to adequate vocabulary and verbal reasoning on the one hand and deficiencies in visual differentiation and perceptual organiz-ation on the other. Similar deficiencies have been reported in children with brain damage [17] as well as in physically handicapped children without cerebral damage [9]. Possible reason for the deficiencies in our children may be a combined effect resulting from minimal brain dysfunction due to hydrocephalus and lack of senso-motor experience. Our data support the notion that children with spina bifida are generally not mentally retarded. Our case studies present evidence for the relative uselessness of a general IQ-score in respect to clinical counselling. Decisions about special training, school and occupational placement should rather be based on a comprehensive evaluation of the child's total situation as well as on its cognitive ability [13]. The children should not be treated in a deficit-oriented manner, but should be supported by broadening and tutoring the cerebral functions and their psycho-social experiences [1].

Summary

In the comprehensive care of children with spina bifida the need arises for a precise assessment of the children's intellectual abilities. In the present paper we have concentrated on the general level of intellectual performance as well as on specific functions. The revised German version of the Wechsler Intelligence Scale for Children was applied to 16 school-aged patients. Whereas the general level of performance was in the subnormal range, the individual test results showed subtest differences requiring individual profile analysis.

References

[1] Ayres, A. J.: Bausteine der kindlichen Entwicklung. Springer, Berlin – Heidelberg – New York 1984.

[2] Brown, J. T., D. G. McLone: The effect of complications on intellectual function in 167 children with myelomeningocele. Z. Kinderchir. **34** (1981) 117 – 121.

[3] Cull, Ch., M. A. Wyke: Memory function of children with spina bifida and shunted hydrocephalus. Dev. Med. Child. Neurol. **26** (1984) 177 – 183.

[4] Frankenberg, I. v., C. M. Kleinert: Anleitungen zur Profilinterpretation beim HAWIK-R. Z. f. Heilpäd. **35** (1984) 357 – 368.

[5] Halliwell, M. D., J. Carr, A. M. Pearson: The intellectual and educational functioning of children with neural tube defects. Z. Kinderchir. **31** (1980) 375 – 381.

[6] Hemmer, R., E. Weissenfels, G. Hänsel-Friedrich et al.: Körperliche und geistige Entwicklung nach Frühoperation der Myelocelen. Neurochirurgia **20** (1977) 7 – 19.

[7] Hunt, G. M.: Spina bifida: Implications for 100 children at school. Dev. Med. Child. Neurol. **23** (1981) 160 – 172.

[8] Hurley, A. D., L. K. Laatsch, C. Dorman: Comparison of spina bifida, hydrocephalic patients and matched controls on neuropsychological test. Z. Kinderchir. **38** (Suppl. II) (1983) 116 – 118.

[9] Jetter, K.: Kindliches Handeln und kognitive Entwicklung. Huber, Bern – Stuttgart – Wien 1975.

[10] Kramer, H. H., W. Mortier, R. Pothmann et al.: Langzeitbetreuung von Spina bifida Patienten. Monatsschr. Kinderheilk. **132** (1984) 43 – 50.

[11] Krisch, K.: Die Intertestvariabilität im HAWIK als Indikator minimaler cerebraler Dysfunktionen. Praxis Kinderpsychol. **27** (1978) 290 – 295.

[12] Kubinger, K. (ed.): Der HAWIK: Möglichkeiten und Grenzen seiner Anwendung. Beltz, Weinheim – Basel 1983.

[13] Leonard, C. O., J. M. Freemann: Spina bifida: A new disease. Pediatrics **68** (1981) 136f.

[14] Lonton, A. P.: Hand preference in children with myelomenigocele and hydrocephalus. Dev. Med. Child. Neurol. **18** (Suppl. 37) (1976) 143 – 149.

[15] Lonton, A. P., K. D. Sklayne: The relationship between social class and educational, psychological and physical aspects of spina bifida and hydrocephalus. Z. Kinderchir. **31** (1980) 369 – 375.

[16] Scherzer, A. L., G. G. Gardner: Studies of the school age child with meningomyelocele: I. Physical and intellectual development. Pediatrics **47** (1971) 424 – 430.

[17] Schneider, R., H. Remschmidt: Der Einfluß des Schädigungszeitpunktes auf Wahrnehmung, kognitive und soziale Entwicklung hirngeschädigter Kinder. Z. Kinder-Jugendpsychiat. **5** (1977) 317 – 345.

[18] Tew. B., K. M. Laurence, A. Richards: Inattention among children with hydrocephalus and spina bifida. Z. Kinderchir. **31** (1980) 381 – 386.

[19] Tewes, U. (ed.): HAWIK-R, Hamburg-Wechsler-Intelligenztest für Kinder. Revision 1983. Huber, Bern – Stuttgart – Wien 1983.

[20] Titze, I., U. Tewes: Messung der Intelligenz bei Kindern mit dem HAWIK-R. Huber, Bern – Stuttgart – Wien 1984.

[21] Tromp, C. N., W. van den Burg, A. Jansen et al.: Nature and severity of hydrocephalus and its relation to later intellectual function. Z. Kinderchir. **28** (1979) 354 – 360.

Developmental problems in children and adolescents with spina bifida (educational and psychological support)

U. Haupt

Introduction

When dealing with developmental problems in children and adolescents with spina bifida, qualified medical treatment and the training and cooperation of children and parents, are of major importance. Especially a meeting like this demonstrates what is possible to-day and how much progress already has been made.

Concerning my experiences with severely handicapped children and their parents I would like to survey their entire life-situation. This implies attempting to understand developmental problems in a holistic way. Such an approach can facilitate further progress in rehabilitation. Questions of integrated support and holistic rehabilitation shall be discussed in three areas of major importance:

- the beginning of rehabilitation after birth of a severely handicapped child with spina bifida,
- training for independence,
- problems of social development, problems concerning partnership and sexual development in handicapped adolescents.

Rehabilitation of a severely impaired child with spina bifida

In order to give these children a chance of survival, immediate and frequently numerous surgical procedures are necessary. Parents are often uncertain whether the child might survive. Immediately after birth they have to share in the decision whether the child is going to be operated on or not. Emotionally, this is an extremely difficult situation for them. The parents are not familiar with the handicap. When they are informed about possible consequences of the malformation most of them react with a lot of insecurity. There is little time left to come to terms with this situation, as the first surgical procedure has to be performed within the first two days of the child's life. The situation becomes even more difficult when parents are encouraged to repress their intense feelings of fear, pain, bitterness and anger provoked by rehabilitation specialists, relatives, or friends who say when the child is born: "You must be very rational now", "You should really think of what your child needs now", "You should not let yourself go now". The repression of these intense feelings is helped by the many tasks parents have to accomplish in terms of nursing the child and training of its movements. In addition there are many necessary medical consultations, to attend to. However, observations in psychosomatic medicine and psychotherapy have established that the repression of intense feelings has a negative influence, not only on a person's emotional condition, but also on his communicative behavior.

It is possible that these repressed feelings lead to an ambivalence towards the child and the rehabilitation programme. A mother once said to me: "I reproach myself that the child is still alive, it is such a torture." When a further brain-operation was necessary she said: "I am scared to lose the child, but she never has belonged to me." And some time later: "On the other hand I wish she were dead; then finally, she would be through with it."

During the extremely difficult first time, important consequences for the entire rehabilitation process emerge and essential support can be given with physicians, psychologists, or other trained persons. These contacts should culminate in the acceptance of parents and child as full partners in the rehabilitation. The acceptance of the child's situation by the mother, father and child is not dependent on any type of performance or pattern of behaviour. In addition to this acceptance, good counselling, warmth, and deep understanding are vital [5]. It is important that parents from the time of the very first diagnosis are encouraged to express their sadness, fear, pain and anxieties when they feel it. It is helpful when they are assured that they are accepted, not rejected, and when the feelings are not interpreted as criticism or lack of understanding.

A relationship based on total understanding is a secure basis for recommending instructions concerning nursing the child and encouraging support by the parents. These instructions should respect the individual situation of child and parents. It is important that from the very beginning the parents are encouraged not only to care for the child and his development, but also to ask for help, to be able to relax and to care for their own needs. Experts should offer help and support where parents feel unable to care for all the child's needs.

Even when children with spina bifida have very good medical treatment and training, many of them show difficulties regarding their emotional and social adjustment. Problems include such as anxiety, fear, difficulties in playing, social contact and tendency to overcompensate in the intellectual sphere.

Therefore, especially the degree of support during the very early period of childhood is most important. It is essential that the basic needs of young children are met in the hospital and during intensive care. This includes the need for loving physical contact, for emotional and physical closeness with a familiar person who is constantly present, and the need for verbal contact and for sensory stimulation. In this context, I would like to mention that there are indications that basic patterns of experience remain possible even during states medically diagnosed as "unconsciousness". Even very young children are able to experience agony when their life is in danger. Accordingly, loving care, meeting the needs of the child, during and also after extremely difficult situations are most important. The younger a child is, the more holistic are his development and his ways of experiencing. He is unable to differentiate between his personal experience and the intention of another person. For the young child, physical contact, bonding, and experiences with his body are essential for obtaining basic experiences of himself, with other persons, and for developing self-esteem. It follows that co-workers in rehabilitation have the task to facilitate being-touched, being-examined, being-cared, being-trained, being-moved, physiotherapy, occupational therapy as good body and social experiences [1].

Education for independence

Independence means much more than just mastering patterns of movement and action for daily life activities. Independence also means, learning to find out what one's own needs are, taking reponsibility for one's own body and its needs, for the own possibilities and energies, but also for dangers. It implicates taking responsibility for one's own input in social interactions [2].

The main basic condition on which independence can be developed is the experience of trustworthy fulfilment of a child's needs during early life (warmth, food, nursing, bonding, attachment, verbal contact, movement, stimulation of senses, rest). On that basis it is necessary to encourage the child to make use of his growing abilities in expressing himself and moving, and to learn how to contribute to the fulfilment of his needs. At the same time the child has to become familiar with the needs of the other persons in his surroundings in order to become able to react to them. These are the conditions for the development of self-acceptance in a child. Self-esteem is dependent on one's own potentialities, one's own body and social experiences dating from the early childhood on wards. Experiencing satisfying social contacts by being recognized, accepted and understood is the main condition for the development of a positive self-esteem. For a child able to love itself, seeing itself in a positive way it is much easier to develop independence even under the difficult condition of a physical handicap than for a child with a more negative attitude less motivated to cooperate actively in favour of its own development.

The child with spina-bifida [4] needs qualified guidance and instructions to be able to learn the movement patterns necessary for independence. It is of major importance to adapt these instructions to the actual physical and emotional situation of the child, and to find a way to integrate the child's own experiences and interests.

One has to be aware how difficult it is, i.e. to learn movement patterns if parts of the body are not only paralyzed but at the same time are insensitive e. g. person is able to put his feet on the floor but cannot feel a real "grounding". This can be compared to standing and walking as if on stilts. It is difficult to take responsibility for wet dipers or decubiti if you cannot feel them. Several children have additional difficulties due to cerebral dysfunctions and hydroce-phalus such as insecurities in spatial perception, in orientation, in equilibrium, and in the coordination of movements.

Education for independence also includes asking for help and accepting help. It is important to adjust the training of the child to his emotional situation, to the way he lives and the place where he lives as well as to his needs for positive social contacts. The child needs good development in all areas to be able to develop independence and self-responsibility.

Children who react with fear or protest, who cling to relatives signal inner conflicts or interaction — conflicts arising in the family. Sometimes children also block their development when their therapy and support does not fully meet their needs. Forced training is seldom a solution for emotional and social conflicts. In such difficult situations it is important to understand the child and his parents in order to find a solution of the conflicts [3].

Sometimes a situation becomes easier by guidance or advice that really refers to the actual situation of the family. However, if emotional and social tensions are high, only in rare cases can advice or instructions can provide adequate help.

It is important that every day each child has enough time to itself without any duty or exercises. Only under these conditions will a child be able to play and to digest its experiences, to develop its own ideas and be creative.

Questions of social development, of partnership and of sexual development in handicapped adolescents

Concerning social development, partnership and sexuality, plans for the future are of great importance, but the cooperation of the child is the essential point. This cooperation is achieved through attachment, bonding and trustworthy care for its needs. A loving relationship with other persons including physical contact will help the child towards this aim.

References

[1] Haupt, U.: Überlegungen zu einer komplexen Entwicklungsförderung körperbehinderter Säuglinge und Kleinkinder. Zeitschrift für Heilpädagogik **31** (1980) 483 – 492.

[2] Heslinga, K.: Not Made of Stone. Noordhoff, Leyden 1974.

[3] Jansen, G. W.: Die Einstellung der Gesellschaft zu Körperbehinderten. 3rd ed. Schindele, Heidelberg 1976.

[4] Kundert, J. G. (ed.): Wir haben ein Kind mit Spina bifida. Schwabe, Basel 1982.

[5] Tausch, R.: Gesprächspsychotherapie. 7th ed. Hogrefe, Göttingen 1979.

Psychological and educational aspects of spina bifida (from babyhood to adulthood)

B. Schnitger

When asked which factors constituted a normal human being Freud [1] gave the lapidary reply: "A human is able to love and to work." The American psycho-analyst Erik H. Erikson [2] shows how a new-born child has to develop into an adult, conscious and accepting his own identity, capable of building up relation-ships with others, creatively active, experiencing and living out crises and solving them without resorting to despair. In order to be "normal" four vital pre-requisites are necessary whether the child is physically disabled by a spina bifida or not disabled.

The child must possess a primary feeling of *confidence* in others and itself. This feeling originates primarily but not exclusively in the first year of life and becomes endangered or made impossible by experiences of loss, separation and of being forsaken.

In my therapeutic work, the aquaintance of a young disabled woman was made whose admittance to hospital as an in-patient was necessary for an examination of her heart. On account of a deep depression and fears of committing suicide, although being rationally aware that an operation was necessary she was, nevertheless seized by such a strong panic at the thought of having to enter hospital, that she feared for her sanity. The patient was incapable of explaining her fears and regarded them as being abnormal and part of a mental illness, having had previous experience of hospitals. She had always been well cared for by the doctors, sisters and other specialists. In spite of this, she broke down after ten minutes, crying convulsively, feeling defenceless, deserted and helpless. Medical measures, which were objectively essential (such as not to drink anything after the operation) posed such a threat to her as a child, that she lost all confidence. From then on, adults were people capable of inflicting pain and causing harm, whereas she was somebody exposed to them without protection, hopelessly vulnerable.

In the course of a series of therapeutic sessions the patient was taught that her fears were not a sign of insanity but a consequence of her earlier feelings of being deserted and left at the mercy of others. Eventually she was able to understand and to accept that the investigations carried out were essential to her. She felt secure whilst in hospital, as her husband, in whom she had complete confidence, was allowed to stay with her overnight if the need should arise.

There are children who endure tedious and stressing periods in hospital with no detrimental effects. This is dependant upon the parent/child relationship, upon trustworthiness, upon the psychological structure of the child. It is important to make her aware of being treated as a person as well as being liked by the doctors and medical staff.

A disabled child in particular needs the fundamental and deep conviction — also from the medical staff — that he or she is basically not a deficient person.

Seen from a psycho-analytical point of view, cleanliness training is responsible partially for a possible estrangement of a child from its own body, for feelings of shame and doubts of its *independence and security* particularly in a spina bifida child.

For a spina bifida child, as well as other disabled children, bodily contact is of primary importance above all therapeutic, examining, helping, supportingly essentialised and in part simply not perceptible due to loss of sensibility. Spontaneous, emotional, warm and affectionate physical contact however is the exception rather than the rule and even then it concerns the non-disabled limbs.

The following consequences arise as a result: How many people suffering from physical disabilities are overweight and disregard or hide their bodies. How many tirelessly emphasize that the actual value of a person lies in his personality. At some stage, the body or the disabled part of the body will be looked upon with hate, something inconvenient that has to be carried about.

Watson and Hewston reported in Link 7/8, 84 [3] an investigation in which the causes of sores in spina bifida children were examined. After having shown the causes and suggested new therapeutic treatment, astonishment arose that these common-sense measures were unknown to the children, adolescents and parents concerned.

Sores exibited by spina bifida children and adults are not however, only caused by loss of sensibility and ignorance concerning protective measures. It is partially a matter of indifference towards them, and rejection of a body that doesn't function well. It is a vicious circle. The neglected limbs develop sores which temporarily intensify the effects of the disablement, for example by limiting the scope of free play. This in turn enhances or maintains the sense of rejection thus leading to further negligence. It would be an unconventional measure, belonging not only to the sore prophylaxis but also to the neurosis prophylaxis, not to cushion a child more and more in its seat, but to convey to it a feelingful awareness that its body may well be handicapped but that it is nevertheless important and worthy of love, deserving to be protected affectionate and not by a sense of duty only.

Towards the end of its third year of life, a child begins to become steadily more active in overcoming its environment. It has long since mastered the art of walking and is becoming more and more confident at running about. The world has to be conquered, with physical strength and numerous questions. This stage, so far as it has been successfully mastered, gives the child, in addition to a feeling of confidence and autonomy, a feeling of *initiative* as security in being able to overcome the unknown. To do something is the motto.

In this situation, the danger for the disabled child lies in its own anxiety and inhibitions which were, aquired during the first two years, and by having been confined to those closest in relationship, the family, the therapist, and the environment.

I was consulted by an independent practising pediatrician about a young patient, suffering from a progressive degeneration of the muscles of the Duchenne type. The boy was able to walk fairly well and until now, only showed signs of getting tired easily. He was attending a pre-schooling kindergarten and the problem arose whether he should enter a regular school or a special school. The teacher reported that the child had diffulties in learning, and his mother was alarmed whether it would be possible for a disabled child to successfully adapt to a normal primary school. The child knew that it had to visit a physiotherapist because it was weaker than other children, but was otherwise unaware of a disablement. I made contact with the teacher who reported less conspicuous forms of behavior. I than invited the mother and child to see me and intended to test the child. Against all my expectations, the tests revealed that the boy could be placed in the upper third of his matched group as far as intelligence and maturity were concerned. A child, having attained such high marks would, more than likely go to a grammar school. The problem of schooling having been cleared up, I went on to talking over with the parents the reasons why such slightly conspicuous reactions had led to the mother being so concerned and overprotective, discussing which alternative actions could be more appropriate.

They decided not to exert such a strong hold on him, to have confidence in his abilities, and to understand his environment and disablement. The boy had long since known by intuition the reality of his situation and had spent many months praying for his life, learn to speak more openly about his disablement should it become more apparent. In this manner the parents would expose the child to a burdensome reality which would however, be less threatening than his fantasies. In any case providing a less protective attitude and a cautious frankness would allow him to grasp the initiative himself, and to take his life into his own hands.

The feeling of confidence, autonomy and initiative, the child of school age to experience the fourth stage, which Erikson paraphrases with the expression, "*activity*". I personally prefer to use the term, "acquisition of competence" for it clearly illustrates that it deals with the acquisition of skills and knowledge. In unfavourable circumstances, at school, failures produce feelings of inferiority whereas success favours the insight, "I am somebody capable of grasping interrelations and constructing, and making things function". As far as spina bifida children are concerned, this phase appears to me to be the least dangerous one. Provided that the first three difficult years are adequately taken care of, and that the child is given appealing and manageable objects, the feeling is surely one of: "I can cope with the material world."

Depending on the child and the severity of its disablement the offer available ranges from intellectual knowledge, e.g. from books, handicraft skills, e.g. from tools and materials to artistic skills. The aquisition of abilities is important as the disabled persons are given credit for it.

The awareness of identity begins to develop during adolescence. Idols and ideals which are at first of transient value but which later take on an everlasting and concrete form, are developed during this phase and the search for a professional, social and sexual identity is initiated.

The therapy of a sixteen-year-old, disabled by spina bifida, was passed on to me by a colleague. Since entering adolescence, she withdrew increasingly from her family and friends. She developed spells of depression, thoughts of suicide, and psychically induced cramps in her extremities. More and more of her girlfriends entered relationship with members of the opposite sex, causing her to become isolated; an isolation further enhanced by the relatively restricted scope of movement imposed by her disablement. Not having an apprenticeship, she was completely without professional perspectives. This in turn meant that she could neither develop, nor attempt to achieve vocational, social or sexual aims in life. Therapeutic contact was maintained over a period of three years, and continually revolved around dealing with the following questions:

"What do you like about yourself?"
"What do you like about your body?"
"What do you wish yourself?"
"Which of it is now attainable, and what can you do to achieve it?"
"Which unchangeable limitations are there for you at the moment, and what do you need to be able to cope with them?"
"What does it mean to you to be disabled, and why do you allow your disablement to leave you helpless?"

Talks with the parents were held at the same time. The parent, understandably, were overtaxed by the problems of their daughter, and were tending to react steadily towards pity and overprotection.

With the exception of occasional depressive moods, the patient is, after three years, free of symptoms. Although, unfortunately not receiving full professional education, she is being trained to become an office clerk. Having passed her driving test, she has a car and is able to move around. She is, once again able to approach people, build up and maintain relationships. She is still fighting to achieve a sexual identity – wishing for a partnership, and yet at the same time having an immense fear of searching for and constructing such a relationship. Living space, work, and leisure are the spheres around which the lives of disabled adolescents and adults revolve. These areas are not entirely free from difficulties but are nevertheless easier to satisfy and regulate than those concerning sexuality and partnership. Nearly all disabled people desire a relationship to a non-handicapped partner although many are, as yet incapable of fulfilling the provisions needed for such a relationship. As long as such aims are not achieved, only resignation will prevail.

References

[1] Freud, S.: Gesammelte Werke I – XVIII. Fischer Verlag, Frankfurt 1964 – 68.
[2] Erikson, E. H.: Jugend und Krise. Klett-Cotta, Stuttgart 1980.
[3] Watson, S. J., J. E. Hewson: Sores (ulcers) in anaesthetic skin-causes and prevention. Link, July/August 84, pp. 8 – 19.

V Summary of the present state of diagnostics and treatment of dysraphic malformations

Summary and overview

D. Voth

The main and basic intention of our 5. Autumn Meeting in Mainz has been the analysis of the changing epidemiology of spinal malformations and their various morphological presentations. This analysis included detailed information on the presently used pre- and post-natal diagnostics and methods of treatment with special reference to neurosurgery. It seems at present that a decrease in morbidity of spina bifida is noticeable, despite the fact that better statistical evidence from numerous countries is still lacking. Looking at this superficially one could assume that improved pre-natal diagnosis and the resulting interruption of pregnancy is responsible for a decrease in the number of spina bifida cases. However a critical analysis shows no clear evidence for this view. It is therefore advisable to draw no optimistic conclusions as the trend may be reversed in the years to come.

Pathology and morbidity of dysraphic malformations

Observations by comparative pathologists have shown that dysraphic malforma-tions do occur frequently in animals and are not limited to man. Examples of these genetically caused malformations can be found in the Manx-cat and the Weimaraner dog. The neurospinal dysraphia of this dog however shows features not present in man. Smaller animals too have spina bifida malformations, mainly in the lumbo-sacral region and similar to man show distinct neurological signs. Observations in the field of experimental neuropathology, *experimental ter-atology*, are important contributions for the understanding of dysraphia and the formation of the axial skeleton. Disturbances in the formation and folding of the neural plate and in neural tube closure are the basis of dysraphic malformations.

It may be possible that after the closure of the neural tube a re-opening of the tube occurs. Many factors indicate that the problem of dysraphia is not simply its splitting but that mesenchymal influences may contribute. All those substances, causing dysraphia are most effective during the stage of neural tube formation. Experimental observations and findings of human pathology favour a secondary neuro-schisis. It is even possible that the pressure of the cerebro-spinal fluid might be responsible for the opening of the previously faulty closure of the neural tube. It appears at present that a number of factors may be responsible. as the definition of the various spinal dysraphias is difficult and their conjunction with very severe malformation in head, neck and brain makes the whole range of occuring malformations most complicated to understand. Malformations of the eyes and eye muscle abnormalities which can be combined with a failure of the cortico-callosal fibres to cross the midline, which was demonstrate in separate communications.

These mainly morphological observations showed that midline failure of closure or the acallosal joining of both hemispheres is associated with complex neurological abnormalities, which can be investigated with experimental methods and are accessible to comparative neuro-embryological studies.

Epidemiology, antenatal diagnostics and prevention of dysraphias

In a largish survey including the observations from the University Hospital Giessen the frequency of dysraphias in Germany is discussed. This paper supports the impression that morbidity is decreasing although conflicting views about the validity of German studies do exist in particular in relation to studies abroad.

The numbers given in this retrospective study are one to two cases of spina bifida per 100 births, while prospective studies refer to an incidence of $0,5-1.0$ for 100 births. The incidence for anencephalus is similar. The expectance of recovery for a child already ill shows ethnic differences brought out in previous publications. It is pointed out, that the numbers for the FRG in relation to the total population are $1.0-1.5\%$ and slightly above the numbers for Poland and Switzerland, however below those of London, South Wales and Belfast.

A detailed contribution from Britain deals with the problem of folic acid medication for the prevention of neural malformations. This pilot study was to start with randomised and double blind. The results indicate that folic acid therapy reduces re-occurence significantly and a further project for studying the frequences of dysraphic malformations with and without prophylactic treatment with folic acid. The results available now have been communicated by the team of Laurence but were challenged by Lorber, who pointed out that some aspects of their planing could be improved upon.

Lorber further criticised the planing of the study and believes that benificial effect of multi-vitamin preparations had been proved and possibly too of folic acid alone. Bearing this in mind he stated that further studies in this direction were unnecessary, if not unethical. However investigations into all nutrional factors contributing to malformations appear still very necessary.

A series of lectures were devoted to antenatal diagnostics and biochemical investigations into the level of Alpha-1-feto-protein (AFP) in the amniotic fluid. The measurement of AFP in the maternal serum as a screening method is valuable in particular as only 10% of dysraphias are born into families prone to malformations. The reliability of determining AFP in maternal serum in cases of anencephaly is 90% and about 80% in spina bifida aperta. To verify this further AFP can be measured in the amniotic fluid. It is important also to look for evidence of amniotic acetyl-cholin-esterase as false negative findings with this method occur much more seldom than is the case for AFP measurements. The significance of antenatal sonographic exploration can be well documented in malformations of vertebral column and skull but the method has to be used by an experienced examiner. The post-natal diagnostic in particular in cases of hydrocephalus was demonstrated in a number of clinical studies (fontanelle-window) by the University Paediatric Hospital in Erlangen.

A contribution by Lorber deals extensively with the prognosis of encephaloceles. While the occipital meningocele has a favourable prognosis, a treatment of the occipital encephalocele has given mixed results. Besides good prospects for some patients, others have shown severe impairments, in particular when the un-favourable combination of microcephalus and hydrocephalic dilatation of the ventricles occurs. A further complication is the inclusion of brain tissue into the encephalocele.

The team of Laurence has analysed and presented the results of investigations on about 3500 patients suspect of malformations after exploring their amniotic fluid. These investigations showed evidence for 100 cases of anencephalus and the same number of spina bifida aperta. The series included 3 false-positive AFP values, resulting into the abortion of two normal foetuses.

The emotional reactions has been studied in women after interruption of their pregnancy for genetic reasons. This controlled study was based on a standard interview and with control groups of patients having had a spontaneous abortion, a premature birth resulting in a still birth, and those of an early therapeutic abortion. 77% of the 48 women showed distress, still persisting in 45% after 6 months. These distressful signs were not present in the control groups. While biochemical and sonographic methods are dominant in antenatal examinations, other tests in particular the computer tomography are preferred. Especially computer assisted cysternography and myelography are important for future neuro-surgical intervention.

Surgical treatment of spinal dysraphias — techniques and results

In this aspect the results of the Paediatric Neurosurgery of Mainz University served as a baseline. It has been found to be essential that a very careful investigation is carried out of the neurological status using all modern methods including evoked potentials. The exact localisation and the extent of the myelo-dysplasia is very important. The careful documentation of sensory − motor and autonomic defects in the pre- and post-operative period is of equal importance and has been communicated.

Concerning the indication for operations, very different opinions and procedures have been put forward during the last decades. These indications were either very strict and limited or wide in their scope and as far reaching as it seemed technically feasible. The neurosurgical team of Mainz refrains from operating in cases suffering from severe concomitant malformations or disturbances, which worsen the prognosis considerably. However we are prepared to operate in cases of a large meningomyelocele even at thoracic level. The Mainz team believes that not carrying out an operation does not abolish the problem due to an early death of the child, but considerably enhances the burden of nursing.

The operational procedure should have the aim to preserve neural tissue, even when electrical stimulation reveals no functional response. This aim demands microsurgery and careful repositioning of neural tissue into the neural canal, followed by carefully executed covering of the neural canal in several layers to prevent CSF leakage, if possible the first layer should be the dura.

The closure of the spinal canal can be made with non-neural tissue such as specially prepared heterologous dura, a covering by a fascial muscle graft from the erector trunci with connecting vessels as a third layer. The covering of the skin defects can be carried without difficulties, in particular by using the technique of split skin preparations.

The Mainz team paid special attention to a number of complications resulting from surgical intervention such as CSF leaks, skin necrosis, local or general infections. The team recommends a well planned and unified surgical procedure and the most conscientious follow up. Attention should be paid to the tethered spinal cord syndrome which can be present in rudimentary forms of spinal dysraphias, or the combination of a lumbo-sacral lipoma with spina bifida. The latter malformation was reported to have been present in 14 patients by the Cologne University Neurosurgical Hospital team.

A further contribution from Mainz has been a detailed study of the diagnostic and therapeutic problems arising from the treatment of 14 cases of encephaloceles collected from the last ten years. The neuropathological examinations showed that 13 from the 14 cases had suffered from a true encephalocele localised predominantly in the occipital region.

It was necessary to operate at once in cases with open encephalocele and CSF leakage, while closed encephaloceles can be operated on at a later stage. The most important post-operative complication is the development of a hydrocephalus which has to be drained, although it can appear after a long delay.

The last contribution dealing with operational aspects concerns itself with the possibilities of corrective spinal operations for severaly impaired patients suffering from meningoceles. Experience, good techniques and a clear concept how to achieve a marked improvement are essential.

Interdisciplinary problems in spina bifida

The frequency of occurence of spina bifida occulta was examined in a group of unselected orthopaedic patients. Split vertebral arches in males were found in 17.3% and in women in 9.4%. Asymetrically formed vertebral arches were present in 8.5% of males and 7% of females. Both malformations were found to be associated with significantly greater distances of vertebral arches at level S1. A clinical correlation of spina bifida occulta to pes excavatus and an increased incidence of spondylolisthesis. Operative orthopaedic measures are often required to improve the use of legs, but the operative efforts must be matched by functional gains and by insight and understanding of the patient. These operations involve either soft tissues or bones. In view of a future fitting with a walking aid which includes pelvic support, it is advisable to restrict the operation to soft tissue only. A combination of both is preferable if stabilisation of the hip joint can be expected without external support. Operative intervention at the knee joints are necessary, if impairment in walking is present or the fitting of an aid difficult. A similar indication is valid for operative foot corrections.

Secondary problems of spina bifida and its associated neurological signs are lumbar kyphosis and instability of the hip joint leading to luxation. To alleviate this condition the ventral plate embracing techniques of Mackay can be recommended. In case hip joint instability prevails it may be advantageous to transpose the abdominal external oblique muscle to serve as hip abductor.

A further malformation, well known to urologists is the caudal dysplasia (sacral dysgenesis). This clinical picture shows besides bony anomalies neural signs related to the involved levels. These are a neurogenic bladder and in combination with lumbar dysraphia further sensory and motor deficiencies. The diagnostic aspects have been fully discussed. The implantation of an artificial sphincter for the control of micturition is an important aspect. It appears that the technical side has been solved satisfactorily, but the complications resulting from reactions to foreign material cannot be excluded. It was emphasised in the ensuing discussion that this operation should only be performed in the older patients, as the consent for this repair should be given by the patient himself. The method itself has promising prospects. A neurosurgical and paediatric team of the Hannover Medical School reported their investigations on intelligence development of school children having spina bifida. The results of the Wechsler test for these children were in the lower regions of normality but some interesting differences were noted. In larger groups of patients the IQ is lower than in a healthy control, but hydrocephalic children treated carefully achieve IQ values comparable to normal controls.

The possibility of educational and psychological aids in caring for developing spina bifida children has been extensively discussed. The rehabilition of those children demands careful consideration of complex developmental processes, not only in view of being incapacitated but also by the difficult relationship to parents, other siblings and environmental reactions towards their illness. One contributor spoke very clearly and emphatically on these basic problems which need to be overcome in order to mature. A spina bifida child separated from its mother and to be operated on will undergo an acute increase of her psychological sufferings. In these circumstances psychological support is most important.

The organisers of the 5. Autumn Meeting in Mainz believe that the scientific and clinical exchange between the various disciplines such as experimental pathology, embryology, human and veterinary pathology in their close discourse and contact with neurosurgery and paediatry has been of great value for interdisciplinary collaboration. This exchange will greatly benefit the spina bifida patient in particular if the results of this meeting promote the greatest possible integration of all these working for the welfare of these unfortunate children.

List of contributors

Al-Hami, S., Abt. für Neuropathologie, Institut für Pathologie der Univ. Mainz, Langenbeckstr. 1, D-6500 Mainz 1

Becker, K., Dr. med., Abt. für Kinderpathologie, Institut für Pathologie, der Univ. Mainz, Langenbeckstr. 1, D-6500 Mainz 1

Bergh, van den P., Dr. med., Neurochirurg. Univ.-Klinik, Joseph-Stelzmannstr. 9, D-5000 Köln 41

Bohl, J., Dr. med., Abt. für Neuropathologie, Institut für Pathologie der Univ. Mainz, Langenbeckstr. 1, D-6500 Mainz 1

Brito, J. N., Dr. med., Neurochirurg. Univ.-Klinik, Langenbeckstr. 1, D-6500 Mainz 1

Büsse, M., Dr. med., Akad. Rätin, Univ.-Kinderklinik, Josef-Schneider-Str. 2, D-8700 Würzburg

Collmann, H., Dr. med., Freie Universität Berlin, Univ.-Klinikum Charlottenburg, Abt. für Neurochirurgie, Spandauer Damm 130, D-1000 Berlin 19

Correll, J., Dr. med., Orthopädische Univ.-Klinik, Schlierbacher Str. 200a, D-6900 Heidelberg-Schlierbach

Deeg, K. H., Dr. med., Univ.-Kinderklinik, Loschgestr. 15, D-8520 Erlangen

Dew, J. O., Dr. med., University Hospital of Wales, College of Medicine, Heath Park, Cardiff CF4 4XN (UK)

Dick, W.-, Dr. med., Univ.-Kinderklinik, Loschgestr. 15, D-8520 Erlangen

Düsterbehn, G., Dr. med., Neurochirurg. Klinik, Ev. Krankenhaus, Marienstraße 2 – 14, D-2900 Oldenburg

Dyer, C., Dr. med., Child Health Laboratory, University Hospital of Wales, Heath Park, Cardiff CF4 4XN (UK)

Glees, P., Prof. Dr. med., Department of Anatomy, University of Cambridge, Downing Street, Cambridge CB2 3DY (UK)

Goldhofer, W., Dr. med., Univ.-Frauenklinik, Langenbeckstr. 1, D-6500 Mainz 1

Grey, R.,. Dr. med., Südwestdeutsches Reha-Zentrum, Abt. Orthopädie, D-7516 Karlsbad 1

Hänsel-Friedrich, G., Dr. med., Neurochirurg. Klinik der Med. Hochschule, Postfach 610180, D- 3000 Hannover 61

Härle, A., Prof. Dr. med., Orthopädische Univ.-Klinik, Hüfferstr. 27, D-4400 Münster

Hanefeld, F., Dr. med., Freie Universität Berlin, Abt. Pädiatrie, Schwerpunkt Neurologie im K.A.V.H. Klinikum Charlottenburg, Spandauer Damm 130, D-1000 Berlin 19

Harms, J., Prof. Dr. med., Südwestdeutsches Reha-Zentrum, Abt. Orthopädie, D-7516 Karlsbad 1

Haupt, U., Frau Prof. Dr. phil., Prof. an der Erziehungswiss. Hochschule Rheinland-Pfalz, Fachbereich Sonderpädagogik, Spessartweg 13, D-6095 Ginsheim-Gustavsburg 2

Heller, R., Dr. med., Neurochirurg. Klinik, Krankenhaus Merheim, Ostmerheimer Str. 200, D-500 Köln 91

Henn, M., Dr. med., Neurochirurg. Univ.-Klinik, Langenbeckstr. 1, D-6500 Mainz 1

Hoffmann, G., Dr. med., Univ.-Frauenklinik, Langenbeckstr. 1, D-6500 Mainz 1

Janzer, R. C., Dr. med., Abt. Neuropathologie, Institut für Pathologie, Universitäts-Spital Zürich, Schmelzbergstr. 12, CH-8081 Zürich

Kaufmann, M. H., Dr. med., Department of Anatomy, University of Cambridge, Downing Street, Cambridge CB2 3DY (UK)

Keßel, G., Dr. med., Neurochirurg. Univ.-Klinik, Langenbeckstr. 1, D-6500 Mainz 1

Kiwit, J. W., Dr. med., Neuropathologisches Institut der Universität, Moorenstraße 5, D-4000 Düsseldorf

Koch, M., Dr. med., Zentrum für Kinderheilkunde der Universität, Feulgenstr. 12, D-63000 Gießen

Kreienberg, R., Priv.-Doz. Dr. med., Univ.-Frauenklinik, Langenbeckstr. 1, D-6500 Mainz 1

Laurence, K. M., Prof. Dr. med., Department of Child Health, University of Wales, College of Medicine, Cardiff CF4 4XN (UK)

Lloyd, J., Dr. med., Medical Officer, Welsh Office, Department of Child Health, University of Wales, College of Medicine, Cardiff CF4 4XN (UK)

Lorber, J., Emeritus Professor of Paediatrics, University of Sheffield, 305 Ecclesall Road South, Sheffield S11 9PW (UK)

Mahlmann, E. G., Dr. med., Neurochirurg. Univ.-Klinik, Langenbeckstr. 1, D-6500 Mainz 1

Manz, B., Dipl.-Chem., Univ.-Frauenklinik, Abt. für Experimentelle Endokrinologie, Langenbeckstr. 1, D-6500 Mainz 1

Matthiass, H. H., Dr. med., Orthopädische Univ.-Klinik, Hüfferstr. 27, D-4400 Münster

Menzel, J., Prof. Dr. med., Krankenhaus Merheim, Neurochirurg. Klinik, Ostmerheimer Str. 200, D-5000 Köln 91

Merz, E., Dr. med., Univ.-Frauenklinik, Langenbeckstr. 1, D-6500 Mainz 1

Mielfried, A., Dr. med., Christophorus-Kinderkrankenhaus, Briesingstr. 6, D-1000 Berlin 49

Noll, F., Dr. med., Univ. Witten-Herdecke, Verbandskrankenhaus Schwelm, Urol. Abt., Dr. Möller-Str. 15, D-5830 Schwelm

Pollow, K., Prof. Dr. med., Univ.-Frauenklinik, Abt. für Experimentelle Endokrinologie, Langenbeckstr. 1, D-6500 Mainz 1

Potthoff, P. C., Prof. Dr. med., Neurochirurg. Abt., Universität Ulm, BKH, D-8870 Günzburg

Pozo, J., Dr. med., Neuroradiologische Abt., Ev. Krankenhaus, Marienstr. 2–14, D-2900 Oldenburg

Rating, D., Dr. med., Freie Universität Berlin, Abt. Pädiatrie, Schwerpunkt Neurologie im K.A.V.H. Klinikum Charlottenburg, Spandauer Damm 130, D-1000 Berlin 19

Ratzka, M., Dr. med., Akad. Rat, Neuroradiologische Abt. der Universität, Josef-Schneider-Str. 11, D-8700 Würzburg

Richard, K. E., Prof. Dr. med., Neurochirurgische Univ.-Klinik, Josef-Schneider-Str. 9, D-5000 Köln 41

Rochels, R., Prof. Dr. med., Universitäts-Augenklinik, Langenbeckstr. 1, D-6500 Mainz 1

Roesmann, U., Prof. Dr. med., Division of Neuropathology, Institute of Pathology, Case Western Reserve University, 2085 Adelbert Road, Cleveland, Ohio, 44106 U.S.A.

Rückert, N., Dipl.-Psych., Neurochirurg. Klinik der Med. Hochschule, Konstanty-Gutschow-Str. 8, D-3000 Hannover 61

Rühe, B., Dr. med., Kinderkrankenhaus Neukölln, Mariendorfer Weg 28–38, D-1000 Berlin 44

Sanker, P., Dr. med., Neurochirurg. Univ.-Klinik, Josef-Stelzmann-Str. 19, D-5000 Köln 41

Schmitt, H. P., Prof. Dr. med., Institut für Neuropathologie der Universität, Im Neuenheimer Feld 220, D- 6900 Heidelberg 1

Schnitger, B., Dipl.-Psych., Münsterstr. 8, D-4407 Emsdetten

Schober, R., Dr. med., Neuropatholog. Institut der Universität, Moorenstr. 5, D-4000 Düsseldorf

Schreiter, F., Dr. med., Univ. Witten-Herdecke, Verbandskrankenhaus Schwelm, Urolog. Abt., Dr. Möller-Str. 15, D-5830 Schwelm

Schrott, B., Prof. Dr. med., Urologische Univ.-Klinik, Maximiliansplatz, D-8520 Erlangen

Schwarz, M., Dr. med., Neurochirurg. Univ.-Klinik, Langenbeckstr. 1, D-6500 Mainz 1

Sigel, A., Prof. Dr. med., Urologische Univ.-Klinik, Maximiliansplatz, D-8520 Erlangen

Sörensen, N., Prof. Dr. med., Neurochirurg. Univ.-Klinik, Josef-Schneider-Str. 11, D-8700 Würzburg

Sommer, H. M., Dr. med., Orthopädische Univ.-Klinik, Schlierbacher Str. 200a, D-6900 Heidelberg-Schlierbach

Stoeckel, W., Dr. med., Kinderklinik des Rudolf-Virchow-Krankenhauses, Reinickendorfer Str. 61, D-1000 Berlin 65

Vandevelde, M., Priv.-Doz. Dr. med., Institute of Comparative Neurology, University of Bern, P.O. Box 2735, CH-3001 Bern

Vitzthum, H. Gräfin, Dr. med., Edinger-Institut der Universität Frankfurt, Deutschordenstr. 46, D-6000 Frankfurt a. M.

Voth, D., Prof. Dr. med., Neurochirurg. Univ.-Klinik, Langenbeckstr. 1, D-6500 Mainz 1

Wechsler, W., Prof. Dr. med., Neuropatholog. Institut der Universität, Moorenstr. 5, D-4000 Düsseldorf

Weissmüller, J., Dr. med., Urolog. Univ.-Klinik, Maximiliansplatz, D-8520 Erlangen

Wellstein, R., Dr. med., Univ.-Frauenklinik, Langenbeckstr. 1, D-6500 Mainz 1

Wenzel, D., Priv.-Doz. Dr. med., Univ. Kinderklinik, Neuropädiatrische Abt., Loschgestr. 15, D-8520 Erlangen

Wolff, G., Dr. phil., Dipl.-Psych., Kinderklinik der Med. Hochschule, Postfach 610180, D-3000 Hannover 61

Zieger, A., Dr. med., Neurochirurg. Klinik, Ev. Krankenhaus, Marienstr. 2 – 14, D-2900 Oldenburg

Zielke, K., Prof. Dr. med., Skoliosezentrum, Werner Wicker-Klinik, D-3590 Bad Wildungen

Author's index

Subject index